CANCER AND STEM CELLS

Cancer and Stem Cells

Thomas Dittmar
and
Kurt S. Zänker
Editors

Nova Biomedical Books
New York

For permission to use material from this book please contact us:
Telephone 631-231-7269; Fax 631-231-8175
Web Site: http://www.novapublishers.com

Library of Congress Cataloging-in-Publication Data

Cancer and stem cells / Thomas Dittmar and Kurt S. Zander (editors).
p. ; cm.
Includes bibliographical references and index.
ISBN 978-1-60456-478-5 (hardcover)

1. Cancer cells. 2. Stem cells. I. Dittmar, Thomas. II. Zander, Kurt S.
[DNLM: 1. Neoplastic Stem Cells--physiology. QZ 202 C21435 2008]
RC269.7.C36 2008
616.99'4071--dc22

2008012725

Published by Nova Science Publishers, Inc. ✦ New York

Contents

Preface

Obtaining knowledge on the etiopathology of neoplasias and trying to elaborate a consistent explanation of their origin is a scientific and public issue. It is as old as mankind itself. Cancer as a disease has already been described in the earliest medical records found in the history of mankind, dating back to ancient Egypt. The term "cancer" is attributed to the Greek physician Hippocrates and is derived from bizarre "crablike" growth of tumors – "karkinoma (καρκινομα)" is the Greek word for "crab". Today, cancer is the second most prevalent cause of death after heart disease in the industrialized world, but it is assumed that in about 15-20 years from now cancer will be on top of the cause of death.

Although big efforts have been made in the fight against cancer in the recent decades – in particular in early diagnosis of cancer as well as novel anti-cancer strategies such as humanized antibodies or tyrosine kinase inhibitors – considerably less is still known about this disease. Nevertheless, from day-to-day, from month-to-month we learn more about the complexity of this disease, which will help us to find the targets where tumor cells are vulnerable.

In this context, cancer stem cells have now been addressed to be the most effective target cells for novel anti-cancer strategies. Cancer stem cells have been described as a rare population of cancer cells exhibiting stem cell properties such as self-renewing, differentiation, tissue reconstitution, and multiple drug resistance. Thus cancer stem cells might be responsible for all stages of a tumor disease including primary tumor initiation, metastasis formation, and cancer relapse after therapy, which in turn suggests that eradication of this particular cell type, thereby getting down to the root of the trouble, will lead to a complete cure of the disease.

But what are cancer stem cells and what will be a correct definition? What are the mechanisms that lead to cancer stem cell formation and what are the cell types cancer stem cells arise from. And, finally, what are the best strategies to eradicate this pivotal cell type? State of the art answers and visions to these questions will be given in this book.

We are glad that so many internationally recognized experts accepted our invitation to contribute to this exciting book. We sincerely thank them all for their interest in this important topic and that they, despite other duties and responsibilities, found the possibility to present excellent and comprehensive overviews of the most important recent findings in their field of scientific engagement within this topic.

We further thank Mrs. Maya Columbus and Mr. Frank Columbus from Nova Science Publishers for their helpful assistance and excellent collaboration with this challenging project.

We hope that this book may encourage new scientific approaches within the field of oncology and tumor pathology as well as closer interdisciplinary collaborations on this fascinating and important issue on cancer research in the future.

November 2007

Thomas Dittmar
Kurt S. Zänker
Institute of Immunology
Witten/ Herdecke University
Witten
Germany

In: Cancer and Stem Cells
Eds: Thomas Dittmar and Kurt S. Zänker
ISBN 978-1-60456-478-5

Chapter 1

Cancer Stem Cells: A Definition

Jichao Qin[1] and Dean G. Tang[1,2*]
[1]Department of Carcinogenesis, The University of Texas
M.D. Anderson Cancer Center, Science Park-Research Division,
Smithville, TX 78957, USA
[2]Program in Molecular Carcinogenesis,
Graduate School of Biomedical Sciences (GSBS),
The University of Texas Health Science Center, Houston, TX 77030, USA

Abstract

Cancer stem cells (CSCs) are stem-like cells in the tumor that are hypothesized to possess self-renewal ability, unlimited proliferative capacity, and multilineage differentiation potentials. These cells, although generally rare, appear to be highly tumorigenic and may be the cells that drive tumor formation, progression, and metastasis. In this chapter, we provide our insight on how a CSC should be defined, summarize the characteristics of reported putative CSCs, and present several methodologies that can be potentially used to identify them.

Synonyms

Cancer stem cells (CSC)
Cancer Stem-like cells
Stem-like cancer cells
Tumor progenitors
Tumor-initiating cells (TIL)

* Corresponding author: The University of Texas M.D Anderson Cancer Center, Department of Carcinogenesis, Science Park-Research Division, 1808 Park Rd. 1C, Smithville, TX 78957. Phone: (512)-237-9575; Fax: (512)-237-2475; E-mail: dtang@mdanderson.org

Tumor-reinitiating cells
Tumor-repopulating cells

Abbreviations

CAFs	carcinoma-associated fibroblasts
CSCs	cancer stem cells
PCa	prostate cancer
PSA	prostate-specific antigen
LRCs	label-retaining cells
SCs	stem cells
SP	side population
LT-CSCs	long-term cancer stem cells
ST-CSCs	short-term cancer stem cells
HSCs	hematopoietic stem cells
MDR	multi-drug resistance

Definition

CSC is functional rather than a fixed definition [1, 2]. *The least stringent* definition would be that the prospectively purified CSC population is more tumorigenic than the bulk or the marker-negative tumor cell population(s) in a suitable tumor development assay. Using *the most stringent* definition, a CSC should be a cell that, at the single-cell level, can reconstitute, in a recipient animal, a tumor that is *identical to* the parental patient tumor and can be serially xenotransplanted indefinitely [1]. Therefore, in a strict sense, none of the CSCs thus far reported can be truly classified as CSCs and should more appropriately be called tumor-reinitiating cells. In reality, it will be very difficult to identify a tumorigenic cell that can fulfill the most stringent definition of a CSC mentioned above. *Firstly*, a tumor, especially a solid tumor, is made of numerous cell types. To expect one cell or even a population of cells, when transplanted into a foreign host (i.e., mice) in an exotic environment, to fully reconstitute an original patient tumor in its complete composition is very difficult and essentially impossible to prove. *Secondly*, when such experiments are actually done, the best one can do is to co-inject the putative tumorigenic cell population with certain stromal components, such as ‘normal’ fibroblasts [3,4], carcinoma-associated fibroblasts or CAFs [5,6] or urogenital sinus mesenchyme or UGM [6,7], in an extracellular matrix (e.g., Matrigel or collagen; [8, 9]) into an ‘orthotopic’ animal site such as brain, mammary fat pad, or prostate lobes [1,9-12]. These orthotopic sites are considerably different from their human counterparts and tumor establishment would inevitably require the recruitment of various host (i.e., mouse) cells by the tumor-reinitiating cells. Such ‘reconstituted’ tumors could never be *identical to* the original patient tumors. *Thirdly*, during the purification process, the majority of cells are often discarded to obtain marker-positive and -negative populations. These discarded cells would be important in the original tumor composition but they would be very difficult to reconstitute in tumor development assays. Altogether, one can say, at the very best, that the experimental tumor reconstituted from the presumptive CSCs histologically 'resembles' the primary tumor.

Consequently, we probably have to seek a middle ground when making the claim to a CSC. A *functional definition of CSCs* is as follows. *First*, the presumptive CSCs (i.e., the cell population enriched in putative CSCs) must be *prospectively* purified from, e.g., cell cultures, xenografts, and/or primary tumors. When purifying candidate populations of CSCs from tumors, lineage selection must be performed to remove 'irrelevant' cells such as stromal and blood cells that may contain other stem cells (SCs) including mesenchymal and hematopoietic SC, which might have the ability to undergo transdifferentiation [13] and thus confound the interpretation of results. *Second, in vivo* tumorigenicity experiments must be done to show that such cell populations are enriched in tumor-(re)initiating cells. When feasible, serial tumor transplantation should be carried out to determine whether the tumors derived from the putative CSCs could be transplanted for multiple generations. Histologically, the reconstituted as well as serially transplanted tumors should resemble the original tumor. *Third*, the presumptive CSC population, or a subpopulation within, has to be studied to show that they possess certain intrinsic biological properties normally associated with SCs such as self-renewal and multilineage differentiation. Only when these conditions are fulfilled can one confidently claim that the candidate population of tumor cells under investigation is *enriched* in potential CSCs or tumor-initiating cells. Importantly, even such tumorigenic populations are likely heterogeneous with true CSCs representing perhaps only a very small fraction [14].

Characteristics

CSCs identified in different types of tumors or in different patients of the same type of tumor may manifest different biological and functional properties. On the other hand, all CSCs are expected to share certain common properties such as relative dormancy but with extended proliferative capacity, significant clonogenic potential, preferential expression of SC-related genes (e.g., self-renewal genes), the ability to undergo asymmetric cell division [15], enhanced in vivo tumorigenic and metastatic potentials [16] , resistance to radiotherapy [17, 18], and probably resistance to chemotherapy.

Blood-forming SCs and progenitors are organized as a hierarchy with the long-term hematopoietic SCs (LT-HSCs) the only cells that can regenerate differentiated blood cells lifetime [19]. Theoretically, tumor cells in any cancer, depending on their differentiation status, may also be organized as a hierarchy containing LT-CSCs, short-term CSCs (ST-CSCs), early and late tumor progenitors, and differentiating and differentiated tumor cells (Figure 1, next page). The LT-CSCs, analogous to the LT-HSCs, should possess indefinite self-renewal and ST-CSCs some self-renewal properties. The early tumor progenitors may or may not possess any self-renewal activities. The LT-CSCs, localized in the putative CSC niche, likely proliferate slowly although these cells possess the highest proliferative potential.

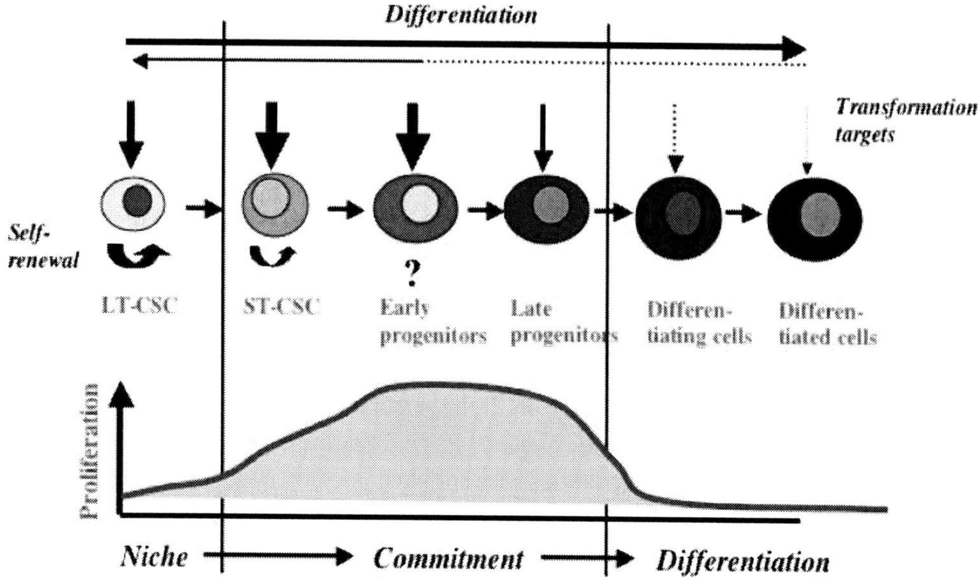

Figure 1. A hypothetical model of tumor cell hierarchy, which hypothetically comprises LT and ST CSCs, tumor progenitor cells, and more mature cells at different stages of differentiation. LT-CSCs localized in putative niches make the commitment to develop into ST-CSCs and tumor progenitors, which in turn differentiate into 'functional' cell types such as PSA-producing PCa cells. In most tumors, tumor progenitors and ST-CSCs may constitute the bulk of proliferating cell compartment and their normal counterparts may represent the major transformation targets. With increasing levels of differentiation, cells may become less susceptible to tumorigenic transformation. See text for more discussions.

By contrast, the cell types that constitute the bulk of the proliferating cell compartment in a tumor are mostly tumor progenitors and ST-CSCs (Figure 1; demarcated by two vertical lines). Differentiating and differentiated tumor cells, which should express tissue-specific differentiation markers such as prostate-specific antigen (PSA) in prostate cancer (PCa), are hypothesized to lack significant proliferative capacity and self-renewal in vivo and might represent poor transformation targets of tumorigenesis. Theoretically, both CSCs and tumor progenitors should have the ability to regenerate tumors although in principle, tumors initiated by CSCs should be able to be passaged indefinitely whereas tumors initiated by tumor progenitors can only be propagated for a limited number of times [1]. At present, there is no sufficient knowledge in any tumor system that allows clear-cut distinctions among putative LT-CSCs, ST-CSCs, and tumor progenitor cells and, in essentially all the cases, only two populations of tumor cells, i.e., tumorigenic vs. non-tumorigenic, have been demonstrated.

Putative CSCs are often thought to be derived from normal SCs, which may or may not be the case [16, 19, 20]. In fact, because normal progenitor cells are the major proliferating cells in a tissue or an organ and they may possess certain self-renewal abilities or they may acquire self-renewal abilities by the transforming events, these cells are more likely the targets of initial tumor transformation (Figure 1). In other words, transformed tissue progenitor cells may actually be the real CSCs. Alternatively, the initial tumor transformation may occur in normal SCs but further genetic mutations and/or epigenetic alterations take place in more mature tumor progenitor cells, which thus represent the real CSCs that drive tumor formation, progression, and recurrence. Both of these concepts have been recently born out in acute and chronic myelogenous leukemia (AML and CML) [21-24]. Finally, although most differentiated cells are thought not to be able to 'dedifferentiate' (i.e., going back along the lineage development; Figure 1), some somatic cells such as hepatocytes and endothelial cells are known to be able to replicate themselves. Therefore, some differentiated cells may also become transformation targets and subsequently become CSCs.

Identification

Putative CSCs that fit the above-discussed functional and realistic definitions of CSCs have now been reported in several human tumors including leukemia [25], glioma [26], and breast [27], prostate [11], colon [28, 29], and pancreatic [30] cancers. Several experimental strategies have been utilized to identify putative CSCs.

1) Marker-based analysis. This is the most widely used and also the most practical approach. A variety of adult tissue SCs are found to express relatively specific markers, which can be cell-surface or intracellular (e.g., nuclear and cytoskeletal). Interestingly, CSCs seem to express various cell surface markers such as CD44 and/or CD133 that identify their normal counterparts [1, 11, 12, 25-31], which allows a relatively simple enrichment procedure by utilizing either flow cytometry-based cell sorting or microbeads-based affinity purification. For intracellular markers such as a nuclear or cytoskeletal protein, a gene promoter-driven reporter construct such as GFP-tagged retroviral or lentiviral vector system can be developed to track down and purify putative (cancer) SCs [32]. Alternatively, transgenic animal models can be made by knocking in the gene promoter-driven reporter (GFP, LacZ, etc) followed by flow purification [33]. The disadvantages associated with using pre-determined marker(s) to identify CSCs include that the marker proteins frequently change during cell development in vivo and cell preparation in vitro and that in most cases the functions of these markers in both normal SCs and stem-like cancer cells are unclear.

2) Side population (SP) analysis Mouse HSCs are found to preferentially express multi-drug resistance (MDR) family proteins such as MDR1 and other membrane transporters such as ABCG2 (also called BCRP for breast cancer resistance protein) [10]. This property allows the HSCs, in an experimental setting, to pump out the Hoechst 33342 dye. Therefore, on dual-wavelength flow cytometry, the CSC-enriched cell population is identified as a 'side' or tail Hoechst^{dim} population at the lower left quadrant of the histogram. By contrast, the major population of cells is displayed as Hoechst^{hi} cells called as non-SP or main population [34, 35]. Recent work reveals that multiple adult tissue SCs can also be enriched by the SP protocol and that the SP from several cancer types are also enriched in stem-like cancer cells [36, 37]. The major advantage of this technique when used to identify putative CSCs is its simplicity. The potential problems associated with the technique are that chronic accumulation of Hoechst dye in non-SP cells may be cytotoxic (thus invalidating suitable controls) and that SP cells isolated from some normal tissues or tumors seem to be enriched in progenitor cells rather than SCs.

3) Sphere-formation assays Many normal SCs such as neural, hematopoietic, and mammary SCs, when maintained under special culture conditions, can form three-dimensional spheres, which are like mini-organs that can differentiate into multiple cell types. Putative CSCs identified in brain and prostate tumors as well as in melanoma also have the ability to form anchorage-independent spheres [1, 26, 38]. The advantage of using sphere-forming assays to enrich for CSC is its initial independence of specific markers. The disadvantages include the empirical nature of finding culture conditions suitable for sphere formation and the necessity of finding ways later to identify and purify the real CSCs from the spheres.

4) Label-retaining properties Mammary SCs and normal keratinocyte SCs in interfollicular epidermis and hair follicle bulges are quiescent and can be identified with a pulse label with the thymidine analog BrdU (bromodeoxyuridine) followed by a long-term 'chase' (i.e., removal of the label). Fast proliferating progenitor cells dilute out the BrdU label after several cell divisions whereas the slow-dividing SC retain BrdU and thus identified as 'label-retaining cells' or LRCs by either immunohistochemistry or flow cytometry analysis [39, 40]. Interestingly, the LRCs in human breast tumors co-express mammary epithelial SC markers and seem to have certain SC properties [41]. Human PCa [11] and nasopharyngeal carcinomas also possess slow-cycling LRCs [42]. The main challenge of this approach is that the LRCs have to be purified out *live* to show they indeed represent slow-cycling CSCs, which generally is difficult to do without a suitable genetic-tracking system. Furthermore, recent studies in HSCs suggest that not all LRCs may represent SCs [43].

Acknowledgements

We thank all current and past Tang lab members for their support and helpful discussions. We apologize to those colleagues whose original work could not be cited in this review due to space constraint. This work was supported in part by grants from NIH (CA90297, AG023374, and CCSG-5 P30 CA166672), NIEHS (ES07784), American Cancer Society (RSG MGO-105961), Department of Defense (DAMD17-03-1-0137), Prostate Cancer Foundation, and M.D Anderson Cancer Center (PCRP and IRG). J. Qin was supported in part by a postdoctoral fellowship from Department of Defense (W81XWH-07-1-0098 01).

References

[1] Tang, D. G., Patrawala, L., Calhoun, T., Bhatia, B., Choy, G., Schneider-Broussard, R., and Jeter, C. (2007). Prostate cancer stem/progenitor cells: identification, characterization, and implications. *Mol. Carcinog., 46:* 1-14.

[2] Clarke, M. F., Dick, J. E., Dirks, P. B., Eaves, C. J., Jamieson, C. H., Jones, D. L., Visvader, J., Weissman, I. L., and Wahl, G. M. (2006). Cancer stem cells--perspectives

on current status and future directions: AACR Workshop on cancer stem cells. *Cancer Res., 66*: 9339-9344.

[3] Kalluri, R. and Zeisberg, M. (2006). Fibroblasts in cancer. *Nat. Rev. Cancer, 6:* 392-401.

[4] Mueller, M. M. and Fusenig, N. E. (2004). Friends or foes - bipolar effects of the tumour stroma in cancer. *Nat. Rev. Cancer, 4:* 839-849.

[5] Orimo, A. and Weinberg, R. A. (2006). Stromal fibroblasts in cancer: a novel tumor-promoting cell type. *Cell Cycle, 5:* 1597-1601.

[6] Hayward, S. W., Wang, Y., Cao, M., Hom, Y. K., Zhang, B., Grossfeld, G. D., Sudilovsky, D., and Cunha, G. R. (2001). Malignant transformation in a nontumorigenic human prostatic epithelial cell line. *Cancer Res., 61:* 8135-8142.

[7] Zhau, H. E., Hong, S. J., and Chung, L. W. (1994). A fetal rat urogenital sinus mesenchymal cell line (rUGM): accelerated growth and conferral of androgen-induced growth responsiveness upon a human bladder cancer epithelial cell line in vivo. *Int. J. Cancer, 56:* 706-714.

[8] Kleinman, H. K. and Martin, G. R. (2005). Matrigel: basement membrane matrix with biological activity. *Semin. Cancer Biol., 15:* 378-386.

[9] Yamada, K. M. and Cukierman, E. (2007). Modeling tissue morphogenesis and cancer in 3D. *Cell, 130:* 601-610.

[10] Patrawala, L., Calhoun, T., Schneider-Broussard, R., Zhou, J., Claypool, K., and Tang, D. G. (2005). Side population is enriched in tumorigenic, stem-like cancer cells, whereas ABCG2+ and ABCG2- cancer cells are similarly tumorigenic. *Cancer Res., 65:* 6207-6219.

[11] Patrawala, L., Calhoun, T., Schneider-Broussard, R., Li, H., Bhatia, B., Tang, S., Reilly, J. G., Chandra, D., Zhou, J., Claypool, K., Coghlan, L., and Tang, D. G. (2006). Highly purified CD44+ prostate cancer cells from xenograft human tumors are enriched in tumorigenic and metastatic progenitor cells. *Oncogene, 25:* 1696-1708.

[12] Patrawala, L., Calhoun-Davis, T., Schneider-Broussard, R., and Tang, D. G. (2007). Hierarchical organization of prostate cancer cells in xenograft tumors: the CD44+alpha2beta1+ cell population is enriched in tumor-initiating cells. *Cancer Res. 67:* 6796-6805.

[13] Raff, M. (2003). Adult stem cell plasticity: fact or artifact? *Annu. Rev. Cell Dev. Biol., 19:* 1-22.

[14] Hope, K. J., Jin, L., and Dick, J. E. (2004). Acute myeloid leukemia originates from a hierarchy of leukemic stem cell classes that differ in self-renewal capacity. *Nat. Immun*ol., *5:* 738-743.

[15] Morrison, S. J. and Kimble, J. (2006). Asymmetric and symmetric stem-cell divisions in development and cancer. *Nature, 441:* 1068-1074.

[16] Lobo, N. A., Shimono, Y., Qian, D., and Clarke, M. F. (2007). The Biology of cancer stem cells. *Annu. Rev. Cell Dev. Biol., 23:* 675-699.

[17] Bao, S., Wu, Q., McLendon, R. E., Hao, Y., Shi, Q., Hjelmeland, A. B., Dewhirst, M. W., Bigner, D. D., and Rich, J. N. (2006). Glioma stem cells promote radioresistance by preferential activation of the DNA damage response. *Nature, 444:* 756-760.

[18] Phillips, T. M., McBride, W. H., and Pajonk, F. (2006). The response of $CD24^{-/low}CD44^{+}$ breast cancer-initiating cells to radiation. J Natl Cancer Inst, *98:* 1777-1785.
[19] Passegue, E., Jamieson, C. H., Ailles, L. E., and Weissman, I. L. (2003). Normal and leukemic hematopoiesis: are leukemias a stem cell disorder or a reacquisition of stem cell characteristics? *Proc. Natl. Acad. Sci. USA, 100:* 11842-11849.
[20] Tavil, B., Cetin, M., and Tuncer, M. (2006). CD34/CD117 positivity in assessment of prognosis in children with myelodysplastic syndrome. *Leuk. Res., 30:* 222-224.
[21] Huntly, B. J., Shigematsu, H., Deguchi, K., Lee, B. H., Mizuno, S., Duclos, N., Rowan, R., Amaral, S., Curley, D., Williams, I. R., Akashi, K., and Gilliland, D. G. (2004). MOZ-TIF2, but not BCR-ABL, confers properties of leukemic stem cells to committed murine hematopoietic progenitors. *Cancer Cell, 6:* 587-596.
[22] Jamieson, C. H., Ailles, L. E., Dylla, S. J., Muijtjens, M., Jones, C., Zehnder, J. L., Gotlib, J., Li, K., Manz, M. G., Keating, A., Sawyers, C. L., and Weissman, I. L. (2004). Granulocyte-macrophage progenitors as candidate leukemic stem cells in blast-crisis CML. *N. Engl. J. Med., 351:* 657-667.
[23] Jamieson, C. H., Weissman, I. L., and Passegue, E. (2004). Chronic versus acute myelogenous leukemia: a question of self-renewal. *Cancer Cell, 6:* 531-533.
[24] Krivtsov, A. V., Twomey, D., Feng, Z., Stubbs, M. C., Wang, Y., Faber, J., Levine, J. E., Wang, J., Hahn, W. C., Gilliland, D. G., Golub, T. R., and Armstrong, S. A. (2006). Transformation from committed progenitor to leukaemia stem cell initiated by MLL-AF9. *Nature, 442:* 818-822.
[25] Bonnet, D. and Dick, J. E. (1997). Human acute myeloid leukemia is organized as a hierarchy that originates from a primitive hematopoietic cell. *Nat. Med., 3:* 730-737.
[26] Singh, S. K., Hawkins, C., Clarke, I. D., Squire, J. A., Bayani, J., Hide, T., Henkelman, R. M., Cusimano, M. D., and Dirks, P. B. Identification of human brain tumour initiating cells. *Nature, 432:* 396-401, 2004.
[27] Al-Hajj, M., Wicha, M. S., Benito-Hernandez, A., Morrison, S. J., and Clarke, M. F. (2003). Prospective identification of tumorigenic breast cancer cells. *Proc. Natl. Acad. Sci. USA, 100:* 3983-3988.
[28] O'Brien, C. A., Pollett, A., Gallinger, S., and Dick, J. E. (2007). A human colon cancer cell capable of initiating tumour growth in immunodeficient mice. *Nature, 445:* 106-110.
[29] Ricci-Vitiani, L., Lombardi, D. G., Pilozzi, E., Biffoni, M., Todaro, M., Peschle, C., and De Maria, R. (2007). Identification and expansion of human colon-cancer-initiating cells. *Nature, 445:* 111-115.
[30] Li, C., Heidt, D. G., Dalerba, P., Burant, C. F., Zhang, L., Adsay, V., Wicha, M., Clarke, M. F., and Simeone, D. M. (2007). Identification of pancreatic cancer stem cells. *Cancer Res., 67:* 1030-1037.
[31] Pardal, R., Clarke, M. F., and Morrison, S. J. (2003). Applying the principles of stem-cell biology to cancer. *Nat. Rev. Cancer, 3:* 895-902.
[32] Mazurier, F., Gan, O. I., McKenzie, J. L., Doedens, M., and Dick, J. E. (2004). Lentivector-mediated clonal tracking reveals intrinsic heterogeneity in the human hematopoietic stem cell compartment and culture-induced stem cell impairment. *Blood, 103:* 545-552.

[33] Barker, N., van Es, J.H., Kuipers, J., Kujala, P., van den Born, M., Cozijnsen, M., Haegebarth, A., Korving, J., Begthel, H., Peters, P.J., and Clevers, H. (2007). Identification of stem cells in small intestine and colon by marker gene Lgr5. *Nature*, *449*: 1003-1007.

[34] Clarke, R. B., Spence, K., Anderson, E., Howell, A., Okano, H., and Potten, C. S. (2005). A putative human breast stem cell population is enriched for steroid receptor-positive cells. *Dev. Biol., 277:* 443-456.

[35] Kondo, T., Setoguchi, T., and Taga, T. (2004). Persistence of a small subpopulation of cancer stem-like cells in the C6 glioma cell line. *Proc. Natl. Acad. Sci. USA*, *101:* 781-786.

[36] Hadnagy, A., Gaboury, L., Beaulieu, R., and Balicki, D. (2006). SP analysis may be used to identify cancer stem cell populations. *Exp. Cell Res*., *312:* 3701-3710.

[37] Ho, M. M., Ng, A. V., Lam, S., and Hung, J. Y. (2007). Side population in human lung cancer cell lines and tumors is enriched with stem-like cancer cells. *Cancer Res*., *67:* 4827-4833.

[38] Fang, D., Nguyen, T. K., Leishear, K., Finko, R., Kulp, A. N., Hotz, S., Van Belle, P. A., Xu, X., Elder, D. E., and Herlyn, M. (2005). A tumorigenic subpopulation with stem cell properties in melanomas. *Cancer Res., 65:* 9328-9337.

[39] Fuchs, E., Tumbar, T., and Guasch, G. (2004). Socializing with the neighbors: stem cells and their niche. *Cell, 116:* 769-778.

[40] Tumbar, T., Guasch, G., Greco, V., Blanpain, C., Lowry, W. E., Rendl, M., and Fuchs, E. (2004). Defining the epithelial stem cell niche in skin. *Science*, *303:* 359-363.

[41] Clarke, R. B., Anderson, E., Howell, A., and Potten, C. S. (2003). Regulation of human breast epithelial stem cells. *Cell Prolif, 36:* 45-58.

[42] Zhang, H. B., Ren, C. P., Yang, X. Y., Wang, L., Li, H., Zhao, M., Yang, H., and Yao, K. T. (2007). Identification of label-retaining cells in nasopharyngeal epithelia and nasopharyngeal carcinoma tissues. *Histochem. Cell Biol*., *127:* 347-354.

[43] Kiel, M.J., He, S., Ashkenazi, R., Gentry, S.N., Teta, M., Kushner, J.A., Jackson, T.L., and Morrison, S.J. (2007). Haematopoietic stem cells do not asymmetrically segregate chromosomes or retain BrdU. *Nature*, *449*: 238-242.

In: Cancer and Stem Cells
Eds: Thomas Dittmar and Kurt S. Zänker

ISBN 978-1-60456-478-5

Chapter 2

Mathematical Modeling of Stem Cells Related to Cancer

Monika Joanna Piotrowska[1,2], Heiko Enderling[3], Uwe an der Heiden[1] and Michael C. Mackey[4]

[1]Institute of Mathematics, University of Witten/Herdecke, Stockumer Str. 10, 58448 Witten, Germany

[2]Institute of Applied Mathematics and Mechanics, Department of Mathematics, Informatics and Mechanics, Warsaw University, Banacha 2, 02–097 Warsaw, Poland

[3]Center of Cancer System Biology, Caritas St. Elizabeth's Medical Center, Tufts University School of Medicine, 736 Cambridge Street, Boston, MA 02135, USA

[4]Departments of Physiology, Physics and Mathematics and Centre for Nonlinear Dynamics, McGill University, 3655 Promenade Sir William Osler, Montreal, QC, H3G 1Y6, Canada

Abstract

In this chapter we present an overview of different mathematical and numerical approaches to describe stem cell proliferation and differentiation and the development of small cancer stem cell populations that are origins of neoplasm disease. The purpose of this chapter is not to scare the reader with complex mathematical and numerical analysis. Instead we aim to summarize the wide range of possibilities that mathematics and computer sciences can offer to experimentalists and theoretical biologists.

We briefly introduce recently developed models that address different aspects of stem cell dynamics and cancer development. First we focus on models of periodic hematological diseases having origin in abnormal behavior of hematopoietic stem cells in bone marrow. We also present models, less organ specific, describing the differentiation and possible mutation of stem cells which can give rise to cancer. We introduce a simple model which simulates the crucial interplay of proliferating and quiescent stem cells, and we discuss its potential application to treatment design. One of the presented models illustrates in detail the role of nuclear factor κB-complex in proliferation of adult neural stem cells. Finally the reader will become acquainted with a computational model approach able to simulate stem cell dependent tissue development, homeostasis, and recovery from external perturbations.

Introduction

Recent research confirms that many neoplastic diseases like breast cancer [1], [2], prostate cancer [3], liver cancer [4], or leukemia [5], can occur because of mutations in normal stem and/or early progenitor cells. Moreover, it has been shown that various genes regulating the self-renewal in normal cells are also found in cancer cells [6]. It is known that most cancers are not clonal, but consist of heterogeneous sub-populations with distinct characteristics within a single neoplasm. These sub-populations are similar to the hierarchical tree of stem cell lineages. These results manifest the so-called stem cell cancer hypothesis, claiming that some cancers have stem cell origin. Moreover, it is known that the self-renewal ability in cancer stem cells (CSCs) is poorly controlled, leading to abnormal differentiation and faster proliferation in cancer tissue [7]--[9]. Hence, it appears likely that CSCs are often responsible for recurrences of the disease after treatment.

It is well known that key to tumor control is early detection of neoplasmatic changes in healthy tissue. It is important to understand the mechanism of carcinogenesis and the complexity of its progress and development. Modern life sciences, such as biology, molecular biology, medicine or oncology, are based primarily on experiments and clinical observations. Scientists try to understand the dynamics and particular function of selected signaling pathways, proteins and drugs focusing mainly only on statistical results of experiments. Although necessary, this knowledge does not reveal the general dynamics and the complexity of the problem even in case of single cell. It is crucial for future research and application in medicine to understand the 'engine' that drives the whole biochemical machinery.

Mathematical modeling and computational approaches have become more accepted by experimentalists and clinicians in recent years as contributing to new understandings of complicated cell mechanisms and tissue physiology. Indeed, even a single cell or small tissue samples are complex dynamical systems that adapt to environmental challenges in space and time - which renders them suitable to modeling. Mathematical models and numerical simulations can explain and uncover some still unknown aspects of cell behavior and tissue function. Models based on key biological mechanisms can give interesting insights and formulate predictions that cannot be derived from specific experiments or statistical data alone. Therefore, novel research approaches should incorporate interdisciplinary dialogs between biology, mathematical modeling and computer simulations to validate experimental data and non-intuitive scenarios such as the stem cell hypothesis (Figure 1).

Mathematical models can be classified into macroscopic and microscopic models depending on their level of description. Macroscopic models usually describe the evolution of sub-populations and interactions (competition and/or cooperation) between them rather than between individual entities.

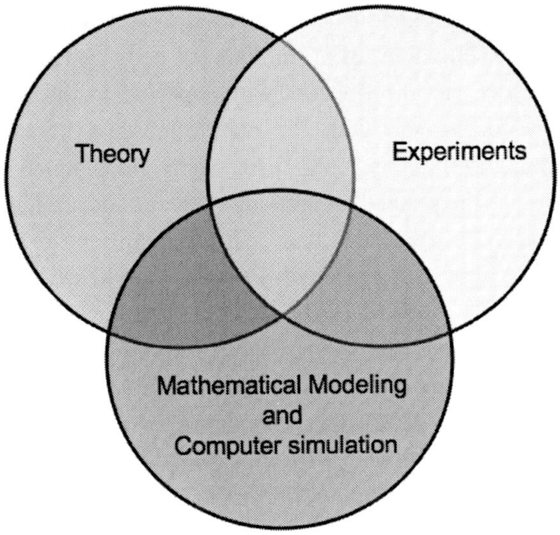

Figure 1. The schematic representation of modern biology, which should base on experiments run in laboratories, theory and should be also supported by mathematical models and computer simulations.

Microscopic models describe cellular and sub-cellular interactions between cells, and are based on processes like (a) chemical signaling between cells, and between cell and surrounding environment through the emission of activating or/and inhibiting cytokine signals; (b) protein and cyclin synthesis; (c) molecular interactions between proteins and protein complexes which can take place in the cell cytoplasm, in the nucleus or at the membrane.

From a mathematical and numerical point of view we furthermore distinguish between continuous and discrete models with respect to time. Continuous models describe the rate of change of for example cell density or protein concentrations over time. On the other hand in discrete models individual entities such as cells in populations or molecules in chemical concentrations are described at fixed separated time points. According to this distinction, in the following we first present some continuous modeling approaches that discuss stem cell dynamics in terms of cell populations or protein concentrations. Later on we discuss discrete models and develop an agent-based model of cell dynamics.

Continuous Mathematical Models

Continuous Models of Periodic Hematological Diseases

All blood cells arise from a common origin in the bone marrow, the hematopoietic stem cells. These stem cells can differentiate into one of three major cell lines: leukocytes, platelets, and erythrocytes. The exact details of how the numbers of circulating cells of each type are regulated remain somewhat obscure, though the broad outlines are clear. Interestingly, mathematical modeling of periodic hematological diseases has allowed us great insight into these regulatory processes.

In periodic chronic myelogenous leukemia (PCML) the leukocyte count varies periodically, typically between values of 30 to 200×10^9 cells/L. This is far above the normal value of 6×10^9 cells/L. The variation occurs with a period in the range of 40 to 80 days, which is very long in comparison with the maturation and lifespan of stem cells and leukocytes. In addition, oscillations may also occur in platelets and occasionally in reticulocytes. In these cases the platelet and reticulocyte periods are the same as the leukocyte periods [29] [30]. It has been argued that this, in addition to the occurrence of the Philadelphia chromosome in all differentiated lineages, is indicative of the stem cell origins of PCML [30].

Cyclical neutropenia (CN) is characterized by oscillations that are most prominent in neutrophils. Neutrophil numbers fall from normal or above normal levels to almost zero, and rise again, with a period of about 19-21 days in humans [31]--[33]. The disease also occurs in grey collies, with a shorter period of 11-16 days [34]. Interestingly, the platelet numbers typically oscillate as well, with the same period as neutrophils, but with a mean around the normal platelet level. Reticulocyte levels may also oscillate, again with the same period as neutrophils and platelets.

In both PCML and CN, the hypothesis that oscillations originate in stem cells is related to the fact that oscillations occur in different lines. However, in many earlier mathematical models, only one cell line, or one line coupled to the stem cells, is represented. In this context it is not possible to examine the effects of a destabilization in one line or in the stem cell compartment on whole system. For example, while Pujo-Menjouet et al., ([35]) explored how long period oscillations (as seen in PCML) could arise within the context of a G_0 stem cell model, the stem cell model alone could not predict whether leukocytes and platelets would oscillate at the levels observed in PCML. Similarly, Bernard et al., ([36]) were able to duplicate various features of cyclical neutropenia with an integrated mathematical model of the HSC and peripheral neutrophil control. However, since their model did not include platelet and erythrocyte regulation it is unknown if their simulated neutropenic conditions would be consistent with observed platelet and erythrocyte data in CN.

Cyclical thrombocytopenia (CT) is a rare hematological disorder described mostly in adults and characterized by periodic platelet count fluctuations of unknown etiology. The incidence of the statistically significant periodic platelet data is equally distributed between men and women. Sometimes this disease is associated with bleeding symptoms which have no apparent cause other than thrombocytopenia. Although, in general, human platelet levels remain relatively stable for years (150×10^9 - 450×10^9 platelets/L with an average of 290×10^9 platelets/L), many factors can influence an individual's platelet count (e.g. exercise, racial origin, some diseases, pregnancy). In CT the platelet counts oscillate from very low (1×10^9 platelets/L) to normal or very high levels (2000×10^9 platelets/L). This hematological disorder was reviewed by Go ([37]), Swinburne and Mackey ([38]), Cohenand Cooney ([39]), and has been the subject of mathematical modeling (Santillan et al. ([40]), Von Schulthess and Gessner ([41])).

In previous work leukocyte ([42], [43], [36]), erythrocyte ([44]--[46]) and platelet ([47], [40]) dynamics have been modelled separately, with the goal of building quantitative understanding of cellular production within the context of periodic hematological disorders. Colijn and Mackey [48] linked these models together, connecting models for the three distinct cell lines to a mathematical model of the stem cell population ([49]--[51], [35]). The model has four distinct compartments representing hematopoietic stem cells and circulating leukocytes, platelets and erythrocytes. The stem cells are pluripotential and self-renewing, and can differentiate into the leukocyte, erythrocyte or platelet lines. Alternatively, stem cells may re-enter the proliferative phase of the stem cell compartment. The stem cell and leukocyte compartments are modelled using the stem cell model connected to a neutrophil population as in [36]. The platelet and erythrocyte compartments are simplified approximations of earlier modelling efforts. The full model is described by a system of five highly nonlinear differential delay equations, cf. [48], [52] for full details of the model development as well as its usage in understanding PCML and CN.

In [48] Colijn and Mackey analyzed data taken from published studies of periodic chronic myelogenous leukemia. These data were previously analyzed for significant periodicity using Lomb periodogram ([53]) techniques by Fortin and Mackey ([30]). Each primary study presented time series of patient leukocyte counts, and some also provided platelet and reticulocyte data. Based on estimates of parameters for a typical normal human, they systematically explored the changes in some of these parameters necessary to account for the quantitative data on leukocyte, platelet and reticulocyte cycling in these PCML patients.

Their results indicate that the oscillatory nature of PCML is probably generated through a bifurcation in the dynamics of the coupled hematopoietic stem cell compartment and the regulation of differentiated leukocytes. Based on the simulations, the critical model parameter changes required to simulate the periodic chronic myelogenous leukemia patient data are the amplification in the leukocyte line, the differentiation rate from the stem cell compartment into the leukocyte line, and the rate of apoptosis in the stem cell compartment. There was a suggestion that changes in the numbers of proliferating stem cells may be important in generating PCML.

In [52] Colijn and Mackey used the model from [48] to understand the dynamics of CN in nine grey collies and 27 CN patients and the effects of treatment with granulocyte colony stimulating factor (G-CSF). Their results lend credibility to the hypothesis that the origins of oscillation in cyclical neutropenia are a destabilization in the stem cell compartment, induced by changes in the neutrophil line; the oscillations are then transmitted to the other lines. A biological interpretation of their model simulations is that CN is due to a decreased amplification (increased apoptosis) within the proliferating neutrophil precursor compartment, and a decrease in the maximal rate of re-entry into the proliferative phase of the stem cell compartment.

An analysis of data from the grey collies as well as human patients under treatment with G-CSF implies that G-CSF leads to an increased amplification (lower rate of apoptosis) in the proliferating neutrophil precursors, and there was on average a higher rate of differentiation into the neutrophil line than without the treatment. As in the untreated subjects all of these changes are consistent with laboratory and clinical findings.

Recently Apostu and Mackey ([54]) used the model presented in [48] to elucidate the nature of cyclical thrombocytopenia. They concluded that the platelet fluctuations in amegakaryocytic CT are caused by a cyclic inhibition of megakaryocytopoiesis, accentuated by an increased platelet maturation time and a reduced release of platelets per megakaryocyte. Their results suggest that the onset of oscillations in autoimmune CT can be explained by an accelerated peripheral destruction of platelets, exacerbated by an increased maturation of megakaryocytes and a slow relative growth rate of megakaryocytes.

A Continuous Model of Stem Cell and Cancer Stem Cell Proliferation, Differentiation and Maturation

The hypotheses and implications of mathematical models describing population dynamics of CSCs and their differentiation have recently been discussed [10]. In this paper a predictive model concerning self-renewing brain CSCs has validated principles according to which cancers can occur as a result of mutations in normal stem cells, early progenitor cells and even mature cells.

The model, a large system of ordinary differential equations, contains many nonlinear terms. We refrain from discussing the mathematics in detail, and refer to the original publication [10]. However, in the following we describe the model assumptions, present the main results and their biological interpretation. Ganguly and Puri distinguish seven main types of cells - stem cells (SC); early progenitor cells (EP); late progenitor cells (LP); mature cells (MC); abnormal stem cells (SC_A); abnormal early progenitor cells (EP_A) and abnormal progeny (tumor) cells (AP). Each cell type is considered as a separate model compartment, with cell population growth being modeled by considering individual rate expressions for each given cell type. Figure 2a shows a schematic representation of the model. SCs can self-renew with probability P_{SC} (both daughter cells retain stem cell features) or differentiate and transfer to the EP compartment. Stem cell DNA can mutate during the replication with probability M_{SC} such that the daughter cell which inherits the mutated gene is transferred into the SC_A population. EP cells, as well as EP_A cells, undergo only a limited number (*k*) of self-renewal steps. Thus, cells with identical self-renewal capacity are grouped into *k* sub-compartments. However, cells belonging to the kth compartment can not self-renew any more. If EP_i ($EP_{A,i}$) cells undergo cell division they self-renew into a subgroup EP_{i+1} ($EP_{A,i+1}$) with given probability P_{EP} ($P_{EP,A}$), which is assumed to be equal for all sub-populations, respectively. Dividing cells that do not supply the EP_{i+1} ($EP_{A,i+1}$) compartment differentiate into LP (AP, in case of abnormal cells) cells. Moreover, at each division EP_i cells are subject to mutations defined by mutation probability M_{EP}, which is assumed to be identical for each EP_i compartment. Naturally, the AP compartment is supplied by EP_A cells. Finally, cells that reach the MC or AP compartment die due to apoptosis.

Without mutations SC, EP and LP populations converge to a steady state, and for specific apoptosis rates the MC population remains constant. A sudden damage to the mature tissue (caused for example by acute radiation or surgery) activates tissue healing signals resulting in increased SC and EP cell proliferation rates. If mutations are enabled, SC and EP cells can produce SC_A or EP_A cells, respectively, that eventually form the AP compartment. Stochastic numerical simulations of this model show that an oncogenic event in SC leads to faster enrichment in AP cells, compared to the case of mutations in EP cells. Hence, the increase of the growth rate of EP_A cells leads to faster proliferation and increased cancer risk.

It has been also concluded that AP cell growth rate increases as the mean time between two consecutive insults decreases.

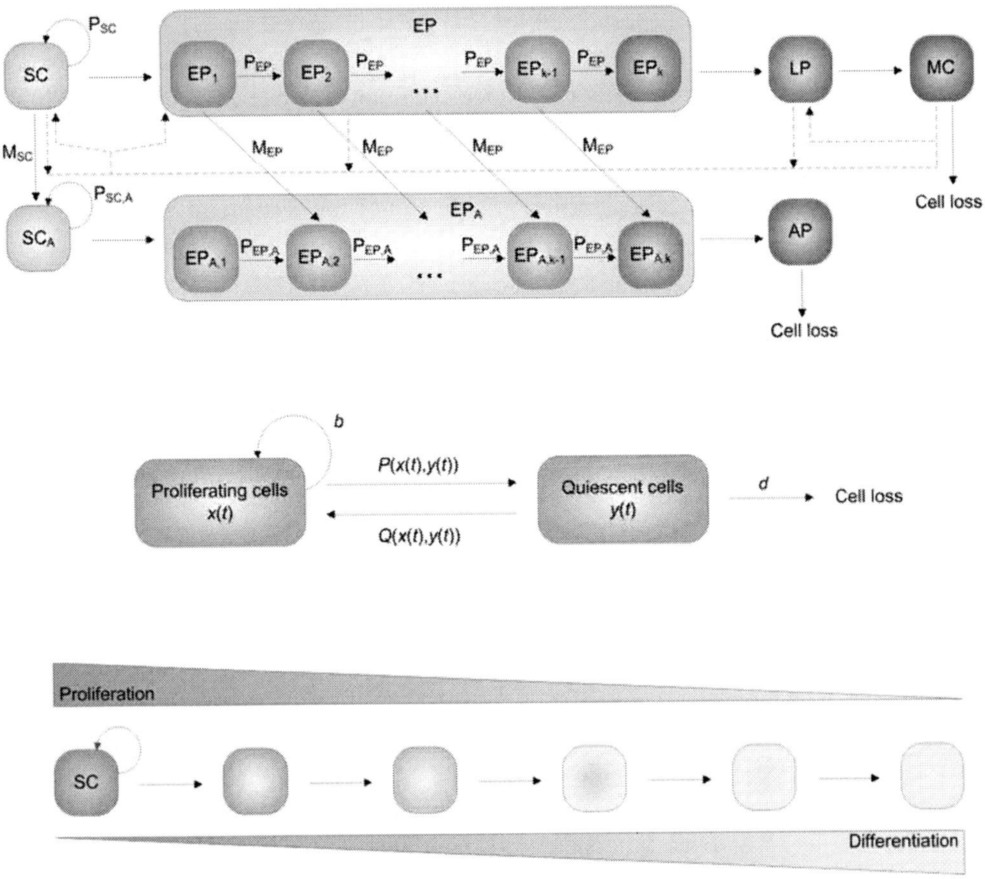

Figure 2. a) Multi compartment block diagram of a mathematical model developed by Ganguly and Puri, [10]. Here: SC represents the population of stem cells; EP early progenitor cells; LP late progenitor cells; MC mature cells; SC_A abnormal stem cells; EP_A abnormal early progenitor cells and AP abnormal progeny (tumor) cells. The EP cells as well as EP_A cells are split into k sub-compartments that contain identical cells regarding the type, which differ only with respect to the number of times they have undergone self-renewal. For more details see text. The solid lines indicate the direct transition from one compartment to another one, while dashed lines stand for feedback interaction loops. b) Two compartment block diagram of the mathematical model developed by Solyanik et al., [9]. Here $x(t)$ is the fraction of proliferating cells given at time t; $y(t)$ is the fraction of quiescent cells given at time t; b is the cell division rate of the proliferating cells and d is the cell death rate of quiescence cells. $P(x(t),y(t))$ and $Q(x(t),y(t))$ describe the intensity of cell transition from proliferating to quiescent compartment and vice versa, respectively. c) Stem cells and differentiated cells defined by their proliferation capacity and differentiation level. Non-differentiated stem cells have unlimited replicative potential and self-renewing ability. Stem cell progeny will differentiate with each proliferation and lose replication capacity.

Interaction between Quiescent and Proliferating Stem Cells Described by a Continuous Mathematical Model

Another interesting model postulated by [11], later discussed by [12], investigates the behavior of proliferating ($x(t)$) and quiescent cancer cell ($y(t)$) populations, based on experimental data. Proliferating cells can divide with constant rate β or lose their division ability and therefore transit to the resting phase. Resting cells can either return to the proliferating state or die with constant rate δ (Figure 2b). The interactions between these two cancer cell sub-populations are described by the following system of coupled ordinary differential equations

$$\begin{aligned} \frac{d}{dt}x(t) &= \overbrace{\beta x(t)}^{\text{cell proliferation}} - \overbrace{P(x(t),y(t))x(t)}^{\substack{\text{transition from proliferating}\\ \text{to quiescent compartment}}} + \overbrace{Q(x(t),y(t))y(t)}^{\substack{\text{transition from quiescent to}\\ \text{proliferating compartment}}}, \\ \frac{d}{dt}y(t) &= \overbrace{P(x(t),y(t))x(t)}^{\substack{\text{transition from proliferating}\\ \text{to quiescent compartment}}} - \overbrace{Q(x(t),y(t))y(t)}^{\substack{\text{transition from quiescent to}\\ \text{proliferating compartment}}} - \overbrace{\delta y(t)}^{\text{cell death}}, \end{aligned} \tag{1}$$

where $P(x(t),y(t))$ and $Q(x(t),y(t))$ describe the intensity of cell transition from proliferating to quiescent state per day and vice versa. It is additionally assumed that the transition from the quiescent to the proliferating state depends on the number of proliferating cells only. Moreover, the transition of quiescent cells into the proliferating compartment $Q(x(t),y(t))$ increases with increasing $x(t)$ at low levels, but decreases when the number of proliferating cells becomes very large. It has been experimentally observed that cells can only proliferate in the sufficient presence of biological and physical factors. Hence, $P(x(t),y(t))$ depends on the number of all cells, and the authors proposed the following function

$$P(x(t),y(t)) = \gamma[x(t) + \alpha y(t)],$$

where α and γ describe the proliferating and quiescent cells' nutrient consumption, respectively.

With negligible transition form quiescent to proliferating compartment due to the large duration of growth delay i.e. $Q(x(t),y(t)) = 0$ [11] the system goes to a stable equilibrium at $(r/(a+r),\ a/(a+r))$. If $Q(x(t),y(t)) \neq 0$ a mathematical analysis of (1) becomes more difficult, and numerical simulations have to be used to reproduce the experimental data [12]. The experiments were done by Wallen et al., [13], [14], who cultivated the three unfed mouse mammary tumor cell lines 66, 67 and 68H for two weeks. In both, simulations and experiments it has been shown that more than 98% of unfed cells where alive after two weeks (initially the population grew exponentially before reaching a plateau), and only a small fraction of cells was still proliferating (for details see [13], [14]). We understand that a certain ratio of cells dies over time. However, the overall cell population remains constant as long as there is a sufficient fraction of proliferating cells.

The advantage of this kind of modeling approach is the estimation of treatment success prior to clinical application, as most cancer treatment protocols mainly eradicate proliferating cells. It seems to be possible to fit experimental data for a potential two weeks trial to estimate the long-term behavior of proliferating and quiescent populations such as cancer stem cells.

A Continuous Mathematical Model for Nuclear Factor κB Complex Determinating the Proliferation of Adult Neural Stem Cells

The mathematical models described above simulate macroscopic properties of tissues or cell cultures, and neglect details of molecular mechanisms governing cell proliferation and cancer development. Since molecular biology can only investigates subsets of mechanisms that determine the cell behavior, mathematicians should develop multi-scale models that link different levels of complexity, for example, overexpression of proteins at the cellular level with the proliferation of cells at tissue level. The next model we would like to discuss in more detail focuses on the role of sub-cellular processing on single stem cell dynamics.

In a recent study it has been shown that the nuclear factor κB (NF-κB) plays an essential role in proliferation of neural stem cells (NSCs) [15]. In fact, most substances or conditions positively modulate proliferation of NSCs via the NF-κB pathway. Following these findings, Piotrowska et al., [16] have proposed a simple continuous mathematical model (containing two ordinary differential equations) for NF-κB dependent proliferation of NSCs.

NF-κB protein is a transcription factor, crucially involved in many biological and physical processes such as regulation apoptosis and survival genes, inflammation, cancer, innate immunity [17], [18], as well as memory formation and learning [19]. Furthermore, NF-κB is directly responsible for cell growth and proliferation [20]. The most frequent form of NF-κB is a heterodimer composed of two subunits: p50 and p65. Activation of NF-κB is mainly controlled at the posttranscriptional level by complex formation with the inhibitory protein IκB in the cytoplasm. After binding of the stimulating agent (e.g., tumour necrosis factor (TNF) or erythropoietin (EPO)) to a receptor in the cell membrane, the signal is transduced via intermediate kinases to the IKKα/β/γ complex (Figure 3a). This leads subsequently to phosphorylation of IκB and its proteasome degradation. This degradation triggers the translocation of NF-κB into the nucleus followed by binding to regulatory DNA-sequences and initiation of a transcription process [21].

The changes of active NF-κB concentration in a cell ($x(t)$) can be described by a nonlinear ordinary differential equation, such as

$$\frac{d}{dt}x(t) = \overbrace{\alpha\frac{1-x(t)}{J_1+1-x(t)}}^{\text{actvation of NF-}\kappa\text{B}} - \overbrace{\beta\frac{\delta(t)x(t)}{J_2+x(t)}}^{\substack{\text{deactvation of NF-}\kappa\text{B}\\ \text{due to I}\kappa\text{B binding}}} - \overbrace{kx(t)}^{\substack{\text{proteasomal}\\ \text{degradation of}\\ \text{NF-}\kappa\text{B}}}, \qquad (2)$$

where $1 - x(t)$ and $\delta(t)$ denote the scaled concentrations of inactive NF-κB and IκB at time t, respectively, and J_1, J_2, k, α and β are nonnegative constants [16]. The first term in Eq. (2)

represents the activation of NF-κB via phosphorylation of IκB by the IKK complex due to the stimulus represented by α; while the second term models the deactivation of active NF-κB by NF-κB driven autoregulatory expression of IκB. Both terms are governed by so-called Michaelis-Menten kinetics, with J_1 and J_2 being the Michaelis-Menten constants [22]. The last term in Eq. (2) corresponds to the degradation of active NF-κB.

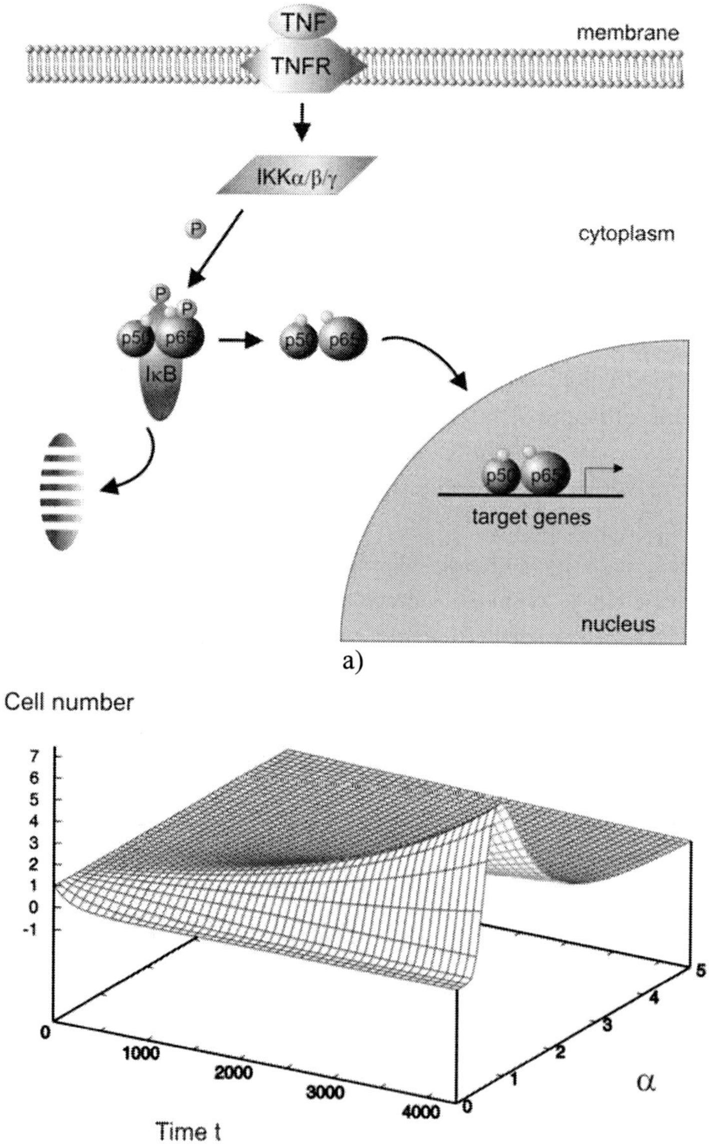

Figure 3. a) Schematic representation of signal transduction leading to NF- B driven proliferation. After binding of an NF- B activator (i.e. TNF or EPO) to its receptor (TNFR), the signal is transduced to the IKK complex. This complex phosphorylates inhibitory protein I B, which is then ubiquitinated and proteosomally degraded. The degradation triggers the translocation of NF- B into the nucleus of the cell, followed by initiation of transcription by binding to regulatory DNA sequences. It

leads to transcription of specific target genes and finally to proliferation of NSCs. Figure modified after Piotrowska et al. [16]. b) Graph of $y(t)$-solutions to Eqs. (2)–(5) proposed in [16] for different values of parameter $\alpha \in [0,5]$, which represents the relative cell number. Here α stands for relative concentration of the NF-κB activator such as TNFα or EPO. Simulation has been performed for the initial data $x(0) = 0.1$, $y(0) = 1$. All other model parameter values are as in Table 1 in [16]. Figure is reproduced from [16] by permission.

Experiments have shown a negative correlation between active NF-κB and IκB [23]. Therefore, the concentration of IκB (denoted by $\delta(t)$) is assumed to be a decreasing function of active NF-κB (denoted by $x(t)$), which can be modelled by a Hill function:

$$\delta(t) = \delta_0 \frac{\theta}{\theta + x(t)}, \tag{3}$$

where δ_0 and θ are positive constants.

Piotrowska et al. were able to relate the cellular concentration of active NF-κB with NSC proliferation speed. Since *in vitro* cultivated cells are not affected by factors that limit proliferation, the change of cell number $y(t)$ can be described by

$$\frac{d}{dt} y(t) = \overbrace{\gamma \underbrace{f[x(t)]}_{\substack{\text{dependence}\\ \text{on NF}-\kappa\text{B}}} y(t)}^{\text{proliferation}}, \tag{4}$$

with positive constant γ. Both, low and pathologically high NF-κB concentrations (hyperactivation) lead to cell death in the NSC population and only for intermediate values of active NF-κB cells are stimulated to proliferate [19] (compare with Figure. 3 in [16]). Based on these observations a reproduction function such as

$$f(x(t)) = b^2 - (x(t) - d)^2, \tag{5}$$

can been assumed, where b and d are positive constants to mark the physical level of NF-κB needed for cells to proliferate, with $d > b$ and $d + b < 1$. The local and global existence, non-negativity and boundness of solutions for bounded initial data as well as the analytical analysis of steady state existence and stability can be found in [16]. The solutions of the system (2-5) strongly depend on the constants d and b, and parameter α (the stimulus) as well. For fixed parameter values (see Table 1. in [16]) and $\alpha \neq 0.5244$ or $\alpha \neq 3.408$ there is only one biologically relevant steady state of the system (2-5). For $\alpha \in (0.5244, 3.408)$, the population of in vitro cultivated NSCs will either grow infinitely, or the population will die out, otherwise.

Figure 3b visualizes the change of cell number over time ($y(t)$-solution to Eqs. (2-5)) for α parameter values in the interval [0,5]. Recall that α is the stimulus for the activation of NF-κB via phosphorylation of IκB by the IKK complex. For a very small stimulating signal there is a little activation of NF-κB, insufficient for cells to proliferate (compare to Figure 5 and Figure 9 in [16]). As α increases the concentration of active NF-κB increases, and after reaching a threshold level the cells will start to proliferate. However, increasing α above another critical threshold results in hyperactivation of NF-κB and subsequent cell apoptosis. The model was compared with *in vitro* experimental data of NSCs after exposure to 0 (control) and 10 ng/ml TNF [16]. In the model as well as in experiments presented in [16], adult NSCs respond to TNF with significantly increased proliferation compared to untreated cells, see Figure 10 in [16].

The discussed model differs from previous models describing the NF-κB activation in fibroblasts [23]--[25]. For simplicity, only interactions between IKK complex and inactive NF-κB, IκB and active NF-κB, and proteasomal degradation of active NF-κB are considered. Focussing only on these crucial interactions reduces the system to two nonlinear ordinary differential equations, which enables mathematical analysis of the dynamics. For more complex systems (20 equations with more than 30 independent model parameters, [23], [24]) such an analysis is impossible and numerical simulations alone have to be used to study system properties.

So far we have discussed NF-κB as a modulator of NSC proliferation. However, the dependence of proliferating cancer stem cells on NF-κB has been observed recently, too [26]-- [28]. With parameter adaptation, the discussed model can be adapted to study cancer cell and cancer stem cell dynamics. Such a simple model could give useful insights into cancer development, as it can provide a potent tool for predicting results of proliferation assays and NSCs expansion.

Discrete Mathematical Models

Systems of coupled differential equations simulate behavior of cells or concentrations of molecules. In discrete models the fate of individual cell or molecule is followed. In fact, many individual events are crucial to determinate the cells' phenotype and behavior. Moreover, the cell phenotype can change depending on the input it receives from the microenvironment according to certain probability distributions. Cellular automaton and agent-based models can treat discrete features of cells and the resulting phenotype variability. Thus, in discrete mathematical and computer models, time is discretized, and at each time step every cell (or agent, for general agent-based models) follows certain defined rules that determine the state of the cell and consequently the whole system at this time point. The rules can, and often do so, include stochasticity and probability distributions giving the system more realistic non-deterministic behavior, which allows to study the impact of varying environmental factors. Dynamics of single cells are combined to populations and a complex system behavior emerges. By virtue of this approach properties of individual agents and their mutation give rise to multiple distinct subpopulations, which in cancer modeling can be interpreted as different cell types such as stem cells or differentiated cells, and more or less aggressive tumor clones.

In a recent interdisciplinary study using a hybrid continuous-discrete model it has been shown that the tumor microenvironment can orchestrate tumor phenotype development and selection [55]. Another automaton model has been designed to predict proliferating and quiescent cell populations and the tumor volume doubling time which is clinically important [56]. It is known that actively proliferating cells are more susceptible to treatment such as radiation and chemicals than quiescent cells, resting in G_0 phase. These cells stay arrested until DNA damage is completely repaired or the cell is sent into apoptosis. Stem cells are surrounded and protected by adjacent cells, and are thought to be quiescent under normal conditions. Resting at the time of an environmental insult, stem cells have a higher chance of surviving and subsequently re-populating the tissue.

A Discrete Cellular Automaton Model of Stem Cells and Tissue Homeostasis

A discrete mathematical model of stem cells and their role in tissue homeostasis has been developed by Agur and co-workers [57]. The model considers: bone marrow stem cells S, differentiated cells D, and null cells N, i.e. empty lattice space. Each cell's behavior is determined by their cell cycle, their internal state and by number and type of cells in the neighborhood. The model is defined as a connected, locally finite undirected graph $G = (V,E)$ where the vertices V describe the cells and the edges E describe their neighborhood. Operators on the set of all states on the graph define the dynamic behavior of the systems.

The rules of the system are defined such that differentiated cells mature until time Φ before they leave the domain (i.e., the bone marrow). Stem cells mature into differentiated cell if their age, i.e. internal counter, exceeds Ψ and its neighbors consist of stem cells alone. Finally, stem cells proliferate into an empty site after time Θ. A detailed explanation of all rules and the proofs can be found in [57].

The model characterizes some universal properties of stem cells to produce mature cells and recover from severe perturbations. The direct stem cell environment modulates the decision to remain quiescent or to proliferate. Eventually the system results in a dense stem cell population and the system never dies out. Stem cell maturation Ψ drives the system dynamics, and stem cell proliferation Θ and differentiated cell maturation Φ play a secondary role only. The disadvantage of such a cellular automaton approach is the necessary simplicity - and due to lack of simulations there is a need to prove the dynamics of the proposed rules.

An Agent Based Model of Stem Cell and Non-Stem Cell Tissue Dynamics

A more complex discrete modeling technique is agent-based modeling. Agents are autonomous entities whose behavior is based on a certain set of rules and in response to the local environment [55], [56]. The agents make non-deterministic decisions independently from large systems or aims of complex populations. However, as many agents not only respond to the environment but also modify it, changes in single cell state and behavior can lead to system catastrophes.

We now construct a small-scale agent-based stem cell and non-stem cell model to simulate single cell dynamics and cell-cell interactions as they occur in the early stages of tissue or tumor development [58]. We define rules from general biological observations to describe individual cell behavior and simulate dynamic patterns of the emerging population system. We distinguish between a stem cell and a non-stem cell phenotype, and allow for variations of some of the implemented rules to discuss aberrations that lead to cancer development.

Key cellular behavior events are cell division and cell death. For both events, a chain of internal and external signals must occur. Tissue homeostasis is a complex dynamic process and cells obey external signals that define cell cycle progression. The environment determines the fate of each cell, for example by diffusion of signals or cell-cell signaling. Cells either proceed through the cell cycle to undergo mitosis, or rest in the so-called G_0 phase. Resting cells may re-enter the cell cycle and proceed into mitosis if nearby cells died and need to be replaced. In a stable tissue the change in cell number over time should be negligible. Whenever a cell dies another one will proliferate, and when a cell proliferates another one is sent into apoptosis. This phenomenon is called Moran Process [59]. To avoid overcrowding we believe there is a contact inhibition between cells i.e. cells are less likely to divide if they are surrounded by other cells, and more likely to undergo mitosis in a microenvironment without spatial constraints. The potential to undergo mitosis is different for stem cells and differentiated cells. Stem cells are undifferentiated cells with unlimited replicative potential and self-renewal capacity. They can divide symmetrically to either form two stem cells or two differentiated cells, or asymmetrically to maintain one stem cell and send the offspring into differentiation. With each cell division non-stem cells become more differentiated and fulfill specific functions. However, these cells lose their replicative potential and die within a short time frame (Figure 2c). We define the proliferative potential $p_s = \infty$ for stem cells and $p_d = 12\pm3$ for differentiated cells. As the non-stem cells divide their proliferative potential decreases, and the daughter cells inherit the potential. Progeny of stem cells with differentiation fate get assigned a random p_d within the above stated interval.

In our simulation, we increment time at discrete 1-hour time steps. Cell age is increased and the cells progress in the cell cycle subject to certain environmental conditions. At the end of mitosis (M phase) proliferation capacity is checked. If the proliferation potential is exhausted, i.e. $p_d = 0$, the cell is sent into apoptosis. The flowchart of the simulation process and the decisions made by every cell at each time point is shown in Figure 4.

Now we present some simulations that show the cellular behavior based on the implemented rules. First we initialize our system with a single non-stem cell with proliferation capacity $p_d = 10$ in the center of the domain. If the cell has passed through the cell cycle it will divide because no neighbors are inhibiting it. As a result of this division, the original cell and its offspring have both now a proliferation capacity of $p_d = 9$. Both cells will cycle and reach mitosis, resulting in four cells all with $p_d = 8$. The emerging population will initially grow exponentially without contact inhibition. As the number of cells increases the available space for each cell decreases. If there is no space available, then the cell ready to proliferate will be sent into G_0 phase and stay there until an adjacent grid point becomes vacant. In Figure 5 proliferation capacity is color-coded, with maximum proliferation potential being red and no cell division left - black. As the population grows a proliferation capacity gradient from the center to the outer rim is formed. Limited proliferation (Figure 5a) results in population number oscillations already at very small cell numbers. Cells in the core of the population are contact inhibited and rest. Cells at the outer rim proliferate until all their proliferation capacity is exhausted and subsequently die. Previously resting cells will re-enter the cell cycle and start to proliferate again and occupy the freed space. This 'die off – re-population' process continues until all cells have exceeded their proliferation potential and the cluster vanishes. However, if we initialize a single stem cell with unlimited replicative potential, all direct offspring of this stem cell will start to populate the domain with maximum proliferation capacity p_d= 10 (Figure 5b).

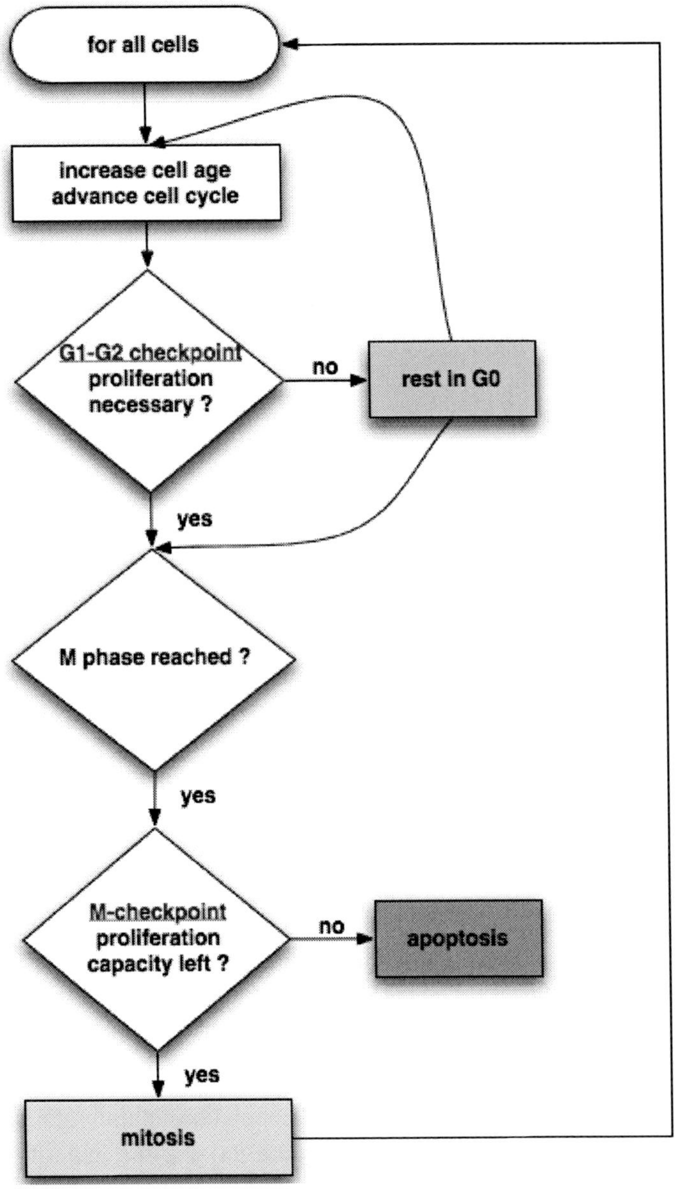

Figure 4. Cell life cycle scheme. At each time step the cell age increases. The cell will rest in G_0 if the microenvironment is saturated. If there is space for the cell to divide it will proceed into mitosis (M phase). If the proliferation capacity is exhausted the cell will undergo apoptosis; otherwise it will produce a daughter cell.

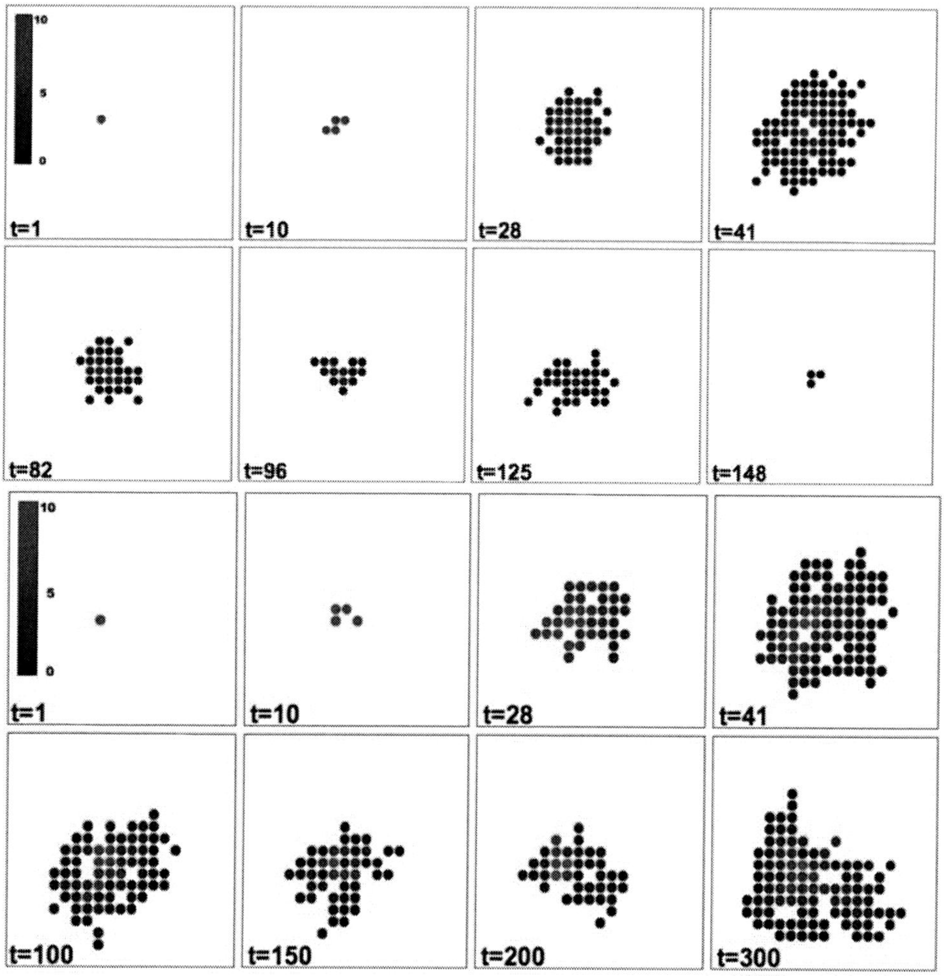

Figure 5. Cell cluster formation from non-stem cells and stem cells. As cells divide they lose proliferation capacity (red→black). Initially the populations grow exponentially as each cell experiences sufficient space. As the number of cells increases, cells in the core of the population cluster get contact inhibited and sent to rest. When the outer cells die off, cells in the interior will re-enter the cell cycle and start proliferating again until their proliferation capacity is exhausted, too. a) The cell number in populations arising from single cells with limited replicative potential $pd = 12$ (red, $t = 1$) oscillate over time with cells at the outer rim dieing and cells in the interior re-enter proliferation. After $t = 148$ days no cells with proliferation capacity is left, and at day $t = 150$ days all cells are dead. b) Populations emerging from a stem cell have initial similar behavior than those arising from non-stem cells. However, more cells are produced, as the core of the population is direct offspring of the stem cell with maximum proliferation capacity. As cells die off the stem cell will generate more potent offspring re-populating the cell cluster.

This results in a larger number of cells in the population. Initially the population growth is similar to the population described above (Figure 5a). As the majority of cells die off, however, the stem cell will again produce potent progeny that repopulate the domain as before. Hence a population that arises from a stem cell will persist despite intermediate oscillations in cell number.

Tissues and organs are complex, heterogeneous structures with many cells that fulfill specific functions. Different stem cell ratios have been estimated or identified for different tissues. The fraction of stem cells in the breast, for example, has been reported to be between 0.2% and 5% [60]. Tissue homeostasis, a 'stable and constant' number of cells in the population, is assured by the interplay of stem cells and non-stem cells. Differentiated cells die off due to normal tissue turnover or when their proliferation capacity is exhausted. Those cells have to be replaced by potent cells to maintain tissue integrity. In a theoretical domain of constant size, say 100×100 grid points, each cell can occupy one grid point. Furthermore, at any time at most one cell can reside on a single grid point. With a small number of stem cells arbitrarily distributed in the domain, the size of each of the resulting cell clusters is not sufficient to occupy all the space in the domain and single cluster dynamics result in large variations in overall cell number. As the stem cell ratio increases multiple clusters arise that eventually compete for space. If progeny of stem cells in one cluster die, cells from adjacent clusters can replace the vacant space. If these cells later die, the original cells can populate this space again and the number of cells in the tissue is maintained. Figure 6a shows a sample simulation of 100 initial stem cells forming individual clusters of cells, each of which follows the growth dynamics as presented above. Despite of oscillations in cell numbers over time the overall tissue structure is preserved. Figure 6b shows plots of cell numbers obtained from simulations with 0.2% stem cell ratio, 1% stem cell ratio, and 5% stem cell ratio for five different simulations each. With increasing number of stem cells the variation of cell numbers in the tissue reduces as discussed.

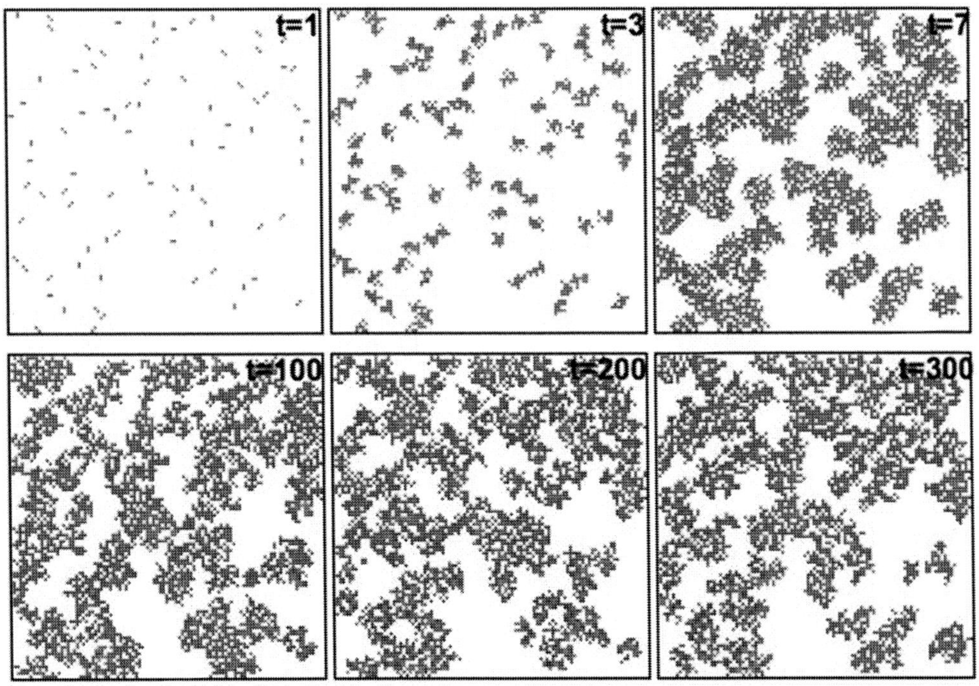

a)

Figure 6. (Continued).

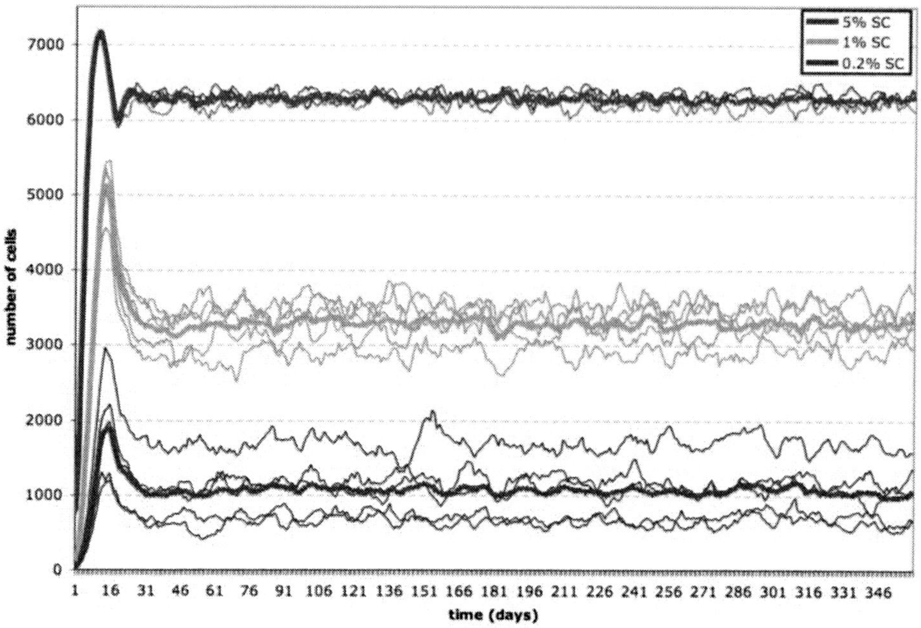

b)

Figure 6. Simulation of tissue homeostasis in a domain of 100×100 grid points holding at the most 100,000 cells. a) An initial arbitrary distribution of 1% stem cells, i.e. 1000 cells, results in cell cluster formation within the first 7 weeks. Despite oscillations in cell numbers the tissue structure is overall preserved. b) Plot of cell numbers obtained from simulations with 0.2% stem cell ratio (blue), 1% stem cell ratio (green) and 5% stem cell ratio (red). Shown are five different simulations for each stem cell ratio and an average over those runs (thick line). With increasing number of stem cells the variation of cell numbers in the tissue reduces.

So far we have only discussed asymmetric stem cell division. For functional tissue it is crucial to maintain homeostasis especially after sudden loss of cells and stem cells e.g. during exposure to acute radiation or other cellular catastrophes. Symmetric stem cell division is needed to preserve a constant stem cell compartment and the tissue integrity. We assume that stem cells fate is determined by diffusion of signals in the extracellular matrix [61]. Figure 7 shows the development of a tissue from initially about 400 stem cells. Very quickly about 7.200 cells get produced and the domain gets populated to an arbitrarily set density of 75%. We simulate at time $t = 100$ steps a cellular catastrophe by randomly killing 50% of all cells, both stem and non-stem cells. The surviving stem cells start immediately to divide symmetrically until the pre-catastrophe stem cell compartment is re-established. The newly produced stem cells move away arbitrarily and start repopulation of the tissue by asymmetric division. Without symmetric stem cell division, the reduced number of stem cells cannot produce the cell numbers that have been in the domain previous to the perturbation resulting in a less dense tissue (Figure 7b).

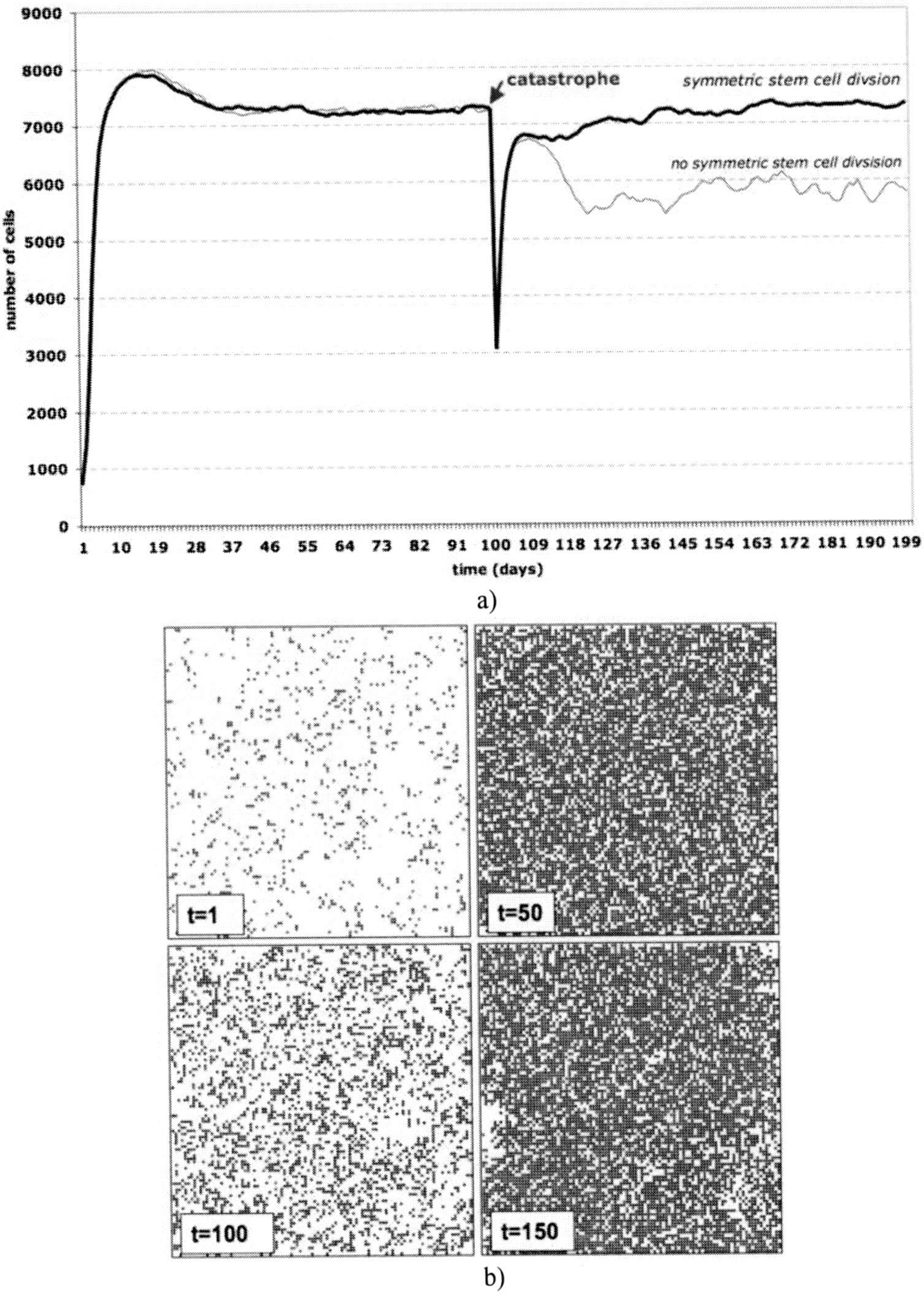

Figure 7. Impact of symmetric stem cell division on recovery to homeostasis after catastrophe. Stem cell ratio is 5%. At time $t = 100$ a catastrophe destroys randomly 50% of the cells. a) If stem cells cannot divide symmetrically (thin plot) pre-catastrophe cell number cannot be established. Only symmetric stem cell division (thick plot) and random cell migration enables quick recovery after a disaster. b) Sample simulation for development of a tissue from 5% stem cells with cell migration enabled and recovery from a disaster at time $t = 100$.

Conclusion

Mathematical models applied to biology and medicine describe and simulate possible not yet know scenarios. Complex biological dynamics, for example cell behavior, tissue recovery or cancer development, are reduced to key mechanisms which enable the analysis of how the system changes if any of these mechanisms are interrupted. In this chapter we have tried to discuss a small selection of representative modeling approaches that can have significant implications for stem cell study. Some describe stem cell differentiation and maturation [10], interactions between proliferative and quiescent stem cells [11], [12], or cell proliferation controlled by signaling pathways [15], while others focus on tissue homeostasis for healthy tissue [57], [58]. Most, if not all of the mathematical models of stem cell dynamics have subsequent implications to cancer development and treatment. For example, from the last presented agent based model [58] and simulations it seems obvious that each tumor reaching the clinical significance must contain cancer stem cells to drive the development up to a malignant size. Without stem cells, the tumor cell cluster would remain small and be doomed to die out. *In vivo* tumors are known to be heterogeneous in terms of clonogenicity. Using a model in which human breast cancer cells were grown in immunocompromized mice, it was shown that only a minority of the cancer cells had the ability to form new tumors [62]. The disability to form new tumors by the majority of the cancer cells can be explained by a model with limited proliferation capacity such as seen in normal cell populations in Figure 5a, which are likely to die after a certain number of proliferations [58]. Cancer stem cells have been successfully identified in acute myelogenous leukemia [63], [64], breast cancer [62], and brain tumors [26], [65], [66], and recently pancreas cancer [67].

Current cancer treatment is aimed to eradicate as many cancer cells as possible. A treatment protocol that eliminates 99% of the tumor cells may be considered successful. However, if only parts of the residual 1% of cancer cells have stem-cell properties, i.e. unlimited proliferation capacity, then the tumor will recur. More and more research focuses on this small clonogenic sub-population, as tumor treatment may provide better tumor control if the cancer stem cells are eradicated [68]. Recently, it have been shown that breast cancer initiating cells are more radiosensitive compared to the bulk of cancer cells [69]. Moreover, it also has been experimentally proven that glioblastoma stem cells are radioresistant and may therefore contribute to treatment failures [70].

A major advantage of mathematical models and computer simulations is their ability to make predictions of biological systems and their behavior that would be difficult to conduct experimentally. As an obvious example, it is challenging to maintain an unfed cell line longer than approximately 2 weeks and conducting counts. Moreover, mathematical models give the advantage to perform 'virtual' experiments instead of complicated lab experiments, which can be costly and time consuming. Furthermore, models are reproducible and not subject to biological variation, possibly induced by constantly changing external conditions. Mathematical/numerical experiments can give many answers since large numbers of variables and their dependence on time, space, and each other can be measured. Using mathematical models and computer simulations that incorporate new molecular findings may provide a platform to improve understanding of spatio-temporal tumor and cancer stem cell dynamics. Models can be developed to investigate the effect of treatment sensitizing or cell-cycle synchronizing drugs on treatment outcome, which may subsequently lead to improved tumor control.

In summary, mathematical models have a huge potential in biomedical research, which has not yet reached acceptance in many laboratories. We hope that this chapter gives a flavor of how models can help developing new hypotheses or testing existing theories. To use models as a predictive tool, future research needs to incorporate a dialog between biologists, clinicians and mathematicians. We believe that such an interdisciplinary effort will eventually lead to insights that can be translated into the clinic to the ultimate benefit of patients.

Acknowledgments

This work was supported by: the EU project 'Modelling, Mathematical Methods and Computer Simulation of Tumour Growth and Therapy', MRTN - CT - 2004 – 503661; MITACS (Canada) and the Natural Sciences and Engineering Research Council of Canada.

References

[1] Dick, J. E. (2003). Breast cancer stem cells revealed. *Proc. Natl. Acad. Sci. USA*, 100 (7), 3547 - 3549.

[2] Dontu, G., Al-Hajj M., Abdallah, W .M., Clarke, M. F. and Wicha, M. S. (2003). Stem cells in normal breast development and breast cancer. *Cell Prolif.*, 36, 59 - 72.

[3] Brown, M. D., Gilmore, P. E., Hart, C. A., Samuel, J. D., Ramani, V. A., George, N. J., Clarke, N. W. (2007). Characterization of benign and malignant prostate epithelial Hoechst 33342 side populations. *Prostate.*, 67(13), 1384 - 1396.

[4] Alison, M. R. (2005). Liver stem cells: implications for hepatocarcinogenesis. *Stem Cell Rev.*, 1(3), 253 - 60.

[5] Warner, J. K., Wang, J. C. Y., Hope, K. J., Jin, L., Dick, J. E. (2004). Concepts of human leukemic development. *Oncogene*, 23, 7164 - 7177.

[6] Clarke, M. F. (2004). Neurobiology: at the root of brain cancer. Nature, 432, 281 - 282.

[7] Pardal, R., Clarke, M.F. and Morrison, S.J. (2003). Applying the principes of stem-cell biology to cancer. *Nature Rev. Cancer*, 3, 895 – 902.

[8] Reya, T., Morrison, S.J., Clarke M.F. and Weissman, I.L. (2001). Stem cells, cancer, and cancer stem cells. *Nature,* 414, 101-115.

[9] Sell, S and Pierce, G.B. (1994). Maduration arrest of stem cell differentiation is a common pathway for the cellular origin of teratocarcinomas and epithelial cancers. *Lab Invest.*, 70, 6-22.

[10] Ganguly, R. and Puri, I. K. (2006). Mathematical model for the cancer stem cell hypothesis. *Cell Prolif.*, 39, 3 - 14.

[11] Solyani, G. I., Berezetskaya, N. M., Bulkiewicz, R. I., and Kulik, G. I. (1995). Different growth patterns of a cancer cell population as a function of its starting growth characteristics. Analysis by mathematical modelling. *Cell Prolif.*, 28, 263 - 278.

[12] Garner, A. L., Lau, Y. Y., Jordan, D. W., Uhler, M. D. and Gilgenbach, R. M. (2006). Implications of a simple mathematical model to cancer cell population dynamics. *Cell Prolif.*, 39, 15 - 28.

[13] Wallen, C. A., Higashicubo, R. and Dethlefsen, L. A. (1984). Murine mammary tumour cells in vitro. I. The development of a quiescent state. *Cell Tissue Kinet.*, 17, 65 - 77.

[14] Wallen, C. A., Higashicubo, R. and Dethlefsen, L. A. (1984). Murine mammary tumour cells in vitro. II. Recruitment of quiescent state. *Cell Tissue Kinet.*, 17, 79 - 89.

[15] Widera, D., Mikenberg, I., Kaus, A., Kaltschmidt, C. and Kaltschmid, B. (2006). Nuclear factor-kappaB controls the reaggregation of 3D neurosphere cultures in vitro. *Eur. Cell Mater.*, 11, 76 - 84.

[16] Piotrowska, M. J., Widera, D., Kaltschmidt, B., an der Heiden, U. and Kaltschmidt, C. (2006). Mathematical model for NF-κB–driven proliferation of adult neural stem cells. *Cell Prolif.*, 39, 441 - 455.

[17] Bonizzi, G. and Karin, M. (2004). The two NF-kappaB activation pathways and their role in innate and adaptive immunity. *Trends Immunol.*, 25, 280 - 288.

[18] Ghosh, S. and Karin, M. (2002). Missing pieces in the NF-kappaB puzzle. *Cell*, 109, S81 - S96.

[19] Kaltschmidt, B., Widera, D. and Kaltschmidt, C. (2005). Signaling via NF-kappaB in the nervous system. *Biochim. Biophys. Acta.*, 1745, 287 - 299.

[20] Guttridge, D. C., Albanese, C., Reuther, J. Y., Pestell, R. G. and Baldwin, A. S. Jr. (1999). NF-kappaB controls cell growth and differentiation through transcriptional regulation of cyclin D1. *Mol. Cell Biol.*, 19, 5785 - 5799.

[21] Baud, V. and Karin, M. (2001). Signal transduction by tumor necrosis factor and its relatives. *Trends Cell Biol.*, 11, 372 – 377.

[22] Michaelis L., Menten M. (1913). Die Kinetik der Invertinwirkung, *Biochem. Z.* 49:333-369.

[23] Hoffmann, A., Levchenko, A., Scott, M. L. and Baltimore, D. (2002). The IkappaB-NF-kappaB signaling module: temporal control and selective gene activation. *Science*, 298, 1241 - 1245.

[24] Cheong, R., Bergmann, A., Werner, S. L., Regal, J., Hoffmann, A. and Levchenko, A. (2006) Transient IkappaB kinase activity mediates temporal NF-kappaB dynamics in response to a wide range of tumor necrosis factor-alpha doses. *J. Biol. Chem.*, 281, 2945 - 2950.

[25] Lipniacki, T., Paszek, P., Brasier, A. R., Luxon, B., Kimmel, M. (2004). Mathematical model of NF-kappaB regulatory module. *J. Theor. Biol.*, 228, 195 - 215.

[26] Singh, S. K., Hawkins, C., Clarke, I. D., Squire, J.A., Bayani, J., Hide, T., Henkelman, R. M., Cusimano, M. D. and Dirks, P. B. (2004). Identification of human brain tumour initiating cells. *Nature,* 432, 396 - 401.

[27] Hinz, M., Krappmann, D., Eichten, A., Heder, A., Scheidereit, C. and Strauss, M. (1999). NF-kappaB function in growth control: regulation of cyclin D1 expression and G0/G1-to-S-phase transition. *Mol. Cell Biol.*, 19, 2690 - 2698.

[28] Kaltschmidt, B., Kaltschmidt, C., Hehner, S. P., Droge, W. and Schmitz, M. L. (1999). Repression of NF-kappaB impairs HeLa cell proliferation by functional interference with cell cycle checkpoint regulators. *Oncogene*, 18, 3213 - 3225.

[29] Henderson, E. S., Lister, T. A. and Greaves, M. F., eds. (1996). *Leukemia.* Saunders.

[30] Fortin, P. and Mackey, M. (1999). Periodic chronic myelogenous leukemia: Spectral analysis of blood cell counts and etiological implications. *Brit. J. Haematol.*, 104, 336 - 245.

[31] Guerry, D., Dale, C., D., Omine, M., Perry, and S. Wolff, S. M. (1973). Periodic hematopoiesis in human cyclic neutropenia. *J. Clin. Inves.*, 52, 3220 - 3230.

[32] Haurie, C., Mackey, M. C. and Dale, D. C. (1998). Cyclical neutropenia and other periodic hematological diseases: A review of mechanisms and mathematical models. *Blood,* 92, 2629 - 2640.

[33] Hammond, W. P., Price, T. H., Souza, L. M. and Dale, D. C. (1989). Treatment of cyclic neutropenia with granulocyte colony stimulating factor. *New Eng. J. Med.*, 320, 1306 - 1311.

[34] Haurie, C., Person, R., Dale, D. C. and Mackey, M. (1999). Haematopoietic dynamics in grey collies. *Exper. Hematol.*, 27, 1139 - 1148.

[35] Pujo-Menjouet, L., Bernard, S. and Mackey, M. (2001). Long period oscillations in a g_0 model of hematopoietic stem cells. *SIAM,* 4, 312 - 332.

[36] Bernard, S., Belair, J. and Mackey, M. (2003). Oscillations in cyclical neutropenia: New evidence based on mathematical modeling. *J. Theor. Biol.*, 223, 283 - 298.

[37] Go, R. S. (2005). Ideopathic cyclic thrombocytopenia. *Blood Reviews*, 19, 53 - 59.

[38] Swinburne, J. and Mackey, M. C. (2000). Cyclical thrombocytopenia: Characterisation by spectral analysis and a review. *J. Theor. Med.*, 2, 81 - 91.

[39] Cohen, T. and Cooney, D. P. (1974). Cyclic thrombocytopenia. Case report and Review of literature. *Scand. J. Haematol.*, 12, 9 - 17.

[40] Santillan, M., Mahaffy, J., Belair, J. and Mackey, M. (2000). Regulation of platelet production: the normal response to perturbation and cyclical platelet disease. *J. Theor. Biol.*, 206, 585 - 603.

[41] Von Schulthess, G. K. and Gessner, U. (1986). Oscillating platelet counts in healthy individuals: Experimental investigation and quantitative evaluation of thrombocytopenic feedback control. *Scand. J. Haematol.*, 36, 473 - 479.

[42] Hearn, T., Haurie, C. and Mackey, M. (1998). Cyclical neutropenia and the peripherial control of white blood cell production. *J. theor. Biol*, 192, 167 - 181.

[43] Haurie, C. and Mackey, M. (2000). Modeling complex neutrophil dynamics in the grey collie. *J. theor. Biol.*, 204, 504 - 519.

[44] Mackey, M. C. (1979). Periodic auto-immune hemolytic anemia: An induced dynamical disease. *Bull. Math. Biol.*, 41, 829 - 834.

[45] Bélair, J., Mackey, M. and Mahaffy, J. (1995). Age-structured and two-delay models for erythropoiesis. *Math. Biosci.*, 128, 317 - 346.

[46] Mahaffy, J., Belair, J. and Mackey, M. (1998). Hematopoietic model with moving boundary condition and state dependent delay: Applications in erythropoiesis. *J. Theor. Biol.,* 190, 135 - 146.

[47] Bélair, J. and Mackey, M. (1987). A model for the regulation of mammalian platelet. *Ann. N.Y. Acad. Sci.,* 504, 280 - 282.

[48] Colijn, C. and Mackey, M. C. (2005). A mathematical model of hematopoiesis: Periodic chronic myelogenous leukemia, part I. *J. Theor. Biol.*, 237, 117 – 132.

[49] Mackey, M. C. (1978). A unified hypothesis for the origin of aplastic anemia and periodic haematopoiesis. *Blood*, 51, 941 - 956.

[50] Mackey, M. C. (1979). Dynamic haematological disorders of stem cell origin. In: Vassileva-Popova, J. G. and Jensen, E. V., eds., *Biophysical and Biochemical Information Transfer in Recognition*, 373 - 409. New York: Plenum Publishing Corp.

[51] Mackey, M. C.} (2000). Cell kinetic status of haematopoietic stem cells. *Cell Prolif.*, 34, 71 - 83.

[52] Colijn, C. and Mackey, M. C. (2005). A mathematical model of hematopoiesis: Cyclical neutropenia, part II. *J. Theor. Biol.*, 237, 133 - 146.

[53] Lomb, N. R. (1976). Least-squares frequency analysis of unequally spaced data. Astrophysics and space. *Science*, 39, 447 - 462.

[54] Apostu, R. and Mackey, M. (2007, in press). Understanding cyclical thrombocytopenia: A mathematical modeling approach. *J. Theor. Biol.*

[55] Anderson, A. R. A., Weaver, A. M., Cummings, P.T. and Quaranta, V. (2006). Tumor Morphology and Phenotypic Evolution Driven by Selective Pressure from the Microenvironment. *Cell* 127, 905-915.

[56] Kansal, A. R., Torquato S., Harsh GR IV, Chiocca E. A. and Deisboeck T. S. (2000). Simulated Brain Tumor growth dynamics using a three-dimensional cellular automaton. *J. Theor. Biol.*, 203(4), 367-382.

[57] Agur Z., Daniel Y. and Ginosar Y. (2002). The universal properties of stem cells as pinpointed by a simple discrete model. *J. Math. Biol.*, 44(1), 79-86.

[58] Enderling H., Hlatky, L. and Hahnfeldt, P. (2007). Agent-based modeling of stem cell dynamics and tissue homeostasis. in preparation.

[59] Moran P. A. P. (1962). *The statistical processes of evolutionary theory*. Oxford: Clarendon Press. 200 p.

[60] Clarke, R. B. (2005). Isolation and characterization of human mammary stem cells. *Cell Prolif.* 38 (6), 375–386.

[61] Wright E. G., Lord B. I., Dexter T. M. and Lajtha L. G. (1979). Mechanisms of haemopoietic stem cell proliferation control. *Blood Cells*. 1979 Jun 15;5(2):247-258.

[62] Al-Hajj M., Wicha M. S., Benito-Hernandez A., Morrison S. J. and Clarke M. F. (2003). Prospective identification of tumorigenic breast cancer cells. *Proc. Natl. Acad. Sci. USA*. 100(7), 3983-3988.

[63] Bonnet D. and Dick J. E. (1997). Human acute myeloid leukemia is organized as a hierarchy that originates from a primitive hematopoietic cell. *Nat. Med.*, 3, 730–737.

[64] Lapidot T., Sirard C. and Vormoor J. (1994) A cell initiating human acute myeloid leukemia after transplantation into SCID mice. *Nature,* 17, 645–648.

[65] Galli R., Binda E. and Orfanelli U. (2004). Isolation and characterization of tumorigenic, stem-like neural precursors from human glioblastoma. *Cancer Res.*, 64, 7011–7021.

[66] Hemmati H. D., Nakano I. and Lazareff J. A. (2003). Cancerous stem cells arise from pediatric brain tumors. *Proc. Natl. Acad. Sci. USA*, 100, 15178–15183.

[67] Li C., Heidt D. G., Dalerba P., Burant C. F., Zhang L., Adsay V., Wicha M., Clarke M. F. and Simeone D. M. (2007). Identification of pancreatic cancer stem cells. *Cancer Res.*, 1030-1037.

[68] Dingli D. and Michor F. (2006) Successful therapy must eradicate cancer stem cells. *Stem Cells*, 24, 2603-2610.

[69] Phillips T. M., McBride W. H. and Pajonk F. (2006). The response of CD24(-/low)/CD44+ breast cancer-initiating cells to radiation. *J. Natl. Cancer Inst.* 98(24):1777-1785.

[70] Bao S., Wu Q., McLendon R. E., Hao Y., Shi Q., Hjelmeland A. B., Dewhirst M. W., Bigner D. D. and Rich J. N. (2006). Glioma stem cells promote radioresistance by preferential activation of the DNA damage response. *Nature*. 444(7120), 756-760.

In: Cancer and Stem Cells
Eds: Thomas Dittmar and Kurt S. Zänker

ISBN 978-1-60456-478-5

Chapter 3

Where Do Cancer Stem Cells Come From?

Calin Stoicov and JeanMarie Houghton*
University of Massachusetts Medical School,
LRB Second Floor 209
365 Plantation Street, Worcester MA 01635

Introduction

The concept of a cancer stem cell, or a cancer initiating cell has regained attention in recent years. What years ago started as a theory, is now supported by solid experimental data derived from multiple models and multiple cancer types. It is believed that all tumors contain a subset of cells (termed the cancer stem cell or cancer initiating cell) responsible for the growth, differentiation, invasion and metastasis of the tumor. The exact proportion of these cells within the tumor itself is controversial and likely varies widely. The surface marker profile and gene expression pattern of these cells is beginning to be delineated, and while there is seemingly a different signature for each tumor type evaluated, there are significant similarities suggesting a common origin may exist for these cells. Now that we recognize a cancer stem cell as the soul of a tumor- responsible for its very existence- we must address the next question- from where does this cancer stem cell originate? Throughout the history of cancer research, virtually every cell type has at one time or another been considered as a candidate for the cancer initiating cell. Our recent thinking however assigns this task to a cell with inherent progenitor or stem cell function. This chapter will discuss the history of the cancer stem cell hypothesis, and present the arguments and data to support a role for a bone marrow derived cell as an additional candidate cell type to the more widely held peripheral stem cell candidate.

* 508 856 6441 ; FAX 508 856 4770 ; Email: jeanmarie.houghton@umassmed.edu

Cancer Stem Cell Hypothesis

The origin of cancer has remained mysterious for many years. More than 150 years ago, Rudolf Virchow originally proposed that cancer may arise from "embryonic-like cells" [1]; a concept that was further supported by Cohnheim and Durante [2]. Waldeyer believed that almost any epithelial cell could transform to form cancer [3]. Our understanding of the origins of cancer has undergone a considerable revolution in recent years partly based on the evolving paradigm of cancer stem cells or tumor initiating cells. Once thought of as a homogeneous group of cells, tumors are now thought of as a heterogeneous collection of cells akin to an organ- sustained by a subset of cells similar to organ stem cells- which has the exclusive ability to generate, renew and propagate a tumor.

The origin of the cancer stem cell hypothesis dates back to the discovery of the light microscope in the 19th century. Julius Cohnheim in 1867 proposed that tumors were derived not from normal adult tissues but from "embryonal cell rests" which represented residual embryonic cells that were left behind during the development of the adult organ [4]. Nevertheless, during most of the 20th century, it was believed that the majority of cells in a tumor should be competent for tumor formation. Cohnheim's theory was largely ignored for one hundred years until the 1970s when additional experimental evidence came to light. Studies in leukemia and multiple myeloma showed that only a small subset of cells had the capacity for extensive proliferation and could give rise to colony forming units *in vitro* or splenic colonies in mice [3]. Similarly, work in solid tumors also showed that fewer than 1 in 1,000 cells were clonogenic *in vitro* or *in vivo*. Based on his studies of mouse teratocarcinoma, Pierce speculated that tumors contain a very small number of malignant cells that sustain the tumor and gave rise to daughter cells with varying degrees of differentiation and function [5].

The actual existence of cancer stem cells was first directly demonstrated by John Dick in 1994, when his group proved the hypothesis to be largely true for AML [6]. In these studies, only a small subset of human leukemic AML cells were capable of reproducing the disease in NOD/SCID mice, and these cells were quite similar, if not identical, to hematopoetic stem cells (HSCs) with the CD34+CD38- phenotype. The AML cancer stem cells could be passed from animal to animal consistent with the property of self-renewal. This approach has been used to demonstrate the existence of cancer stem cells (CSCs) in a number of other tumors and to identify a putative collection of cell surface markers is used to identify these cancer initiating cells. Injection of the putative stem cell population, and not the population lacking the markers into NOD/SCID mice recapitulates the original tumor (see Figure 1). Isolation and serial implantation of these stem cells into a secondary host confirms self renewal properties. This procedure has become the "gold standard" for defining a cancer stem cell, but it must be recognized that the phenotype of the cancer stem cell appears to be unique to the organ in which it resides. For example, breast cancer stem cells were shown to be CD44+CD24low/- [7], while brain cancer (glioblastoma) stem cells were enriched by sorting for CD133+ cells [8]. Cancer stem cells have also been demonstrated for prostate cancer [9], melanoma [10], colon cancer [11, 12, 13]; hepatocellular cancer [14] and pancreatic cancer [15]. In these studies, the CSC population has a growth advantage in the in vitro studies as well as in vivo - where only the CSC population is able to give rise to tumors. It must be realized however that these phenotypic determinants enrich for a population- but do not precisely define the stem cell (see Figure 1).

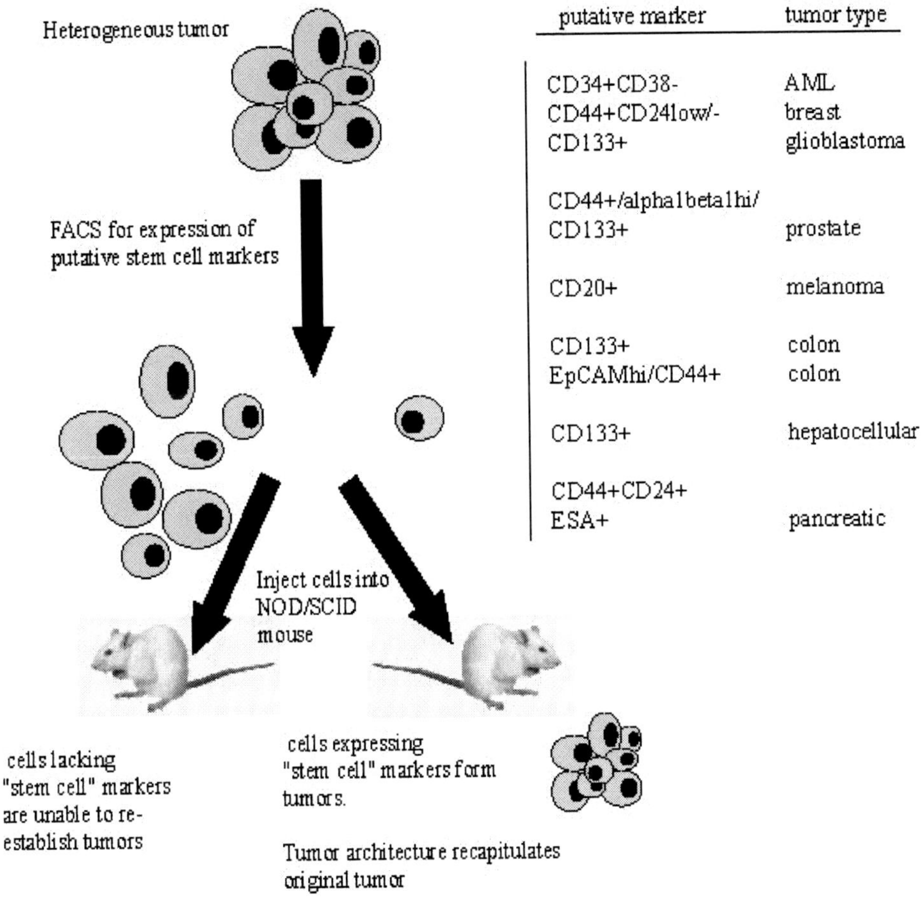

Figure 1. Tumor initiating cells. Populations of cells enriched for the tumor initiating cells have been isolated from solid tumors using a variety of surface markers. These putative cancer stem cell populations form tumors in immunocompromised mice, whereas the population of cells lacking the chosen markers fails to form tumors.

Even though as few as 100 cells in some assays are capable of tumor formation (in other words 1:100 cells has CSC capabilities) - clearly, there are cells with the same phenotype (i.e., the other 99 cells) which are incapable of tumor formation. While the bulk of experimental data to date suggests that the CSC is a rare cell within a tumor, comprising the minority of cells, recent data challenging the notion of the cancer stem cell being a rare cell type suggest that at least in some models (the authors report on preB/Blymphoma cells from three independent Eμ-myc transgenic mice) the majority of cells within a tumor may retain the cancer stem cell phenotype [16]. These findings further stress the heterogeneity between different types of tumors, and the difficulty in extrapolating findings from one model to another.

While the precise signature of surface markers identifying the CSC is not yet delineated-clearly, research in the field is rapidly closing in on identifying more stringent criteria. Based on this data, an AACR workshop agreed upon the definition of cancer stem cells as "cells within a tumor that possess the capacity for self-renewal and that can cause the heterogeneous lineages of cancer cells that constitute the tumor" [17].

The present studies must be interpreted with caution. The assays used to define CSCs may simply test for the ability of cells to grow under specific conditions (e.g. immunodeficient mice), and the demonstration that ablation of a specific cellular subset prevents tumor survival has for the most part not been achieved. Despite these limitations, a growing consensus suggests that cancer can now be viewed much like differentiated tissues and organs, a heterogeneous collection of cells sustained by a small number of progenitors that may represent 1 in 10 to 1 in 1,000,000 cells, depending on the model system and tumor type analyzed. In the cancer stem cell model, it is thought that only these CSCs are able to propagate the tumors and give rise to invasive lesions and metastases. The model has tremendous implications for cancer therapy since currently most of our therapies are successful in eradicating non-CSCs but not the CSCs, and consequently most solid tumors that shrink in response to therapies recur within a few years after therapy is stopped [18].

The traditional model of cancer development suggests that genetic instability and/or environmental factors affect the normal cells of the tissue, inducing mutations that will lead to a cancinogenesis. The tumor cells progress through preneoplastic into a neoplastic stage that may, at later times, metastasize [7, 19]. The majority of cancer research in the last century has focused on tumor cell properties, with less attention dedicated to understanding what type of cells are affected by these mutations, leaving the question – what is the source of the cancer stem cell- unanswered.

In order to understand where cancer stem cells come from, we must first understand the potential sources for this cell, and the growth properties inherent in each of these cell types.

Adult Tissue Stem Cells

Most tissues in the mammalian body have a population of adult stem cells. Tissue specific stem cells have two main properties: the ability of self-renewal and the ability to differentiate into all cell types of the tissue of origin. Adult stem cells are believed to be capable of an unlimited number of cell divisions. During cell division, the stem cell is thought to divide asymmetrically, producing an identical daughter stem cell which remains relatively quiescent, and a transit amplifying cell. The transit amplifying (TA) cell is highly proliferative and gives rise to various differentiated mature cell types specific to the tissue they reside in. These unique biological properties of the adult stem cell allows it to supply the tissues indefinitely with mature differentiated cells, ensuring homeostatic control in the face of continuous turnover, such as occurs in the gut, skin, blood etc. [20], yet delegating the actual work of proliferation to a more "transient" cell (TA). The majority of DNA damage is acquired during cell replication, putting a replicating cell population at risk for malignant transformation. This burst of proliferative activity in a cell with a finite life span may ensure cell proliferation while maintaining the safe guard of TA elimination prior to accumulating genetic damage. In most tissues the true stem cells are rare and relatively quiescent, making them less likely to accumulate genetic damage, but also making them difficult to prospectively identify and study.

To date, experimental evidence suggests that adult stem cells are located in specific locations or stem cell niches within organs [21]. The stem cell niche consists of a combination of a specific location, cell- cell contacts and stromal environment which creates a unique milieu necessary for the functioning of the stem cells. Many stem cell niches are defined- such as the bulge region of the hair follicle, while the majority of stem cell niches remain elusive.

Stem Cells within the Bone Marrow Have the Ability to Regenerate Multiple Tissue Types

Within the bone marrow are at least two populations of stem cells, hematopoietic and mesenchymal stem cells. The hematopoietic stem cell is responsible for producing all the formed elements of the blood. The mesesenchymal stem cell was originally recognized as essential for the production of stromal support cells necessary for hematopoiesis, and later recognized as having tri-lineage potential, with the ability to differentiate to bone, cartilage and fat. More recently the mesenchymal stem cell has been shown to possess the plasticity to differentiate down most all cell lineages in the body and participate in tissue restoration and healing as epithelial cells as well as stromal cells. Under normal physiologic conditions, multiple types of epithelial cells have been shown to be derived from bone marrow cells including epithelium of the lung, gastrointestinal tract and skin [22, 23]. Single bone marrow derived stem cells have been shown experimentally to expand within the host and transdifferentiate into diverse epithelial lineages. These data strongly support the existence of a single pluripotent stem cell rather than multiple committed progenitor cells as the cell of origin [23]. Within the gastrointestinal tract, isolated BM-derived epithelial cells in the gastric pits of the stomach, the small intestinal villi, the colonic crypt, and rarely in the esophagus appear as single differentiated epithelial cells, and do not appear to engraft into the stem cell niche. These cells can be recovered months after transplantation so it appears that either the cells are long lived, or engraftment is an ongoing process. Their role within the peripheral tissue is not clear. Human studies which take advantage of patients receiving gender mismatched organs/marrow also demonstrate this phenomenon on BMDC residing in the peripheral tissues as tissue specific cells. In these studies, BMDC have been found in increased numbers within the inflammed epithelium, and the level of engraftment correlates to some degree with the level of graft verses host disease present [24, 25].

Similarity between the Somatic (Tissue) Stem Cells and Cancer Stem Cells

One of the most important properties of the stem cells is self-renewal. Self-renewal is vital for stem cell function, because it will allow their survival for the duration of the host's life. Stem cell self-renewal is a well regulated process whereby a stem cell divides asymmetrically to give rise to another stem cell (self renewal) and a more differentiated daughter cell. This daughter cell has a high proliferative capacity and is responsible for producing the cells needed to replenish and repair the tissue. This rapidly dividing daughter cell gives rise to multiple cell types within the tissue, has a finite life span, and requires periodic replacement by the true stem cell. Because cancer is considered to be a disease of unregulated self-renewal, the understanding of stem cell self-renewal may facilitate our understanding of cancer cell proliferation. Cancer stem cells and the normal stem cells share self-renewal ability, one may extrapolate that the cancer stem cells use the pathways and regulation mechanisms to control cell division [26]. Indeed, the Notch and Wnt signaling pathways regulate normal stem cell self-renewal, and are also implicated in carcinogenesis.

Wnt signaling regulates development and the cell differentiation in many different tissues [27]. Beta-catenin signaling is fundamental in stem cell lineage determination in epithelial tissues as evidenced by studies in mice which show that mice deficient in the components of this pathway (Tcf4, Tcf3, Lef1, Lef4, beta catenin) do not develop hair follicles, mammary glands or teeth, and in the postnatal period there is a loss of the follicle stem cell niche. Additionally, only differentiated, nondividing villus cells are recovered in the intestinal epithelium [28, 29, 30, 31]. Similarly, inhibition of the Wnt ligand Dkk1 results in the loss of the intestinal crypts and a failure to develop mammary glands and hair follicles [32, 33, 34]. Because of the important role the wnt signaling plays in stem cell function it is not surprising to find that mutations in wnt/beta-catenin are associated with human epithelial cancers: colon adenocarcinoma [26] and mammary adenocarcinoma [35, 36].

Notch signaling controls selective cell-fate determination in a large variety of tissues. The Notch pathway is highly conserved in eukaryotic systems where it regulates cell-fate decisions through local cell-cell interactions [37]. In the gut Notch signaling regulates cell fate in the crypt as evidenced by studies performed in the Hes1 knock-out mouse (a Notch target gene). Mice deficient in Hes1 have an increased pool of paneth and goblet cells at the expense of intestinal enterocytes [38, 39]. By blocking the Notch end target (gamma-secretase), intestinal tumors in APC mutant mice differentiate into goblet cells [40]. Notch signaling also promotes proliferation and differentiation in mammary epithelium. Overexpression of Notch4 leads to mammary cancer [41], but skin deficient in Notch1 has a higher susceptibility to chemically induced cancer [42].

The Niche and Stem Cell's Fate

One area of increasing interest is the effect of chronic inflammation on the stem cell niche. Recent work has demonstrated that the behavior and lineage-specific differentiation patterns of stem cells are governed primarily by the local microenvironment, also known as the stem cell niche, a concept first proposed by Schofield (1978). This niche consists of a variety of cell types, including stromal cells (fibroblasts and myofibroblasts), endothelial cells, macrophages, and other cell types. Stromal cells are believed to generate instructive regulatory signals constituting a microenvironment that governs stem cell behavior. The understanding of these relationships may offer new direction for cancer therapeutic strategies. The microenvironment influence on the stem cell fate is epigenetic and does not affect the DNA sequence, rather the environment induces reversible modifications in transcription and cell signaling [43].

Studies in Drosophila, particularly with Drosophila germline cells, have shown the importance of niche signals in lineage determination. These studies indicate that stem cells may be somewhat interchangeable, and germline stem cells that are lost can be efficiently replaced by secondary cell types, with the niche (e.g. cap cells) playing the crucial role in the ultimate behavior of the cell that occupies the niche [44]. This concept of the empty niche, and an appreciation of the cell types that can replace resident tissue stem cells and occupy the niche may be fundamental to understanding the pathogenesis of cancer stem cells. To this end, changes to the stem cell niche that occur in the setting of inflammation in the gastrointestinal tract [45, 46], may lead to changes in stem cell behavior.

Cancer Stem Cells Originating from Bone Marrow

To begin to evaluate BMDC activity in an inflammatory model, we used the well-described *H. felis*/C57BL/6 mouse model of gastric inflammation and injury [47, 48]. The C57BL/6 model of *Helicobacter felis* induced gastric cancer is ideal to address this question because C57BL/6 mice do not develop gastric cancer under control conditions, but they reliably develop cancer with Helicobacter felis infection [47, 48]. The process and pathological changes within the stomach recapitulate human disease, where gastric cancer in the absence of *Helicobacter* infection is unusual, while longstanding infection carries a significant (up to 1-3%) risk of gastric cancer [49] making this a very useful animal model. This mouse model provides a continuum of disease from the initial acute inflammation with minimal mucosal damage, through atrophy metaplasia and dysplasia, culminating in gastric adenocarcinoma. For these studies, C57BL/6 mice transplanted with marked bone marrow were infected with *Helicobacter felis*, and evaluated at various time points for the presence of BMDC within the gastric mucosa. Acute *Helicobacter* infection resulted in an influx of bone marrow derived inflammatory cells into the gastric mucosa, but not to differentiation of BMDC as epithelial cells. At between 8 and 20 weeks of infection there is loss of specialized cells and a reorganization of the gastric architecture. Metaplastic and dysplastic cell changes are prominent reflecting the effects of an abnormal tissue milieu on rapidly proliferating cells [48]. Engraftment of BMDC within the mucosa, and differentiation to an epithelial cell phenotype first becomes evident at about 20 weeks of infection, corresponding with the appearance of metaplastic cell lineages. As time progresses, the number of BMD-glands increases dramatically suggesting both an expansion of resident BMDC through proliferation, and/or the recruitment of additional cells [50]. Based on these studies, we believe long standing inflammation and inflammatory mediated damage is required for BMDC engraftment within the gastric epithelium. Long standing inflammation and tissue remodeling is associated with premalignant and malignant conditions, further suggesting to us that this environment may be driving the transformation of the BMDC within inflamed sites.

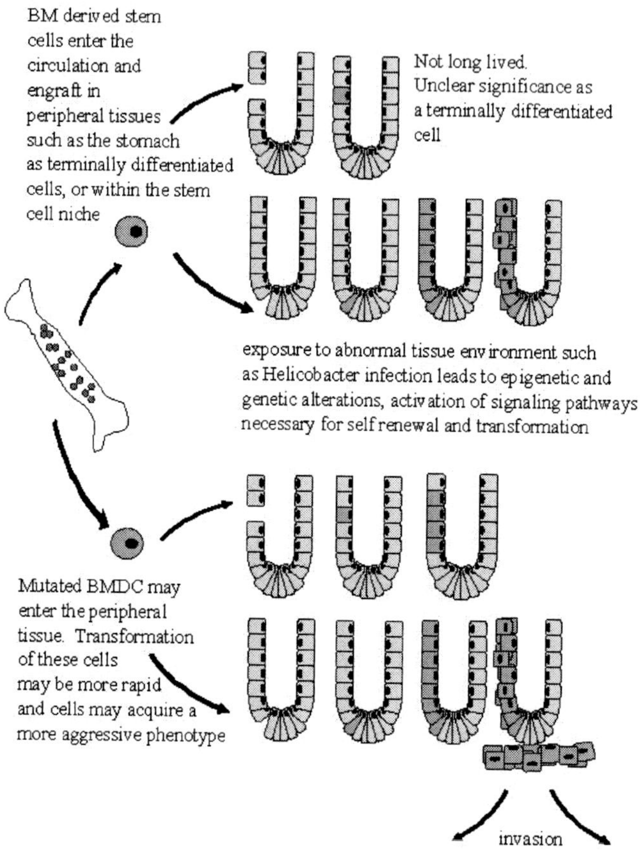

Figure 2. Model of BMDC as the cancer initiating cell. Cells from the bone marrow may engraft in the peripheral tissue and transform as a result of forced proliferation in an inflammatory environment. Conversely, cells carrying mutations may have a selective advantage and contribute to a more aggressive phenotype.

In this model, intraepithelial neoplasia in mice infected for 12 to 16 months arose from donor marrow cells, strongly suggesting an inherent vulnerability of this population of cells to transformation. In addition to epithelial cells within the tumor, BMDCs also comprise a subset of cells within the tumor stroma and within seemingly uninvolved epithelium and subepithelial spaces adjacent to the tumors. Adipocytes, fibroblast, endothelial cells and myofibroblasts derived from bone marrow precursors can be found in areas adjacent to dysplasia and neoplasia [49, 51]. For as many questions these studies answer, there are more that are raised, and remain to be answered. The data from the H.felis induced gastric cancer model implies that BMDC are recruited to the inflammed tissue and there, transform. We do not yet know if BMDC in the tissue regain access to the circulation setting up a scenario where environmental influences at one site could affect the BMDC, which then could grow at a different site. If this were the case, it could be imagined that BMDC which carry mutations could home to and engraft into peripheral tissues possibly resulting in malignancy in a shorter time frame, or with a more aggressive phenotype (Figure 2). Additional work in the animal model is needed to address these points.

Interestingly, analysis of human tissues demonstrates clonal expansion of BMDC and near complete donor origin of some tumors supporting the role of BMDC as the cancer stem cell in certain human tumors by [53, 54]. Other studies clearly demonstrate donor derived cells within malignancy, however their role in initiating malignancy is less clear. Several studied have shown a contribution of BMDC to malignancy as a fraction (<1%) of cells, or as a substantial portion (20% or more) as epithelial cells, tumor cells and stromal support cells [55, 56]. In this setting the precise role of BMDC within tumors is not clear. It may be that the initiating cells in the tumors studied were present within the tissues at the time of transplant and of recipient origin, though the source (peripheral or bone marrow derived) is not clear. What is clear from these studies is that BMDC seem to continually be added to some tumors through a mechanism that is not yet clear. The implications of this phenomenon is also not clear, but these cells as epithelial cells, or stromal cells may provide needed signaling to aid in neoplastic growth. Ongoing studies will like shed light on the many facetted role of BMDC in cancer.

Conclusion

The field of cancer biology has undergone significant shifts in recent years, with a focus on identifying and understanding the cancer stem cell. The evolving picture is one of a rare group of cells with in a tumor with a surface marker profile and gene expression pattern unique to its role as a stem cell. A body of work suggests that the cancer stem cell may arise from the bone marrow, however, more work is needed to determine if this notion can be extrapolated to other models of cancer. In addition the importance of BMDC in human cancer it needs to be clarified. Characterizing and developing markers for the BMDC subpopulations that can contribute to solid tumors is of major importance to facilitate early detection in patients and to develop targeted therapies aimed at the cancer stem cell. It seems likely that some solid tumors may be derived from resident tissue stem cells rather than circulating BMDCs, with the environment, genetic make up of the host and other factors dictating the cell which undergoes transformation. It is extremely important for these two paradigms to be understood- in their similarities, as well as their differences. The possible role of cell fusion by BMDCs has yet to be fully elucidated and research in this area will likely provide novel and exciting insights into the complexity of the relationship of the BMDC and peripheral tissues. Additionally, the concept of an aberrant stem cell niche and its role in contributing to cancer development from BMDCs will need further clarification. Prevention and/or reversibility of preneoplastic lesions (for example by eradication of *H. pylori*) are clearly worth addressing further in the *Helicobacter* mouse model and can be considered in the context of the biology of stem cell differentiation.

Finally, the precise relationship of chronic inflammation to BMDCs needs further investigation. One suspects that future studies will reveal the involvement of many cell types and specific factors – including cytokines, chemokines, hypoxia and oxidative stress – in the mobilization, recruitment, engraftment, and progression of stem cells toward cancer. Understanding these mechanisms offers the exciting hope of new approaches to cancer treatment.

References

[1] Virchow, RLK. *Cellular Pathology*. Hirschwald, Berlin; 1858.

[2] Sell, S. Stem cell origin of cancer and differentiation therapy. *Crit. Rev. Oncol. Hemat*, 2004 51, 1-28.

[3] Houghton, JM; Morozov, A; Smirnova, I; Wang TC. Stem cells and cancer. *Semin. Cancer Biol.*, 2007 17,191-203.

[4] Rather, LJ. *The genesis of cancer: a study in the history of ideas*. The Johns Hopkins University Press, Baltimore; 1978.

[5] Pierce, GB. Neoplasms, differentiations and mutations. *Am. J. Pathol.* 1974 77, 103-118.

[6] Lapidot, T; Sirard, C; Vormoor, J; Murdoch, B; Hoang, T; Caceres-Cortes, J; Minden, M; Paterson, B; Caligiuri, MA; Dick, JE. A cell initiating human acute myeloid leukaemia after transplantation into SCID mice. *Nature.* 1994 367, 645-648.

[7] Al-Hajj, M; Wicha, MS; Benito-Hernandez, A; Morrison, SJ; Clarke MF. Prospective identification of tumorigenic breast cancer cells. *Proc. Nat'l. Acad. Sci. USA*. 2003 100, 3983-3988.

[8] Singh, SK; Hawkins, C; Clarke, ID; Squire, JA; Bayani, J; Hide, T; Henkelman, RM; Cusimano, MD; Dirks, PB. Identification of human brain tumour initiating cells. *Nature.* 2004 432, 396-401.

[9] Collins, AT; Berry, PA; Hyde, C; Stower, M; Maitland, NJ. Prospective identification of tumorigenic prostate cancer stem cells. *Cancer Res.* 2005 65, 10946-10951.

[10] Fang, D; Nguyen, TK; Leishear, K; Finko, R; Kulp, AN; Hotz, S; Van Belle, PA; Xu, X; Elder, DE; Herlyn, M. A tumorigenic subpopulation with stem cell properties in melanomas. *Cancer Res.* 2005 65, 9328-37.

[11] O'Brien, CA; Pollett, A; Gallinger, S; Dick, JE. A human colon cancer cell capable of initiating tumour growth in immunodeficient mice. *Nature.* 2007 44, 5106-110.

[12] Ricci-Vitiani, L; Lombardi, DG; Pilozzi, E; Biffoni, M; Todaro, M; Peschle, C; De Maria, R. Identification and expansion of human colon-cancer-initiating cells. *Nature.* 2007 445, 111-115.

[13] Dalerba, P; Dylla, SJ; Park, IK; Liu, R; Wang, X; Cho, RW; Hoey, T; Gurney, A; Huang, EH; Simeone, DM; Shelton, AA; Parmiani, G; Castelli, C; Clarke, MF. Phenotypic characterization of human colorectal cancer stem cells. *Proc. Natl. Acad. Sci. USA.* 2007 104, 10158-10163.

[14] Ma, S; Chan, KW; Hu, L; Lee, TK; Wo, JY; Ng, IO; Zheng, BJ; Guan, XY. Identification and characterization of tumorigenic liver cancer stem/progenitor cells. *Gastroenterology.* 2006 132, 2542-2556.

[15] Li C; Heidt, DG; Dalerba, P; Burant, CF; Zhang, L; Adsay, V; Wicha, M; Clarke, MF; Simeone, DM. Identification of pancreatic cancer stem cells. *Cancer Res.* 2007 67, 1030-1037.

[16] Kelly, PN; Dakic, A; Adams, JM; Nutt, SL; Strasser, A. Tumor growth need not be driven by rare cancer stem cells. *Science*. 2007 317, 337.

[17] Clarke, MF; Dick, JE; Dirks, PB; Eaves, CJ; Jamieson, CH; Jones, DL; Visvader, J; Weissman, IL; Wahl, GM. Cancer Stem Cells--Perspectives on Current Status and Future Directions: AACR Workshop on Cancer Stem Cells. *Cancer Res*. 2006 66, 9339-9344.

[18] Reya, T; Morrison, SJ; Clarke, MF; Weissman, IL. Stem cells, cancer, and cancer stem cells. *Nature*. 2001 414, 105-11.

[19] Wicha, MS; Dontu, G; Al-Hajj, M; Clarke, MF; Arbor, A. *Stem cells in the normal and cancerous human breast*. Presented at San Antonio Breast Cancer Symposium. 2003 San Antonio, USA.

[20] Tan, BT; Park, CY; Ailles, LE; Weissman, IL.The cancer stem cell hypothesis: a work in progress. *Lab Invest*. 2006 86,1203-7. Review.

[21] Coppock, HA; Clarke, RB. Mammary stem cells: the root of breast cancer? *Breast Cancer Online*. 2004, 7.

[22] Jiang, Y; Jahagirdar, BN; Reinhardt, RL; Schwartz, RE; Keene, CD; Ortiz-Gonzalez, XR; Reyes, M; Lenvik, T; Lund, T; Blackstad, M; Du, J; Aldrich, S; Lisberg, A; Low, WC; Largaespada, DA; Verfaillie, CM. Pluripotency of mesenchymal stem cells derived from adult marrow. *Nature*. 2002 418, 41-9.

[23] Krause, DS; Theise, ND; Collector, MI; Henegariu, O; Hwang, S; Gardner, R; Neutzel, S; Sharkis, SJ. Multi-organ, multi-lineage engraftment by a single bone marrow-derived stem cell. *Cell*. 2001 105, 369-77.

[24] Matsumoto, T; Okamoto, R; Yajima, T; Mori, T; Okamoto, S; Ikeda, Y; Mukai, M; Yamazaki, M; Oshima, S; Tsuchiya, K; Nakamura, T; Kanai, T; Okano, H; Inazawa, J; Hibi, T; Watanabe, M. Increase of bone marrow-derived secretory lineage epithelial cells during regeneration in the human intestine. *Gastroenterology*. 2005 128, 1851-67.

[25] Okamoto, R;Yajima, T; Yamazaki, M; Kanai, T; Mukai, M; Okamoto, S; Ikeda, Y; Hibi, T; Inazawa, J; Watanabe, M. Damaged epithelia regenerated by bone marrow-derived cells in the human gastrointestinal tract. *Nat. Med*. 2002 8, 1011-7.

[26] Reya, T; Clevers, H. Wnt signaling in stem cells and cancer. *Nature*. 2005 434, 843-850.

[27] Logan, CY; Nusse, R. The wnt signaling pathway in development and disease. *Annu. Rev.Cell Dev. Biol*. 2004 20, 781-810.

[28] van Genderen, C; Okamura, RM; Farinas, I; Quo, RG; Parslow, TG; Bruhn, L; Grosschedl, R. Development of several organs that require inductive epithelial-mesenchymal interactions is impaired in LEF-1-deficient mice. *Genes Dev*. 1994 15, 2691-703.

[29] Korinek, V; Barker, N; Moerer, P; van Donselaar, E; Huls, G; Peters, PJ; Clevers, H. Depletion of epithelial stem-cell compartments in the small intestine of mice lacking *Tcf-4*. *Nat Genet*. 1998 19, 379-83.

[30] Huelsken, J; Vogel, R; Erdmann, B; Cotsarelis, G; Birchmeier, W. beta-Catenin controls hair follicle morphogenesis and stem cell differentiation in the skin. *Cell*. 2001 105, 533-45.

[31] Lowry, WE; Blanpain, C; Nowak, JA; Guasch, G; Lewis, L; Fuchs, E. Defining the impact of beta-catenin/Tcf transactivation on epithelial stem cells.*Genes Dev*. 2005 19, 1596-611.

[32] Pinto, D; Gregorieff, A; Begthel, H; Clevers, H. Canonical Wnt signals are essential for homeostasis of the intestinal epithelium. *Genes Dev.* 2003 17, 1709-13.

[33] Andl, T; Reddy, ST; Gaddapara., T; Millar, SE. WNT signals are required for the initiation of hair follicle development. *Dev. Cell.* 2002 2, 643-53.

[34] Chu, EY; Hens, J; Andl, T; Kairo, A; Yamaguchi, TP; Brisken, C; Glick, A; Wysolmerski, JJ; Millar, SE. Canonical WNT signaling promotes mammary placode development and is essential for initiation of mammary gland morphogenesis. *Development*. 2004 131, 4819-29.

[35] Teuliere, J; Faraldo, MM; Deugnier, MA; Shtutman, M; Ben-Ze'ev, A; Thiery, JP; Glukhova, MA. Targeted activation of beta-catenin signaling in basal mammary epithelial cells affects mammary development and leads to hyperplasia. *Development.* 2005 132, 267-77.

[36] Tsukamoto, AS; Grosschedl, R; Guzman, RC; Parslow, T; Varmus, HE. Expression of the int-1 gene in transgenic mice is associated with mammary gland hyperplasia and adenocarcinomas in male and female mice. *Cell.* 1988 55, 619-25.

[37] Artavanis-Tsakonas, S; Rand, MD; Lake, RJ. Notch signaling: cell fate control and signal integration in development. *Science*. 1999 284, 770-6. Review.

[38] Jensen, J; Pedersen, EE; Galante, P; Hald, J; Heller, RS; Ishibashi, M; Kageyama, R; Guillemot, F; Serup, P; Madsen, OD. Control of endodermal endocrine development by Hes-1. *Nat. Genet*. 2000 24, 36-44.

[39] Suzuki, K; Fukui, H; Kayahara, T; Sawada, M; Seno, H; Hiai, H; Kageyama, R; Okano, H; Chiba, T. Hes1-deficient mice show precocious differentiation of Paneth cells in the small intestine. *Biochem. Biophys. Res. Commun*. 2005 328, 348-52.

[40] van Es, JH; van Gijn, ME; Riccio, O; van den Born, M; Vooijs, M; Begthel, H; Cozijnsen, M; Robine, S; Winton, DJ; Radtke, F; Clevers H. Notch/gamma-secretase inhibition turns proliferative cells in intestinal crypts and adenomas into goblet cells. *Nature*. 2005 435, 959-63.

[41] Hu, C; Dievart, A; Lupien, M; Calvo, E; Tremblay, G; Jolicoeur, P. Overexpression of activated murine Notch1 and Notch3 in transgenic mice blocks mammary gland development and induces mammary tumors. *Am. J. Pathol.* 2006 168, 973-90.

[42] Nicolas, M; Wolfer, A; Raj, K; Kummer, JA; Mill, P; van Noort, M; Hui, CC; Clevers, H; Dotto, GP; Radtke F. Notch1 functions as a tumor suppressor in mouse skin. *Nat. Genet.* 2003 33, 416-21.

[43] Hendrix, MJ; Seftor, EA; Seftor, RE; Kasemeier-Kulesa, J; Kulesa, PM; Postovit, LM. Reprogramming metastatic tumour cells with embryonic microenvironments. *Nat. Rev. Cancer*. 2007 7, 246-55. Review.

[44] Xie, T; Spradling, AC. A niche maintaining germ line stem cells in the Drosophila ovary. *Science.* 2000 290, 328-30.

[45] Powell, DW; Adegboyega, PA; Di Mari, JF; Mifflin, RC. Epithelial cells and their neighbors I. Role of intestinal myofibroblasts in development, repair, and cancer. *Am. J. Physiol. Gastrointest Liver Physiol*. 2005 289, G2-7.

[46] Pull, SL; Doherty, JM; Mills, JC; Gordon, JI; Stappenbeck, TS. Activated macrophages are an adaptive element of the colonic epithelial progenitor niche necessary for regenerative responses to injury. *Proc. Natl. Acad. Sci. USA*. 2004 102, 99-104.

[47] Wang, TC; Dangler, CA; Chen, D; Goldenring, JR; Koh, T; Raychowdhury, R; Coffey, RJ; Ito, S; Varro, A; Dockray, GJ; Fox, JG. Synergistic interaction between hypergastrinemia and Helicobacter infection in a mouse model of gastric cancer. *Gastroenterology*. 2000 118, 36-47.

[48] Cai, X; Carlson, J; Stoicov, C; Li, H; Wang, TC; Houghton, J. Helicobacter felis eradication restores normal architecture and inhibits gastric cancer progression in C57BL/6 mice. *Gastroenterology*. 2005 128, 1937-52.

[49] Nomura, A; Stemmermann, GN; Chyou, PH; Kato, I; Perez-Perez, GI; Blaser, MJ. Helicobacter pylori infection and gastric carcinoma among Japanese Americans in Hawaii. *N. Engl. J. Med.* 1991 325, 1132-6.

[50] Houghton, J; Stoicov, C; Nomura, S; Rogers, AB; Carlson, J; Li, H; Cai, X; Fox, JG; Goldenring, JR; Wang, TC. Gastric cancer originating from bone marrow-derived cells. *Science*. 2004 306, 1568-71.

[51] Li, HC; Stoicov, C; Rogers, AB; Houghton, J. Stem cells and cancer: evidence for bone marrow stem cells in epithelial cancers. *World J. Gastroenterol.* 2006 12, 363-71. Review.

[52] Aractingi, S; Kanitakis, J; Euvrard, S; Le Danff, C; Peguillet, I; Khosrotehrani, K; Lantz, O; Carosella, ED. Skin carcinoma arising from donor cells in a kidney transplant recipient. *Cancer Res*. 2005 65, 1755-60.

[53] Arai, F; Hirao, A; Suda, T. Regulation of hematopoiesis and its interaction with stem cell niches. *Int. J. Hematol.* 2005 82, 371-6. Review.

[54] Cogle, CR; Theise, ND; Fu, D; Ucar, D; Lee, S; Guthrie, SM; Lonergan, J; Rybka, W; Krause, DS; Scott, EW. Bone marrow contributes to epithelial cancers in mice and humans as developmental mimicry. *Stem Cells*. 2007 25, 1881-7.

[55] Avital, I; Moreira, AL; Klimstra, DS; Leversha, M; Papadopoulos, EB; Brennan, M; Downey, RJ. Donor-derived human bone marrow cells contribute to solid organ cancers developing after bone marrow transplantation. *Stem Cells*. 2007 25, 2903-9.

In: Cancer and Stem Cells
Eds: Thomas Dittmar and Kurt S. Zänker
ISBN 978-1-60456-478-5

Chapter 4

Mismatch Repair Deficiencies and Origin of Cancer Stem Cells

Minal Garg[*]
Department of Biochemistry,
University of Lucknow – 226007, U.P., India

Abstract

The immortal stem cells characterized with exceptional self-renewal capacity, regulated cell proliferation and differential potential maintain the tissue homeostasis. The continuous exogenous and endogenous genotoxic stress accumulate DNA errors and activate the diverse oncogenic signaling pathways, drive the proliferative expansion with the transformation of normal stem cells into cancer stem cells with a heterogeneous population of tumor cells, a common phenomenon for hematological malignancies and solid tumors as well. In response to genomic insult, several DNA repair mechanisms come into play. DNA mismatch repair is one of the well-described repair systems that not only corrects the miscodings in the genomic DNA but also in absence of repair, directly or indirectly activates the cascade of complex cellular mechanisms including cell cycle arrest, transcription induction of apoptosis. This chapter discusses the recent concept on the biological functions of DNA mismatch repair system and its potential role in sensitizing the cancer cells to cytotoxic drugs. Number of studies identifies the presence of MMR gene defects in hematological malignancies and other tumors. Results of various *in vitro* and *in vivo* experiments suggest the involvement of MMR proteins in stem cell maintenance and its therapeutic implication in complete removal of their malignant counterparts. However, the success of cancer therapy lies in the combinational and targeted treatments against the cancer stem cells, which could help in developing an effective novel therapies leaving residual non-tumorigenic population of cells resulting in potential cancer cures.

[*] Corresponding Author: Dr. Minal Vaish *nee* Garg, Ph.D., Lecturer, Department of Biochemistry, University of Lucknow, Lucknow – 226007, U.P., INDIA. e-mail: minal14@yahoo.com. Phone no.: 91-522- 9335820857.

Keywords: stem cells, cancer stem cells, mismatch repair, malignancies, cancer therapy.

1. Introduction

The cells accumulate errors in their genetic makeup either from environmental factors, which could be the exposure to radiation, chemicals or drugs, viruses and bacteria or DNA replication errors (Dean, 2006). This in turn activates DNA mismatch repair (MMR) pathways that restore the mismatched and unpaired nucleotides and thereby provide the most robust defense for the cell by maintaining the genomic and chromosomal stability.

Stem cells are the indispensable entities with self-renewal property, capability of differentiation and extensive proliferation. Low rate of cell division and active DNA repair are the innate properties of normal development of stem cells The adult stem cells are identified in variety of tissues and organs in humans including – bone marrow, brain, skin/ hair follicles, heart, lung, intestine, liver, pancreas, mammary glands, ovaries, prostrate, and testis (Li et al., 2007a). The expression of transport proteins – ABC (ATP-binding cassette) transporter proteins and multidrug resistant proteins are associated with the efflux of xenobiotic toxins and protect stem cells against toxins. Apart from hormonal stimulation, defective DNA repair plays important role in stem cell activation into its malignant counterparts.

The recognition of lesions or defects in DNA of a cell by MMR proteins may directly activate the cascade of complex cellular responses that include loss of cell cycle G2 arrest or apoptosis to stop cell proliferation and remove the damaged cells from the organ depending upon the severity of the DNA damage. The failure of efficient DNA repair machinery cause the stem cells to accumulate harmful mutations and become resistant to apoptosis resulting in the loss of genome or instability, which ultimately lead to malignant transformation of stem cells (Reese et al., 2003).

This chapter sheds light on the potential role of DNA MMR repair machinery in elimination of the structurally distorted paired and unpaired nucleotides and its impact on the stem cell function.

1.1. DNA Repair Pathways

The primary role of the multiple biochemical processes called DNA repair pathways is the correction of spontaneous and induced mutations due to the exposure of exogenous carcinogens, radiation, endogenous free radicals or replication errors in the genetic constituent of the cell. These mutations have deleterious consequences that include malignant transformation ultimately leading to cell death. The cell utilizes the repair pathways and maintains the genomic integrity and thus the normal functioning of stem cells.

1.1.1. DNA Mismatch Repair (MMR)

Mismatch repair process is common to both prokaryotic and eukaryotic cells and their loss result in mutator phenotype. It is a sensory system that scans DNA and when come across the nucleotide mispair, erases the error and summons DNA polymerase to repeat the synthesis. It provides the genome with 100 – 1000 fold level of protection against mutations and guards genome by preventing recombination between non-homologous regions of DNA, thus maintains the genomic integrity (Marsischky, 1996).

The MMR pathway repairs the defective DNA by eliminating the specific mismatched and/ or unmatched bases and insertion-deletion loops (IDLs) where DNA synthesis is liable to errors, either as a part of DNA replication before cell division, or as part of DNA repair (unscheduled DNA synthesis) (Jiricny, 1998). Although DNA polymerases have the ability to identify and correct their own errors, some mistakes are not identified.

1.1.1.1. Components of the DNA MMR System

MMR genes were first described in bacteria and best characterized in *Escherichia coli.* MMR system originally identified in bacteria consists of four mutator genes: Mut S, Mut L, Mut H and Mut U. Process of MMR is highly conserved in eukaryotes and it is reflected by the existence of multiple homologs of Mut S and Mut L proteins. MSH1, homolog of Mut S is required for normal mitochondrial function in *Saccharomyces cerevisiae* and protects against base substitution (Chi and Kolodner, 1994). However, mammalian MSH1 homolog is not known to date. MSH4 and MSH5 have specialized roles in meiotic recombination in yeast and mice. MSH2, MSH3 and MSH6/ GTBP (G: T binding protein) form two heterodimers – Mut Sα (MSH2/ MSH6) and Mut Sβ (MSH2/ MSH3) that recognize mispairs in DNA (Marsischky et al., 1996). Homologs of Mut S in higher eukaryotes (*Xenopus laevis*, mouse and human) are different from Mut S in binding to the stretches of up to 14 extra helical nucleotides (IDLs) *in vitro*. Mut S and its homolog interact with DNA via their N – termini, while the C – terminal domains house dimerization and ATP binding domains. *In vitro* assays show that Mut S binds with high affinity to substrates containing base – base mispairs and IDLs that escape proofreading by the replicating polymerase (Jiricny, 1998). Heterodimer is formed between hPMS2 (Human post meiotic segregation 2) and hMLH1 (human Mut L homolog) or PMS1 in *S. cerevisiae* forms heterodimer with MLH1 (Li and Modrich, 1995). The precise biochemical role of eukaryotic Mut L homologs in mismatch repair is unclear. The role of *S. cerevisiae* MLH1 – PMS1 complex is identified as to enhance the binding of MSH2/ MSH3 heterodimer to an IDL substrate and in humans Mut L homologs interact with Mut S homologs on a DNA substrate and show ATP dependent activity (Gu et al., 1998). The homologs of both Mut H and Mut U are not known in eukaryotic system. Localization of homologs of Mut genes in humans and their functions in higher eukaryotes is given in Table 1. Recently another eukaryotic mismatch repair endonuclease whose amino terminal domain is involved in binding to fully methylated DNA and carboxyl terminal region is involved in catalysis and complex formation with MLH1. This protein is named as MED1 (methyl – CpG binding endonuclease 1). The properties of MED1 felicitate it to be a functional homologue of Mut H. Recent studies do not support the endonuclease activity of MED1 on double-stranded oligonucleotides and rule out the possible role of MED1 and DNA methylation in MMR strand discrimination *in vitro* (Drummond and Bellacosa 2001). In addition to Mut genes some proteins are found participating in DNA metabolic pathways and these are helicases, endonucleases, polymerases and ligases (Vaish and Mittal, 2002).

Table 1. Components of DNA mismatch repair system in prokaryotes and eukaryotes and their functions

Prokaryote MMR system *E. coli*	Eukaryote MMR system in Yeast	in Human	Chromosomal location in human	Eukaryotic functions
Mut S	MSH1	-	-	Avoids mutation in mitochondria
	MSH2	MSH2	2p21	Heterodimers formation with MSH3 and MSH6 for repair replication errors and miscodings in recombinant intermediates; removal of MSH2 – MSH3 (non homologous tails), inhibition of recombination between non identical sequences and thus activate the system to respond to damage
	MSH3	MSH3	5q	Heterodimers formation with MSH2
	MSH4	-	-	Help in crossing over in meiosis and forms heterodimer with MSH5
	MSH5	-	-	Help in crossing over in meiosis and forms heterodimer with MSH4
	MSH6	MSH6/ GTBP	2p21	Hheterodimers formation with MSH2 and may increase MSH2 affinity with DNA mismatches
Mut L	PMS1	PMS2	7p22	Heterodimers formation with MLH1 to repair replication errors and mismatches in recombinant intermediates; inhibition of recombination between non identical sequences and respond to DNA damage
	MLH1	MLH1	3p21 – p23	Heterodimers formation with PMS1, MLH2 and MLH3 and recruit additional repair factors (not known)
	MLH2	PMS1	2q31 – q33	Heterodimers formation with MLH1 to repair replication errors and mismatches in recombinant intermediates
	MLH3		14q24.3	Heterodimers formation with MLH1 to repair replication errors and promote crossing over in meiosis
Mut H	-	MED1	-	Function in mismatch repair is not clearly defined
Mut U	-	-	-	-

Table 2. Cell markers expressed in normal and cancer stem cells of different organs in humans

Organ type	Cancer type	Stem cell markers	Cancer stem cell markers	References
Hematopoietic	Leukemia	$CD34^{+}CD38^{-}Thy1^{-}Lin^{-}$	$CD34^{+}CD38^{-}$ $Thy1^{-}Lin^{-}$	Bonnet and Dick, 1997, Li et al., 2007b
Bone marrow	Multiple myeloma	$CD138^{+}$(syndecan-1) $IL\text{-}6^{+}CD126^{+}$	$CD138^{-}IL\text{-}6^{-}CD126^{-}$	Jego et al., 1999; Matsui et al., 2004
Breast	Mammary cancer	$CD24^{med}$	$CD44^{+}CD24^{-/low}ESA^{+}Lin^{-}$	Al-Hajj et al., 2003; Al-Hajj and Clarke, 2004;
Brain	Brain tumor	$CD133^{+}$(Prominin) Lin^{-}	$CD133^{+}$ Nestin	Uchida et al., 2000; Singh et al., 2003
Skin	Melanoma cancer	$CD20^{-}CD166^{-}$ $Nestin^{-}$	$CD20^{+}$ $CD166^{+}$ Nestin+	Fang et al., 2005; Klein et al., 2007
Prostate	Prostate cancer	$CD133^{+}\alpha_2\beta_1{}^{hi}$	$CD44^{+}\alpha_2\beta_1{}^{hi}CD133^{+}$	Collins et al., 2005
Tongue, Larynx, Throat and Sinus	Head and neck squamous cell carcinoma (HNSCC)	$CD44^{-}$	$CD44^{+}$	Prince et al., 2007
Pancreas	Pancreatic cancer	$CD24^{-}CD44^{-}ESA^{-}$	$CD24^{+}$ $CD44^{+}ESA^{+}$	Li et al., 2007b

MMR system is an excision/ resynthesis system and divided into four phases – (1) recognition, (2) recruitment of repair enzymes, (3) excision of incorrect sequence and (4) resynthesis by DNA polymerase using the parental strand as the template.

1.1.1.1.0. Mismatch Recognition and Recruitment of Repair Enzymes

Mismatch recognition in eukaryotic DNA is done by two heterodimeric complexes of MSH2/ GTBP (Mut Sα) and MSH2/ MSH3 (Mut Sβ) (Kolodner, 1996). Mut Sα binds to both base – base mismatches and small ID (insertion - deletion) heterologies whereas Mut Sβ recognizes larger ID mispairs (Sia et al., 1997). The affinity of Mut Sα for an oligonucleotide heteroduplex, an effect also observed with bacterial Mut S is markedly decreased in the presence of ATP. Hydrolysis of ATP facilitates protein – protein interactions and or sliding along with DNA (Allen et al., 1997). However, Mut S tightly binds to mismatches and do not slide if ADP is present. Studies identify the feature of newly synthesized DNA strand, which is a single strand nick as gaps are present between Okazaki fragments in the lagging, strand and thus discriminate it with the parental strand. MMR proteins recognize and bind to the mismatches at the lagging strand, nascent daughter strand (Thomas et al., 1991). The DNA-Mut Sα (MSH2/ MSH3) - ATP complex recruits Mut L complex [MLH1/ hPMS2 (PMS1 in yeast)] and converts into high molecular weight structure. It also increases the efficiency of Mut S proteins to recognize the mismatch. MLH1/ PMS2 also form the complex with Mut Sβ and help in repair of ID mispairs (Wheeler and Bodmer, 2000). Mut L binds the repair complex in a mismatch independent manner; interact with Mut S at the site of mismatch. Proliferating cell nuclear antigen (PCNA), identified as DNA polymerase processivity factor, a homotrimeric multifunctional sliding clamp and act as a strand discriminating factor at or prior to excision steps (Gu et al., 1998). Mut L dimmers then displace DNA ploymerase and PCNA from the daughter strand and recruits exonuclease 1 (exo 1) and other proteins required for long patch excision.

1.1.1.1.1. Excision of Mismatch and DNA Resynthesis

Bi - directional threading of DNA through Mut S heterodimer is continued till the arrest of forward movement of replication fork that occurs via an interaction with PCNA in the polymerase complex. After dissociation of MMR complex, PCNA, which still binds at the end of error containing primer strand, recruits replication complex and thus re-initiation starts with the help of DNA polymerase. Exo 1 with 5' to 3' exonuclease activity (activity requires Mut S, Exo 1 and replication protein A, RPA) or 3' to 5' exonuclease activity (also requires Mut L, PCNA and replication factor C, RFC) can mediate the excision of one strand of DNA extending from nick to mismatch, spanning over 1000 nucleotides upto 150 nucleotides past the mismatch. RPA, a strand binding protein stabilizes the remaining strand once the mismatch is removed. RFC is an ATPase that loads and unloads PCNA from DNA. Human homolog DNA pol δ along with α and ε are required for the reconstitution of repair synthesis, observed in cell free extract (Chang et al., 2000) (Figure 1).

In addition to it, MMR system mediates the cytotoxicity of several DNA damaging drugs. In the absence of functional MGMT (O^6-methylguanine DNA methyltransferase) (silence due to promoter methylation as in 40% of sporadic colorectal cancer as well as in other cancers), the repair cycle recognizes and preferentially removes the newly synthesized strand containing erroneous nucleotide miscodings every time the DNA undergoes replication.

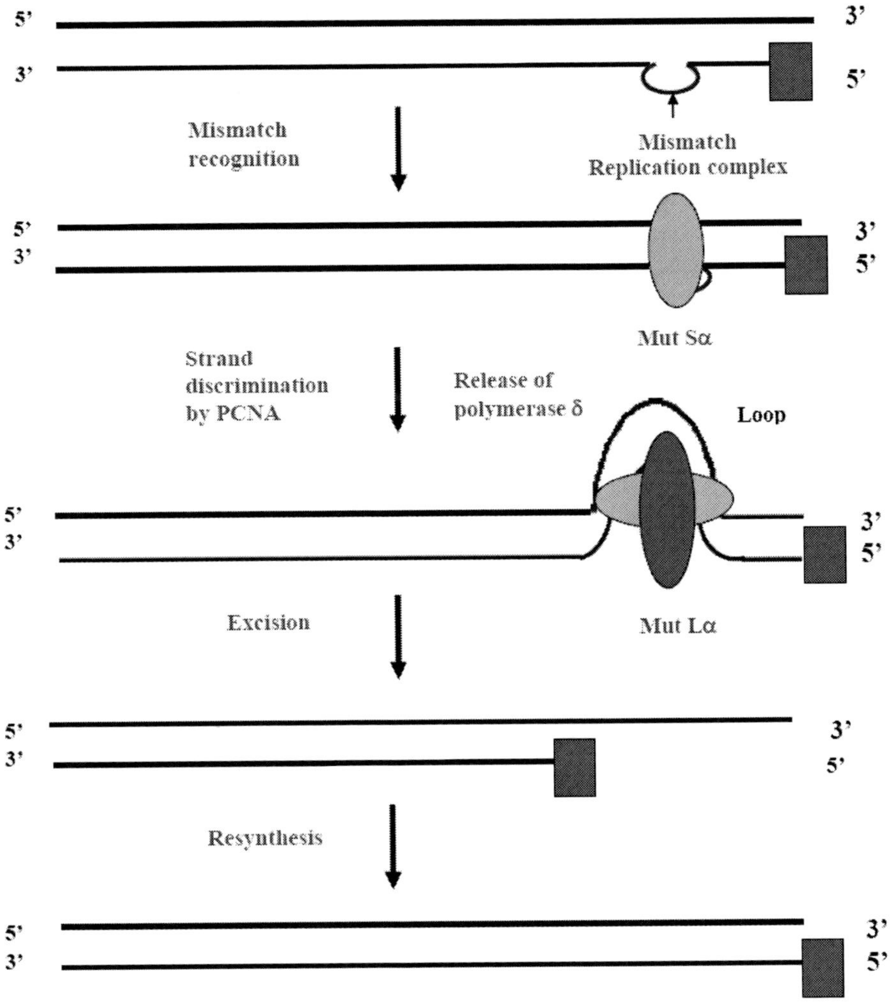

Figure 1. The mismatches in the DNA strand are recognized. The repair enzymes are recruited to excise the incorrect nucleotide patch followed by the resynthesis of DNA strand using the parental DNA as a template.

This leads to strand breaks and correct the mismatches. Following the exposure of cell to low concentration of MNNG (N-methyl-N'-nitro-N-nitrosoguanidine), signal is transduced by MMR proteins evident from direct binding of hMSH2 and checkpoint kinases ATR, arrest the cell in G2 phase (Jascur and Boland, 2006). Cisplatin-treated cells redistribute hPMS2 to the nucleus where, it binds and stabilizes the p53-related protein p73. Increased p73 protein then induces the apoptosis in response to cisplatin (Shimodaira et al., 2003).

Apart from MMR, other DNA repair systems involved and strengthen the defense machinery of the stem cell are discussed below.

1.1.2. O^6- Alkylguanine DNA Alkyl Transferase (AGT) Repair

MGMT encodes DNA repair protein, an AGT repair protein that removes DNA alkyl adducts from O^6 methylguanine and O^4 of thymine leaving normal guanine or thymine. The failure in the repair system results in transition mutation (G to A) and DNA strand break. Methylating agents can methylate the promoter of MGMT and thereby inactivate it, reported in gliomas, lymphomas, hematopoietic tumors, breast, ovarian and retinoblastomas (Shiraishi et al., 2000; Reese et al., 2001). Overexpression of AGT protects stem cells and prevents nitrosourea induced T cell lymphomas.

1.1.3. Nucleotide Excision Repair (NER)

In NER, the oligonucleotide fragments surrounded by the damaged bases are excised. The faulty bases are recognized by XPC (xeroderma pigmentosum complementation group C) and RAD23B whereas XPA, RPA (replication protein A), RNA polymerase II transcription factor IIH and XPG bind to the site of damaged DNA. ERCC1-XPF heterodimer endonuclease binds to it and cuts damaged bases at 5' junction while XPG, a double/ single stranded endonuclease cuts at 3' junction and excises the fragment of 27-30 nucleotides in the vicinity of the damaged bases. DNA polymerases delta and epsilon and other replication proteins (PCNA, RPA and RFC) and ligases fill the gap replace it with the correct sequence. The defect in NER proteins results in xeroderma pigmentosum (skin cancer) (Park and Gerson, 2005).

1.1.4. Base Excision Repair (BER)

It comprises of short and long patch pathways where DNA glycosylases generate apurinic/ apyrimidinic (AP) followed by its 5' excision by AP endonucleases (APE-1) and remove damaged bases. Double-stranded breaks have the potential to be the most disruptive form of DNA damage (Klungland and Lindahl, 1997; Lindahl and Wood, 1999).

1.1.5. Non-Homologous DNA End-Joining (NHEJ) Repair

Double-stranded breaks (DSBs) have the potential to be the most disruptive form of the DNA damage, produced by free radicals generated during oxidative respiration, ionizing radiation, DNA replication, malfunction of recombination activating gene complex during V(D)J (variable region, diversity region-junction region) recombination in T and B lymphocytes. These broken ends are brought in closed proximity by Ku70-Ku80 heterodimer and kinase activity is mediated by DNA dependent protein kinase catalytic subunit (DNA-PKcs) of DNA-PK complex followed by its ligation by XRCC4-DNA ligase IV. About 15% of SCID (Severe Combined Immunodeficiency) is associated with defective NHEJ repair system (Park and Gerson, 2005).

1.1.6. Homologous Recombination (HR) Repair

The DSBs are repaired but may lead to misalignment, deletions, and rearrangement. PI-3 Kinase regulates DSBs repair by binding with DNA and phosphorylating multiple proteins. BRCA1 activated by ATM (ataxia telangiectasia) facilitates BRCA2 and RAD51 binding of the 3' overhang (produced by the nuclease activity of Mre11/Rad50/Nbs1) followed by the attraction of RAD52/RAD54 with the help of BLM/ WRN proteins. The homologous recombination is then facilitated by large protein complexes at the DSBs. High incidence of leukemia, breast-ovarian, Werner and Bloom syndrome with severe premature aging and cancer is seen in defective HR repair system (Valerie and Povirk, 2003; Bakkenist and Kastan, 2003).

1.2. MMR Deficiency and Stem Cell Defects

The maintenance and longevity of stem cell phenotype is characterized by the presence of efficient MMR system. The defective repair systems are unable to cope with normal rates of damage (Anderson, 2001). Early loss of systems results in increased rate of mutagenesis and chromosomal rearrangements (Loeb, 1994). Metastatic phenotype arises from deficiencies in the repair enzymes themselves or from check point defects which fail to halt the cell cycle until repair is effected (Wood, 2001). The mutations characterized by point mutations, insertions or deletions in the length of DNA microsatellite repeat sequences throughout the genome resulting in microsatellite instability (MSI) is a hallmark of defective DNA MMR system (Vaish et al., 2005) may affect transcription, splicing or RNA processing. Since, instability occurs during replication, therefore, it is also known as RER+ phenotype (Peltomaki et al., 1993), (Figure 2).

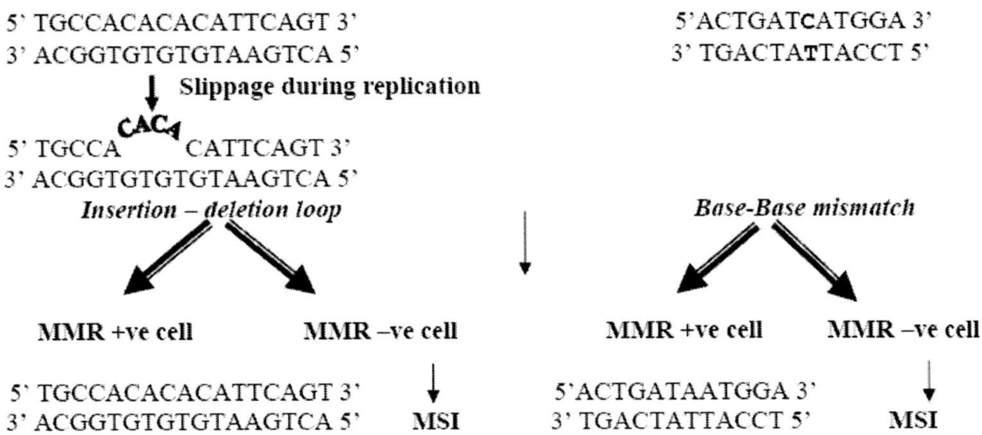

Figure 2. Repair of insertion deletion loop (IDL) or base-base mismatch in MMR proficient cell while MMR deficiency results in microsatellite instability.

Mutations in wild type MMR allele with Msh2$^{-/-}$ and Mlh2h$^{-/-}$ phenotype, mice develop stem cell-derived-lymphoid malignancies and all lymphoid tumors show MSI (Wei et al., 2002). The competitive survival of Msh2$^{-/-}$ primary murine hematopoietic cells was compared with wild type using serial bone marrow transplantation assays. The proportion of MSH2$^{-/-}$ hematopoietic progenitors recovered in the marrow declined with each successive transplant as evident by decrease in Msh2$^{-/-}$ colony forming units (CFUs) and Sca^{+}Kit^{+}Lin^{-} derived clones. MMR deficiency shown by MSI was observed and thus the alteration in growth and survival of hematopoietic stem cells and its long-term repopulation capacity because of accumulation of genomic instability (Reese et al., 2003). In another study, colonogenic survival was assayed in Msh2$^{-/-}$, Msh2$^{+/+}$, Msh2$^{-/+}$ mouse embryonic stem cells following prolonged low level radiation treatment. The cells deficient in active MMR system survive promutagenic genomic insults by alkylating and oxidating agents that contribute to neoplastic transformation as in hereditary non polyposis colorectal cancer (HNPCC) (DeWeese et al., 1998). The six cases of childhood leukemia are reported where patients are homozygous for MSH2, MLH1 or PMS2 loss of function mutations (Whiteside et al., 2002).

The chromosomal translocations, deletions or inversions with deleterious consequences in the adult or during development due to the mitotic homologous recombination further adds up the instability to the genome and this effect is elevated with the loss of MMR, commonly observed in hematological malignancies. High incidence of lymphoma is reported in Msh2 deficient mouse embryonic stem cells (Abuin et al., 2000).

The poor or complete elimination of repair function in Msh2 low and deficient mouse ES (embryonic stem) cells is due to the resistance acquired by the cells against the toxic effects of an ethylating agent, N-ethyl-N-nitrosourea (ENU). The ENU-induced mutagenicity under the fully or partially deficient conditions of MMR proteins exhibits lymphomagenesis (Claij et al., 2003). Toft et al., 1999, showed the increased mutation frequency at Dlb-1 locus due to loss of Msh2 status in normal intestinal cells predispose to malignancy. Msh2$^{-/-}$ mouse ES cells treated with temozolomide shows increased colonogenicity but not with cisplatin, contribute to failed repair mechanism and apoptosis in a p53 dependent manner.

Fink et al., 1997 examined the two-fold resistance to the cytotoxic effects of cisplatin in Msh2$^{-/-}$ mouse ES cells as compared to wild type cells. Study by Claij and Riele, 2004 confirms no relation between the MMR capacity of cells and their response to cisplatin in a colonogenic assay in mouse ES cells. However, certain specific changes like defective p53 (Branch et al., 2000), increased recombinational repair or increased replicative bypass found to be associated with MMR mutator phenotype in affecting the cytotoxicity of cisplatin.

The defective MMR genes directly or indirectly alter signal pathways, loss of strictly regulated expression of cytokine receptors, transcription factors and cell cycle regulation (Reese et al., 2003). Unlike normal stem cells, the presence of damaged DNA inactivate p53 induced G1 cell cycle arrest via inhibiting the functional interaction of repair helicases XPB and XPD with p53 (Nelson and Kastan, 1994; Wang et al., 1996). This contributes to the diminution of stem cells, a proliferative advantage and cancer stem cell formation. Mutations leading to loss of MMR phenotype in the progenitor cells (also known as transit – amplifying cells) arise from normal stem cells have replicative ability but not self-renewal capacity, help in regaining self-renewal property and transform into cancerous cells (Fig 3).

1.2.1. Cancer Stem Cells (CSCs)

In most of the malignancies cancer stem cells constitute less than 1% of total cell population. They were first identified in 1990s in hematological malignancies, mainly acute myelogenous leukemia (AML) as well as in other subtypes like AML M0, M1, M2, M4 and M5. The stem cells are mostly quiescent and have surface markers such as interleukin-3-receptor α chain, not present on the normal stem cells. Chronic myelogenous leukemia (CML), acute lymphoblastic leukemia (ALL) and multiple myeloma have a well-described stem cell phenotype (Pan et al., 2006). CSCs are also known to exist in solid tumors like breast, brain, lung, prostrate, testis, ovary, stomach, colon, skin, liver, pancreas (Al-Hajj and Clarke, 2004; Woodward et al., 2005; Moore and Lemischka, 2006). The key features of

CSCs are self-renewal property but undergo aberrant differentiation and constitute the heterogeneous population of tumor cells and thus the source of all malignant cells in a primary tumor (Vaish, 2007). It is also composed of small reservoir of drug resistant cells responsible for relapse after exposure to chemotherapeutic drugs. These cells are the precursors of distant metastasis and disturb the tissue homeostasis (Figure 3).

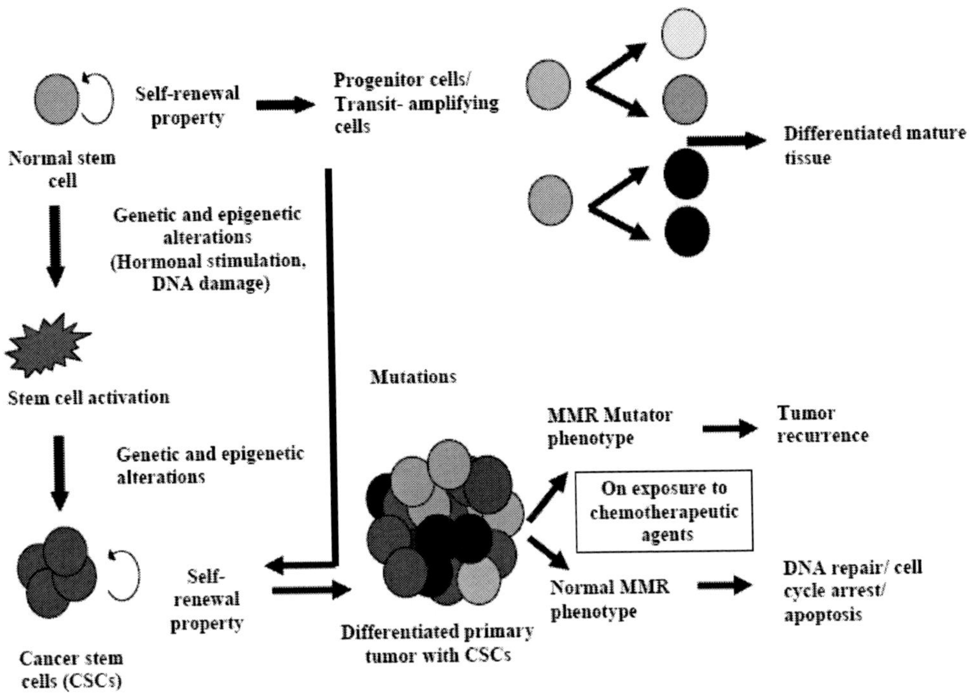

Figure 3. The self-renewal property (indicated by curved arrow), multi-lineage potential (cells shown by different colors) and extensive proliferation give rise to mature differentiated tissue. Accumulation of errors in the genetic makeup of stem cell or progenitor cell activated to generate the cancer stem cells (CSCs). CSCs have self-renewal capacity; proliferate extensively to give rise to heterogeneous population of daughter tumor cells along with small percentage of CSCs. In response to chemotherapeutic agents, the cancerous cells undergo different cellular responses to either rectify the genetic errors or cell cycle arrest or apoptosis (cell death) in presence of normal MMR proteins. MMR mutator phenotype makes cancer cells resistant to such drugs and result in malignant transformation.

CSCs constituting the fraction of total population of cells in the hematopoietic and a solid tumor side population (SP) (identified by the efflux of fluorescent dyes by ABC transporter proteins which are the major multidrug resistant genes) reflects that it is a common phenomenon for all the malignancies.

1.3. Cancer Stem Cell Therapy

Self-renewal capacity at early phases of cancer accumulates oncogenic transformations leads to eventual development of cancer metastasis, a multi-step process. The effective treatment of cancer involves the complete eradication of cancer stem cells. Identifying and characterizing the unique molecular profiles like cell surface antigen markers, mechanisms controlling cell survival and responses to injury of cancer stem cells discriminating them from normal stem cell phenotype may provide opportunities for therapeutic intervention that would spare normal stem cells. Drugs specifically targeting the growth and proliferation of cancer stem cells will undoubtedly help in its complete eradication. Pharmacodynamic assays on mouse leukemia models may help in evaluation of successful anti-cancer agents and future prospects of development of new therapies (Yilmaz et al., 2006).

1.3.1. Elimination of Self-Renewal Capacity

Cancer stem cells exist normally in quiescent state and exhibit chemo- and radio-resistance. Most of the conventional chemotherapeutic drugs are effective in actively dividing cells; therefore, for complete killing of CSCs, the therapeutic agents either should kill cells independently of the cell cycle or selectively induce cycling of cancer cells. The self-renewal capacity is inhibited by hampering the self-renewal pathways likely critical to CSCs with varying level of success. Among the potential therapeutic targets are the oncogenic cascades frequently deregulated in cancer initiating cells including estrogens (ER-α or -β, EGF, TGF-α/EGFR, hedgehog, Wnt/β-catenin, Notch, and/ or signaling elements (telomerase, PI3K, Akt, NF-κB and Myc-1) (Mimeault and Batra, 2007). The use of cyclopamine has been implemented in targeting the hedgehog signaling while exisulind, bromoindirubin-3'-oxime and imatinib target the Wnt/β-catenin pathways (Galmozzi eat al., 2006). The complete success would be achieved by targeting pathways uniquely used by CSCs.

1.3.2. Induction of Differentiation

The self-renewal capability of CSCs can also be eliminated by forcing them to undergo differentiation. These differentiation inducers are *trans*-retinoic acid and synthetic acyclic retenoid NIK-333 for patients with acute premyelocytic leukemia and hepatocellular carcinoma (Fuchs et al., 2004 and Sell, 2004). TPA, DMSO, butyric acid and vitamin D3 are used for solid tumors (Kawamata et al., 2006). These inducers are generally effective against the aggressive cancer forms when they are combined with other conventional treatments.

1.3.3. Inhibition of Drug Transporters

CSCs express high levels of various drug transporter proteins which pump the cytotoxic drugs out of the cell and protect them from damage thus making traditional chemotherapeutic and radiation therapies insufficient to clear the very small population of tumor initiating cells from the body. Inhibitors of these transporters sensitize the CSCs to chemo and radiotherapy thus could revolutionize the way cancer is treated. The fact that normal stem cells also express some of these transporters so non selective inhibition of these multidrug resistant genes makes the treatment ineffective by clearing the normal stem cells out of the body. Previous attempt to inhibit ABCB1 transporter although shows limited clinical success but ABCG2 specific inhibitors could have better results (Dean et al., 2005). Characterization of the stem cell markers (Table 2) would help in distinguishing the cancer stem cell phenotype from the normal stem cells which could selectively eliminate CSCs by specifically targeting the tumor cells (Jordan et al., 2006).

1.3.4. Gain of MMR Function

The absence of DNA repair fidelity helps the drug resistant pluoripotent cells to accumulate mutations and show increased cell survival (Dean, 2005). The susceptibility to cancer is increased as exemplified by hematological malignancies and lymphoma that arise due to chromosomal rearrangements because of loss of MMR proteins (Abuin et al., 2000). Msh2-deficient animals accumulate higher basal levels of mutations and this effect is attributable to increased colonogenicity when exposed to mutagenic effects of temozolomide. It (Msh2) also regulates the *in vivo* initiation of apoptosis after the cytotoxic drugs treatment (temozolomide, N-methyl-N'-nitro-N-nitrosoguanidine and cisplatin). Apoptosis was not influenced by the *in vivo* depletion of O^6-alkylguanine-DNA-alkyltransferase, another repair enzyme after administration of O^6-benzylguanine. This study concludes the requirement of Msh2 in mediating cell death through a p53 dependent pathway (Toft et al., 1999). It is further supported by another study that describes the premature senescence (cellular aging) in hematopoietic stem cells when treated with ionizing radiation or busulfan (Meng et al., 2003). Methylating agent tolerance is evident by the competitive survival advantage of $Msh2^{-/-}$ primary murine marrow progenitors as compared to the wild type (Reese et al., 2003). $Msh2^{-/+}$ and $Msh2^{-/-}$ mice ES cells accumulate more oxidized bases as a consequence of low level radiation than ES cells from $Msh2^{+/+}$ mice and fails to efficiently execute cell death (DeWeese et al., 1998).

In response to alkylation or oxidative DNA damage, MMR proteins are activated and directly or indirectly stimulate signal transduction, transcription factors, loss of cell cycle regulation that derive cell fate decision pathways and eliminate them. Presence of MMR proteins initiates the cisplatin-induced G1 arrest by cyclin D1 degradation (Lan et al., 2002). Functional MSH2 and MLH1 activate c-Abl, one of the proteins of p73-dependent apoptosis pathway (Nehme et al., 1997 and Gong et al., 1999). Defective MMR along with the mutated p53 response contributes to cisplatin resistance (Branch et al., 2000). On the contrary, the study by Claij and Riele, 2004 rules out the possibility of major contribution of MMR deficiency in conferring cisplatin resistance in mouse embryonic fibroblasts. The cooperative effect is shown by hMLH1 and other checkpoint kinases ATR and Chk1 in recruiting the cells with damaged DNA bases to undergo G2 arrest (Wang and Qin, 2003). The hMLH1 also activates stress kinase p38 and its inhibition cause cells to bypass G2 arrest (Hirose et al., 2003).

The wild type MMR expression blocks the homologous recombination between the diverged DNA sequences throughout the genome and thus prevents the stem cell to accumulate further genetic instability. The activation of proficient DNA MMR system would help in inhibiting the survival mechanisms by increasing the sensitivity of cancer cells to therapeutic drugs and reduce its tumor potential by arresting their growth. Oligonucleotide-directed gene modification through homologous recombination in cancer stem cells would help in restoring the wild type functions of MMR proteins thereby engages the cells to undergo apoptosis when DNA is damaged. Owning to mass effect, it is impossible to completely eliminate the progeny cancer cells using single anti-cancer therapeutic approach. Therefore, the combinational therapy involving specific killing of cancer cells, differentiation inducers and gain of mismatch repair function would selectively target the subset of tumor stem cells with undue toxicity of normal stem cells and thus it would be of clinical significance.

1.4. Conclusion

Most of the human cancers are identified having mismatch repair deficiency that result in defect in cell cycle and altered growth. The increased mutation rate and absence of MMR may give rise to stem cell failure, a proliferative advantage and cancer stem cells formation. The defective MMR status in a damaged cell directly contributes to the resistant phenotype against the cytotoxic effects of chemotherapeutic drugs and thus these CSCs survive chemotherapy.

Establishment of specific oncogenic markers expressed by cancer progenitor cells during their malignant transformation helps in improving the diagnostic and prognostic tests for more effective detection and therapeutic intervention against aggressive and metastatic cancers. The process reversing the drug resistance could increase the cure or response rates to chemotherapy. Gain of MMR function hits the proliferative pathways and induces cell death against the cytotoxic treatment to cancer cells. For the full proof cure and complete eradication of cancer stem cells, the anticancer therapy should be shifted from traditional non selective cytotoxic chemotherapy to targeted therapy against the pathophysiological changes of cancer.

References

Abuin, A; Zhang, H; Bradley, A. Genetic analysis of mouse embryonic stem cells bearing Msh3 and Msh2 single and compound mutations. *Mol. Cell Biol.*, 2000 20(1), 149-57.

Al-Hajj, M; Clarke, MF. Self-renewal and solid tumor stem cells. *Oncogene*, 2004 23(43), 7274-82.

Al-Hajj, M; Wicha, MS; Benito-Hernandez, A; Morrison, SJ; Clarke, MF. Prospective identification of tumorigenic breast cancer cells. *Proc. Natl. Acad. Sci. USA*, 2003 100(7), 3983-8.

Allen, D J; Makhov, A; Grilley, M; Taylor, J; Thresher, R; Modrich, P; Griffith JD. Mut S mediates heteroduplex loop formation by a translocation mechanism. *EMBO J.*, 1997 16, 4467-4476.

Anderson, GR. Genomic instability in cancer. *Current Science*, 2001 81, 501-507.

Bakkenist, CJ; Kastan, MB. DNA damage activates ATM through intermolecular autophosphorylation and dimer dissociation. *Nature*, 2003 421(6922), 499-506.

Bonnet, D; Dick, JE. Human acute myeloid leukemia is organized as a hierarchy that originates from a primitive hematopoietic cell. *Nat. Med.*, 1997 3(7), 730-7.

Branch, P; Masson, M; Aquilina, G; Bignami, M; Karran, P. Spontaneous development of drug resistance: mismatch repair and p53 defects in resistance to cisplatin in human tumor cells. *Oncogene*, 2000 19(28), 3138-45.

Chang, DK; Ricciardiello, L; Goel, A; Chang, CL; Boland, CR. Steady-state regulation of the human DNA mismatch repair system. *J. Biol. Chem.*, 2000 275(37), 29178.

Chi, NW; Kolodner, RD. Purification and characterization of MSH1, a yeast mitochondrial protein that binds to DNA mismatches. *J. Biol. Chem.*, 1994 269, 29984-29992.

Claij, N; te Riele, H. Msh2 deficiency does not contribute to cisplatin resistance in mouse embryonic stem cells. *Oncogene*, 2004 23(1), 260-6.

Claij, N; van der Wal, A; Dekker, M; Jansen, L; te Riele, H. DNA mismatch repair deficiency stimulates N-ethyl-N-nitrosourea-induced mutagenesis and lymphomagenesis. *Cancer Res.*, 2003 63(9), 2062-6.

Collins, AT; Berry, PA; Hyde, S; Stower, MJ; Maitland, NJ. Prospective identification of tumorigenic prostate cancer stem cells. *Cancer Res.*, 2005 65, 10946-10951.

Dean, M; Fojo, T; Bates, S. Tumour stem cells and drug resistance. *Nat. Rev. Cancer*, 2005 5(4), 275-84.

Dean, M. Cancer stem cells: Implications for cancer causation and therapy resistance. *Discovery Medicine*, 2005 5, 278-282.

Dean, M. Cancer stem cells: redefining the paradigm of cancer treatment strategies. *Mol. Interv.*, 2006 6(3), 140-8.

DeWeese, TL; Shipman, JM; Larrier, NA; Buckley, NM; Kidd, LR; Groopman, JD; Cutler, RG; te Riele, H; Nelson, WG. Mouse embryonic stem cells carrying one or two defective Msh2 alleles respond abnormally to oxidative stress inflicted by low-level radiation. *Proc. Natl. Acad. Sci. USA,* 1998 95(20), 11915-20.

Drummond, JT; Bellacosa, A. Human DNA mismatch repair in vitro operates independently of methylation status at CpG sites. *Nucl. Acids Res.*, 2001 29, 2234-2243.

Fang, D; Nguyen, TK; Leishear, K; Finko, R; Kulp, AN; Hotz, S; Van Belle, PA; Xu, X; Elder, DE; Herlyn, M. A tumorigenic subpopulation with stem cell properties in melanomas. *Cancer Res.*, 2005 65(20), 9328-37.

Fink, D; Zheng, H; Nebel, S; Norris, PS; Aebi, S; Lin, TP, Nehme, A; Christen, RD; Haas, M; MacLeod, CL; Howell, SB. In vitro and in vivo resistance to cisplatin in cells that have lost DNA mismatch repair. *Cancer Res.*, 1997 57(10), 1841-5.

Fuchs, E; Tumbar, T; Guasch, G. Socializing with the neighbors: stem cells and their niche. *Cell*, 2004 116(6), 769-78.

Galmozzi, E; Facchetti, F; La Porta, CA. Cancer stem cells and therapeutic perspectives. *Curr. Med. Chem.*, 2006 13(6), 603-7.

Gong, JG; Costanzo, A; Yang, HQ; Melino, G; Kaelin, WG Jr; Levrero, M; Wang, JY. The tyrosine kinase c-Abl regulates p73 in apoptotic response to cisplatin-induced DNA damage. *Nature*, 1999 399(6738), 806-9.

Gu, L; Hong, Y; McCulloch, S; Watanabe, H; Li, G M. ATP - dependent interaction of human mismatch repair proteins and dual role of PCNA in mismatch repair. *Nuc. Acids Res.,* 1998 26, 1173-1178.

Hirose, Y; Katayama, M; Stokoe, D; Haas-Kogan, DA; Berger, MS; Pieper, RO. The p38 mitogen-activated protein kinase pathway links the DNA mismatch repair system to the G2 checkpoint and to resistance to chemotherapeutic DNA-methylating agents. *Mol. Cell Biol.*, 2003 23(22), 8306-15.

Jascur, T; Boland, CR. Structure and function of the components of the human DNA mismatch repair system. *Int. J. Cancer,* 2006 119(9), 2030-5.

Jego, G; Robillard, N; Puthier, D; Amiot, M; Accard, F; Pineau, D; Harousseau, JL; Bataille, R; Pellat-Deceunynck, C. Reactive plasmacytoses are expansions of plasmablasts retaining the capacity to differentiate into plasma cells. *Blood,* 1999 94(2), 701-12.

Jiricny, J. Replication errors: challenging the genome. *EMBO J.,* 1998 17, 6427-6436.

Jordan, CT; Guzman, ML; Noble, M. Cancer stem cells. *N. Engl. J. Med.*, 2006 355(12), 1253-61.

Kawamata, H; Tachibana, M; Fujimori, T; Imai, Y. Differentiation-inducing therapy for solid tumors. *Curr. Pharm. Des.,* 2006 12(3), 379-85.

Klungland, A; Lindahl, T. Second pathway for completion of human DNA base excision repair: reconstitution with purified proteins and requirement for DNase IV (FEN1). *EMBO J.,* 1997 16, 3341-48.

Kolodner, R. Biochemistry and genetics of eukaryotic mismatch repair. *Genes Dev.*, 1996; 10, 1433-1442.

Lan, Z; Sever-Chroneos, Z; Strobeck, MW; Park, CH; Baskaran, R; Edelmann, W; Leone, G; Knudsen, ES. DNA damage invokes mismatch repair-dependent cyclin D1 attenuation and retinoblastoma signaling pathways to inhibit CDK2. *J. Biol. Chem.*, 2002 277(10), 8372-81.

Li, F; Tiede, B; Massague, J; Kang, Y. Beyond tumorigenesis: cancer stem cells in metastasis. *Cell Res.*, 2007a 17(1), 3-14.

Li, C; Heidt, DG; Dalerba, P; Burant, CF; Zhang, L; Adsay, V; Wicha, M; Clarke, MF; Simeone, DM. Identification of pancreatic cancer stem cells. *Cancer Res.,* 2007b 67(3), 1030-7.

Lindahl, T; Wood, RD. Quality control by DNA repair. *Science*, 1999 286, 1897-905.

Li, GM; Modrich, P. Restoration of mismatch repair to nuclear extracts of H6 colorectal tumor cells by a heterodimer of human mut L homologs. *Proc. Natl. Acad. Sci. USA*, 1995 92, 1950-1954.

Loeb, LA. Microsatellite instability: Marker of a mutator phenotype of a cancer. *Cancer Res.*, 1994 54, 5059-5063.

Marsischky, G T; Filosi, M; Kane, M F; Kolodner, R. Redundancy of Saccharomyces cerevisiae MSH3 and MSH6 in MSH2-dependent mismatch repair. *Genes Dev.*, 1996 10, 407-420.

Matsui, W; Huff, CA; Wang, Q; Malehorn, MT; Barber, J; Tanhehco, Y; Smith BD; Civin, CL; Richard J. Jones. Characterization of clonogenic multiple myeloma cells. *Blood*, 2004 103(6), 2332-2336.

Meng, A; Wang, Y; Brown, SA; Van Zant, G; Zhou, D. Ionizing radiation and busulfan inhibit murine bone marrow cell hematopoietic function via apoptosis-dependent and -independent mechanisms. *Exp. Hematol.*, 2003 31(12), 1348-56.

Mimeault, M; Batra, SK. Functions of tumorigenic and migrating cancer progenitor cells in cancer progression and metastasis and their therapeutic implications. *Cancer Metastasis Rev.*, 2007 26(1), 203-14.

Moore, KA; Lemischka, IR. Stem cells and their niches. *Science*, 2006 311(5769), 1880-5.

Nehme, A; Baskaran, R; Aebi, S; Fink, D; Nebel, S; Cenni, B; Wang, JY; Howell, SB; Christen, RD. Differential induction of c-Jun NH2-terminal kinase and c-Abl kinase in DNA mismatch repair-proficient and -deficient cells exposed to cisplatin. *Cancer Res.*, 1997 57(15), 3253-7.

Nelson, WG; Kastan, MB. DNA strand breaks: the DNA template alterations that trigger p53-dependent DNA damage response pathways. *Mol. Cell Biol.*, 1994 14(3), 1815-23.

Pan, CX; Zhu, W; Cheng, L. Implications of cancer stem cells in the treatment of cancer. *Future Oncol.*, 2006 2(6), 723-31.

Park, Y; Gerson, SL. DNA repair defects in stem cell function and aging. *Annu. Rev. Med.*, 2005 56, 495-508.

Peltomaki, P; Lothe, RA; Aaltonen, LA; Pylkannen, L; Nystrom-Lahti, M; Seruca, R; David, L; Holm, R; Ryberg, D; Haugen, A et al. Microsatellite instability is associated with tumors that charecterize the hereditary non-polyposis colorectal cancer syndrome. *Cancer Res.*, 1993 53, 5853-5855.

Prince, ME; Sivanandan, R; Kaczorowski, A; Wolf, GT; Kaplan, MJ; Dalerba, P; Weissman, IL; Clarke, MF; Ailles, LE. Identification of a subpopulation of cells with cancer stem cell properties in head and neck squamous cell carcinoma. *Proc. Natl. Acad. Sci. USA*, 2007 104(3), 973-8.

Reese, JS; Liu, L; Gerson, SL. Repopulating defect of mismatch repair-deficient hematopoietic stem cells. *Blood,* 2003 102(5), 1626-33.

Reese, JS; Qin, X; Ballas, CB; Sekiguchi, M; Gerson, SL. MGMT expression in murine bone marrow is a major determinant of animal survival after alkylating agent exposure. *J. Hematother Stem Cell Res.*, 2001 10(1), 115-23.

Sell, S. Stem cell origin of cancer and differentiation therapy. *Crit. Rev. Oncol. Hematol.*, 2004 51(1), 1-28.

Shimodaira, H; Yoshioka-Yamashita, A; Kolodner, RD; Wang, JY. Interaction of mismatch repair protein PMS2 and the p53-related transcription factor p73 in apoptosis response to cisplatin. *Proc. Natl. Acad. Sci. USA*, 2003 100(5), 2420-5.

Shiraishi, A; Sakumi, K; Sekiguchi, M. Increased susceptibility to chemotherapeutic alkylating agents of mice deficient in DNA repair methyltransferase. *Carcinogenesis*, 2000 21(10), 1879-83.

Sia, EA; Kokoska, RJ; Dominska, M; Greenwell, P; Petes, TD. Microsatellite instability in yeast: dependence on repeat unit size and DNA mismatch repair genes. *Mol. Cell Biol.*, 1997 17, 2851-2858.

Singh, SK; Clarke, ID; Terasaki, M; Bonn, VE; Hawkins, C; Squire, J; Dirks, PB. Identification of a cancer stem cell in human brain tumors. *Cancer Res.*, 2003 63(18), 5821-8.

Thomas, DC; Roberts, JD; Kunkel, TA. Heteroduplex repair in extracts of human HeLa cells. *J. Biol. Chem.*, 1991 266(6), 3744-51.

Toft, NJ; Winton, DJ; Kelly, J; Howard, LA; Dekker, M; te Riele, H; Arends, MJ; Wyllie, AH; Margison, GP; Clarke, AR. Msh2 status modulates both apoptosis and mutation frequency in the murine small intestine. *Proc. Natl. Acad. Sci. USA*, 1999 96(7), 3911-5.

Uchida, N; Buck, DW; He, D; Reitsma, MJ; Masek, M; Phan, TV; Tsukamoto, AS; Gage, FH; Weissman, IL. Direct isolation of human central nervous system stem cells. *Proc. Natl. Acad. Sci. USA*, 2000 97(26), 14720-5.

Vaish, M; Mandhani, A; Mittal, RD; Mittal, B. Microsatellite instability as prognostic marker in bladder tumors: a clinical significance. *BMC Urol.*, 2005 5(1):2.

Vaish, M; Mittal, B. DNA mismatch repair, microsatellite instability and cancer. *Ind. J. of Exp. Biol.*, 2002 40, 989-994.

Vaish, M. Mismatch repair deficiencies transforming stem cells into cancer stem cells and therapeutic implications. *Mol. Cancer*, 2007 6:26.

Valerie, K; Povirk, LF. Regulation and mechanisms of mammalian double-strand break repair. *Oncogene,* 2003 22(37), 5792-812.

Klein, WM; Wu, BP; Zhao, S; Wu, H; Klein-Szanto, AJP; Tahan, SR. Increased expression of stem cell markers in malignant melanoma. *Modern Pathology*, 2007 20, 102–107.

Wang, XW; Vermeulen, W; Coursen, JD; Gibson, M; Lupold, SE; Forrester, K; Xu, G; Elmore, L; Yeh, H; Hoeijmakers, JH; Harris, CC. The XPB and XPD DNA helicases are components of the p53-mediated apoptosis pathway. *Genes Dev.*, 1996 10(10), 1219-32.

Wang, Y; Qin, J. MSH2 and ATR form a signaling module and regulate two branches of the damage response to DNA methylation. *Proc. Natl. Acad. Sci. USA*, 2003 100(26), 15387-92.

Wei, K; Kucherlapati, R; Edelmann, W. Mouse models for human DNA mismatch-repair gene defects. *Trends Mol. Med.*, 2002 8(7), 346-53.

Wheeler, JMD; Bodmer, WF. DNA mismatch repair genes and colorectal cancer. *Gut*, 2000 47, 148-153.

Whiteside, D; McLeod, R; Graham, G; Steckley, JL; Booth, K; Somerville, MJ; Andrew, SE. A homozygous germ-line mutation in the human MSH2 gene predisposes to hematological malignancy and multiple cafe-au-lait spots. *Cancer Res.,* 2002 62(2), 359-62.

Wood, RD; Mitchell, M; Sgouros, J; Lindahl, T. Human DNA repair genes. *Science*, 2001 291, 1284-1289.

Woodward, WA; Chen, MS; Behbod, F; Rosen, JM. On mammary stem cells. *J. Cell Sci.*, 2005 118(Pt 16), 3585-94.

Yilmaz, OH; Valdez, R; Theisen, BK; Guo, W; Ferguson, DO; Wu, H; Morrison, SJ. Pten dependence distinguishes haematopoietic stem cells from leukaemia-initiating cells. *Nature*, 2006 441(7092), 475-82.

In: Cancer and Stem Cells
Eds: Thomas Dittmar and Kurt S. Zänker
ISBN 978-1-60456-478-5

Chapter 5

Cancer Stem Cells in Hematological Malignancies

Aniruddha J. Deshpande and Christian Buske [*]
Helmholtz Center for Environment and Health
and the Clinical Cooperative Group- Leukemia
Department of Medicine III, Klinikum Grosshadern,
D-81377 Munich, Germany

Abstract

Leukemia comprises a group of malignancies of the blood system characterized by the abnormal and uncontrolled expansion of white blood cells (leukocytes). The malignant cell population in leukemia, like in many other cancers, is morphologically, phenotypically and functionally heterogeneous. These heterogeneous populations of leukemic cells are now known to emerge from a population of leukemic cells with stem cell characteristics termed leukemic stem cells (LSCs). In many other tumors, the presence of such so called 'cancer stem cells' (CSCs) has been demonstrated. These cells are at the apex of the neoplastic system and can continuously replenish the tumor. They are also believed to be resistant to most currently employed therapies and responsible for tumor relapse after therapy. Leukemias have served as a model disease for studying the concept of CSCs and approaches to target these cells. Significant advances have been made in the understanding of the biology of LSCs and the processes that lead to LSC formation. These insights will be discussed in detail in the following chapter focussing on chronic myeloid leukemia (CML), acute myeloid leukemia (AML) and acute lymphoblastic leukemia (ALL).

[*] Address for Correspondence: Helmholtz Center for Environment and Health, Clinical Cooperative Group-Leukemia, Marchioninistrasse 25, D-81377 Munich, Germany, Telephone + 49 89 7099402, Fax + 49 89 7099400, Email: buske@gsf.de

Keywords: acute myeloid leukemia, AML, cancer stem cells, CSC, leukemic stem cells, LSC, acute lymphoblastic leukemia, ALL, chronic myeloid leukemia, CML, stem cells, tumor stem cells.

Abbreviations

LSC	Leukemic stem cells
CSC	Cancer stem cells
Ph+:	Philadelphia chromosome positive leukemias or cells (The Philadelphia chromosme refers to the chromosome resulting from the t(12;22) translocation expressing the BCR-ABL fusion gene, named after the city in which it was first described).
HSC:	Hematopoietc stem cells
CMP:	Common myeloid progenitor; a non-self-renewing progenitor downstream of the HSC (see Figure 3) that is considered to be the precursors of all myeloid cells and generally restricted in myeloid lineage potential
GMP:	Granulocyte-macrophage progenitor; a non-self-renewing progenitors downstream of the CMP (see Figure 3) that is considered to be the precursors of granulocytes and macrophages
CLP:	Common lymphoid progenitor; a non-self-renewing progenitor downstream of the HSC (see Figure 3) that is considered to be the precursors of all lymphoid cells and generally restricted in lymphoid lineage potential
CML:	Chronic myeloid leukemia
bcCML:	The acute phase of CML
AML:	Acute myeloid leukemia
ALL:	Acute lymphoid leukemia
B-ALL:	Acute lymphoid leukemia of the B cell lineage
T-ALL:	Acute lymphoid leukemia of the T cell lineage
MPD:	Myeloproliferative disease
P210:	The 210 kilidalton form of the BCR-ABL fusion gene
P190:	The 190 kilidalton form of the BCR-ABL fusion gene

1. Introduction

Blood related cancers such as leukemias are now viewed as malignancies arising from a rare subset of cells with stem cell properties. It had been proposed several years ago that cancer is a disease of stem cells reviewed in (Sell 2004). The widely held (Dalerba, Cho et al. 2007) though not unchallenged (Campbell and Polyak 2007; Kelly, Dakic et al. 2007) cancer stem cell hypothesis states that cancer derives from a minor subset of cells with stem cell properties termed cancer stem cells (CSCs) that possess the unique ability to maintain the tumor and to regenerate the heterogeneity of the original tumor. Since the hematopoietic system is the best characterised system as far as the study of tissue stem cells is concerned, the first evidence for this hypothesis came from studies on haematological neoplasia. It had been observed by Bruce and Van der Gaag in 1963 that only 1-4 % of transplanted murine lymphoma cells could generate spleen colonies upon mouse transplantation. In 1973, Earnest McCulloch and colleagues showed that only around 1 in 100 to 1 in 10,000 murine myeloma cells could form colonies *in vitro* suggesting that only a fraction of cells within these tumors had the ability to propagate the tumor. In 1997, it was demonstrated that within the leukemic bone marrow of acute myeloid leukaemia (AML), the ability to generate tumors in recipient mice resided only in a rare subset of cells, which resembled phenotypically normal hematopoietic stem cells (Bonnet and Dick 1997). These results strongly suggested that AML could arise from, and be maintained by this subset of cells with LSC characteristics. The observation that the ability to propagate tumors resides only within a fraction of cells with stem cell properties could subsequently be replicated in multiple human tumor types including tumors of the breast, brain, colon and pancreas (Al-Hajj, Wicha et al. 2003; Singh, Hawkins et al. 2004; Li, Heidt et al. 2007; O'Brien, Pollett et al. 2007). These results showed within tumors, it was this reservoir of cells with stem cell properties that could continuously churn out malignant cells, highlighting the importance of targeting these cells for effective therapeutic intervention.

2. CSCs in Chronic and Acute Leukemias

Leukemias arise as a result of the subversion of normal processes of hematopoiesis. Leukemia can take a chronic or an acute clinical course and the leukemic bulk can display lymphoid or myeloid characteristics. Hence, leukemias are classified into acute and chronic myeloid and lymphoid leukemia. Early studies on hematological malignancies have shown the presence of disease specific cytogenetic aberrations in the primitive cell stem cell like compartments of patients with AML, CML and ALL (Haase, Feuring-Buske et al. 1995; Mehrotra, George et al. 1995; Quijano, Moore et al. 1997; Takahashi, Miura et al. 1998; Deininger, Goldman et al. 2000). These descriptive studies involving the analysis of clonal evolution, multilineage involvement etc, already suggested that hematological malignancies involve early hematopoietic cells. However, more recent studies employing extensive characterization of leukemic populations by prospective isolation of cellular sub-fractions and the use of animal models of leukemia development have shown that leukemias follow the CSC model and are propagated by a rare subpopulation of leukemic cells with stem cell features.

2.1. LSCs in Chronic Myelogeneous Leukemia (CML)

CML is a form of leukemia characterized by an increased and dysregulated growth of myeloid cells and the presence of the BCR-ABL fusion gene generated by the t(9;22)(q34;q11) translocation (also termed the Philadelphia or Ph chromosome). CML is one of the most well characterized neoplastic diseases and can serve as a model for multi-step tumorigenesis seen in different cancers (Melo and Barnes 2007). Decades ago, clonal tracking studies involving chromosomal or isoenzyme markers in cancer suggested that most human tumors were clonal (Fialkow 1974; Fialkow 1979). Interestingly, long before the question of the CSC was addressed, these studies showed that in chronic myeloid leukemia (CML), clonal markers could be observed in cells of multiple lineages suggesting that this disease arose in a multipotent stem cell (Fialkow, Denman et al. 1978). CML is characterized by a latent chronic phase which presents as a myeloproliferative disease (MPD) and usually evolves into an accelerated phase and ultimately into a blast crisis phase. Blast crisis CML (bcCML) is clinically similar to acute leukemia with rapid progression and short survival. The BCR-ABL fusion gene can be detected in the phenotypic HSC compartment in CML patients (Takahashi, Miura et al. 1998). Interestingly, genomic BCR-ABL can also be detected in the bone marrow of some patients in complete remission (Chomel, Brizard et al. 2000) and a very low level of BCR-ABL transcripts can also be detected in blood forming cells of healthy individuals (Bose, Deininger et al. 1998). This suggests that BCR-ABL expressing stem cells are pre-leukemic and the transition to the acute phase requires acquisition of additional mutations. Murine models of CML induced by the BCR-ABL fusion gene have been used since a long time to study BCR-ABL induced transformation (Daley, Van Etten et al. 1990; Van Etten 2001). Importantly, this fusion gene can generate both CML as well as ALL (Li, Ilaria et al. 1999). Interestingly, whereas the retroviral infection of BCR-ABL into 5-fluorouracil enriched bone marrow cells leads preferentially to CML, the introduction of BCR-ABL in steady state bone marrow cells, which includes more differentiated committed progenitors leads to the induction of B-ALL. This suggests that while CML arises in early stem and progenitor cells, BCR-ABL mediated B-ALL development possibly arises from more downstream lymphoid cells (Li, Ilaria et al. 1999). In the mice with the myeloid phenotype, BCR-ABL induces a myeloproliferative syndrome recapitulating chronic phase CML whereas the introduction of additional mutations ('second hits') such as BCL2 (Jaiswal, Traver et al. 2003) induces acute leukemia reflecting bcCML (Cuenco and Ren 2001; Dash, Williams et al. 2002; Mayotte, Roy et al. 2002).

To test whether HSC involvement is necessary for CML development, Jaiswal et al., co-expressed BCR-ABL and BCL2 in myeloid progenitors but not HSCs and showed that leukemia progression could be initiated in these cells. This data showed that bcCML can arise in myeloid progenitors without the need for HSCs involvement in this murine model. Interestingly, another recent study showed that the introduction of BCR-ABL in highly purified HSCs lead to an MPD like disease, but the expression of BCR-ABL alone (unlike in the study from Jaiswal et al.) in non-self renewing myeloid progenitors was not sufficient to initiate leukemia development. These two studies are in line with the notion that even though the BCR-ABL fusion most likely takes place in HSCs, cooperative mutations leading to acute leukemia can occur in BCR-ABL positive HSCs or their progenitors (Figure 1). Consistent with this, in human CML patient samples, Jamieson et al., could show that even though phenotypic HSCs expressed the BCR-ABL fusion gene in all phases of the disease, there was a progressive expansion of the granulocyte-macrophage progenitors (GMP) rather than the HSC compartment with disease progression to the blast crisis phase. These *BCR-ABL* expressing GMPs, unlike their normal counterparts, exhibited a high *in vitro* self-renewal and aberrantly activated ß-catenin (Jamieson, Ailles et al. 2004). These results strongly suggested that the progression of chronic phase CML to blast crisis CML occurs in the highly proliferative GMP compartment which aberrantly acquires 'stem cell' properties.

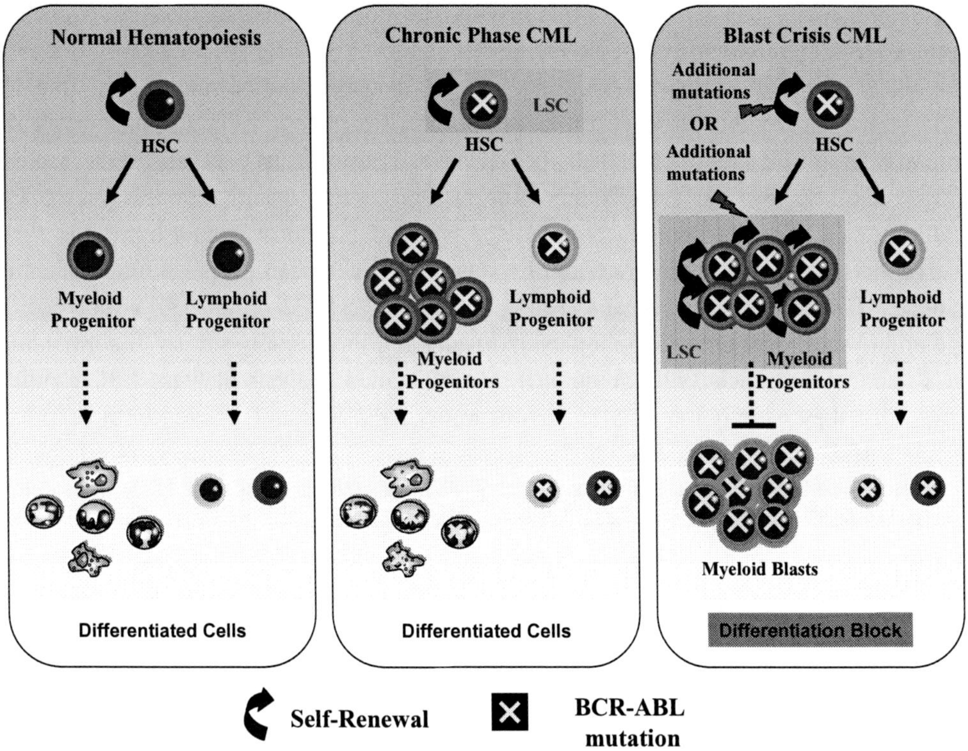

Figure 1. Development of chronic myeloid leukemia. a)The normal hematopoietic scheme: Self-renewing stem cells give rise to myeloid and lymphoid progenitors as well as more differentiated downstream cells. b) BCR-ABL mutations, usually in hematopoietic stem cells, lead to a hyperproliferative myeloid compartment resulting in chronic phase CML. c) CML eventually progresses to an acute phase termed blast crisis CML (bcCML) which seems to involve the acquisition of additional mutations in HSCs or downstream myeloid progenitors. As a result, myeloid progenitors could aberrantly acquire self-renewal capability and act as LSCs in the propagation of the disease.

It also demonstrates that the cell pool which acquires leukemic stem cell characteristics can change during the course of the disease from the HSC compartment to the GMP compartment (Figure 1). This might have clinical implications for the development of therapies which aim at targeting the LSCs, requiring different strategies at different stages of disease. These findings confirm data from AML (see section 2.2) showing that committed progenitors can also aberrantly acquire LSC characteristics.

The findings discussed above are consistent with a model of CML pathogenesis, in which CML is propagated by multipotent HSCs carrying the Philadelphia chromosome and expressing the BCR-ABL fusion gene. The expression of the fusion gene is responsible for the development of myeloproliferation, but insufficient to cause frank leukemia. Subsequently, after several years, this pre-leukemic state of the disease then enters into acute bcCML form after acquisition of additional mutations which inhibit differentiation and/or apoptosis and allow committed progenitors to acquire LSC characteristics (Figure 1).

2.2. LSCs in Acute Myelogeneous Leukemia (AML)

Like CML, AML cells are morphologically and immunophenotypically heterogeneous. This heterogeneity can partly be explained by the observation that these AML cells are organized as a hierarchy of progressively (albeit abnormally) differentiated cells (Bonnet and Dick 1997). The involvement of stem cells in AML has been studied since a long time. Early studies have shown the presence of leukemia specific mutations in the phenotypic HSC compartment of different AML subtypes (Haase, Feuring-Buske et al. 1995; Mehrotra, George et al. 1995) The establishment of qualitative and quantitative assays for HSCs including the use of the immunocompromised NOD/SCID mouse model led to the striking observation that only a minor fraction of human AML cells can propagate the leukemia in recipients (Lapidot, Sirard et al. 1994). Surprisingly, in diverse AML subtypes, this population was shown to be immunophenotypically and functionally similar to normal human HSCs (Bonnet and Dick 1997) (Figure 2). More detailed analysis of these LSC candidates showed that they were not exactly analogous to normal HSCs and differed in the expression of some surface markers (see Section 5). Moreover the CD34+/CD38- fraction from the AML M3 subtype which is associated with the PML-RARα translocation failed to engraft suggesting that the LSCs in some AMLs might reside more downstream of the HSC compartment. An important question in LSC biology therefore, was whether the LSC must arise in the HSC compartment or whether more downstream cells are also targets for LSC formation. This question could be readily answered in experimental AML models due to advances in the prospective isolation of progressively differentiated subsets of the hematopoietic system, relative ease of genetic manipulation, and the availability of disease specific animal models of AML. Therefore, using the murine bone marrow transplantation model and retrovirally induced expression of leukemogenic fusion genes in highly purified hematopoietic subpopulations, it was shown that leukemia could be generated by the retroviral introduction of the leukemogenic *MLL-ENL* fusion gene into highly purified HSC confirming the hypothesis that normal HSCs can become LSCs by the expression of appropriate oncogenes. The same study, however, could also demonstrate that even downstream myeloid progenitors can acquire LSC characteristics when transduced by retroviruses carrying the *MLL-ENL* fusion gene and interestingly, generate a similar leukemia suggesting that myeloid progenitors could also acquire LSC characteristics and initiate leukemia (Cozzio, Passegue et al. 2003). Using the same murine model system, it was subsequently shown that the oncogenic fusion gene *MOZ-TIF2* could generate leukemia from commited myeloid progenitors whereas the fusion gene, *BCR-ABL* could only generate myeloid leukemia when introduced into HSCs (Figure **3**). (Huntly, Shigematsu et al. 2004), showing the distinct abilities of different oncogenes to endow LSC properties to different cell types. Recently, Scott Armstrong and colleagues could elegantly demonstrate in a murine model of the leukemogenic fusion gene *MLL-AF9*, that the potential of this fusion gene to convert committed myeloid progenitors to LSCs was accompanied by the initiation of a leukemic stem cell signature resembling an HSC program in these myeloid cells (Krivtsov, Twomey et al. 2006). This supports the concept that some oncogenes can confer self-renewal properties to non-self renewing committed progenitors and generate LSCs. These studies signal the first steps into uncovering the molecular mechanisms by which *stemness* pathways are subverted for tumor development.

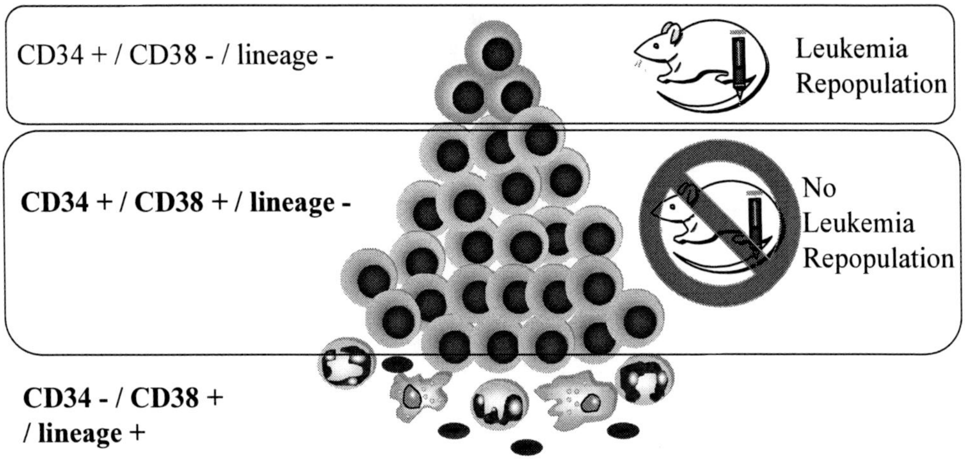

Figure 2. The leukemia initiating cell in AML has an HSC like phenotype. It was observed that the CD34+/CD38- cells from patients of various AML subtypes possessed a high ability to initiate tumors in immunodeficient mouse model of human AML whereas the CD34+/CD38+ cells had no tumorigenicity. These results suggested, for the first time that AML probably originated from HSCs.

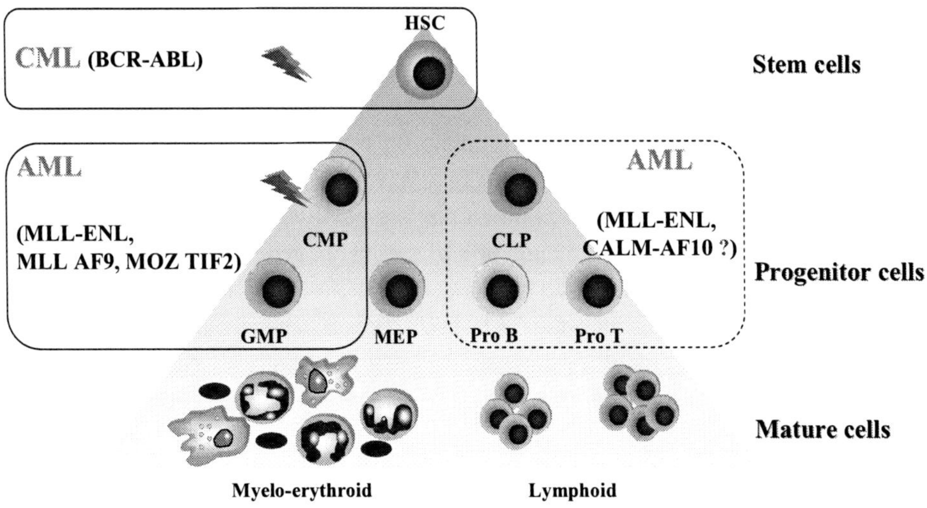

Figure 3. LSCs can arise from HSCs or downstream progenitors. Murine models of leukemia showed that even as oncogenes such as BCR-ABL can only initiate leukemias from HSCs and not downstream myeloid progenitors, MLL-ENL, MLL-AF9 or MOZ-TIF2 do not need HSC involvement and can convert myeloid progenitors into LSCs. Moreover, it is possible that in some AMLs, such as those positive for CALM/AF10 or MLL-ENL, LSCs derive from the lymphoid compartment. These studies highlight the important point that certain oncogenes, but not others, can impart the property of self-renewal to non-self renewing cells and generate LSCs also from cells downstream of HSCs.

Recently, our group generated a murine model of t(10;11) translocation positive AML. Characterization of the LSCs in this model of AML showed that the LSCs harbored lymphoid characteristics such as B220 marker expression and genomic (DJ) rearrangements of the immunoglobulin (IgH) locus (Deshpande, Cusan et al. 2006). We could show that these lymphoid-like LSCs could propagate AML and generate the heterogeneity of the tumor from which it was isolated even at the single cell level. Previously, in a transgenic model of the MLL-ENL fusion gene, it was shown that the fusion gene could induce lineage reassignment in lymphoid precursors and generate a myeloid leukemia. It is therefore likely that AML can also be initiated in progenitors of the lymphoid compartment (Deshpande and Buske 2007).

2.3. Lymphoid LSCs

Although myeloid leukemias have been the proving ground for most of the theories concerning LSCs, recent studies suggest that lymphoid leukemias may also arise from a subset of cells with stem/progenitor cell characteristics. ALL, like AML, is a heterogeneous disease with close to 80 % of ALLs involving B lineage cells. Reports studying the involvement of the HSC compartment in these B-ALLs have failed to provide an unequivocal demonstration that LSCs are derived from normal hematopoietic stem cells, though studies in different types of ALL suggest that ALL originates from a primitive cell rather than from committed progenitors (Quijano, Moore et al. 1997; Cobaleda, Gutierrez-Cianca et al. 2000; George, Franklin et al. 2001; Cox, Evely et al. 2004; Cox, Martin et al. 2007).

A large proportion of pediatric B-ALLs (roughly 25%) harbour the t(12;21) translocation and the resultant *TEL-AML1* fusion gene (Golub, Barker et al. 1995; Romana, Poirel et al. 1995). This translocation is thought to initiate early in life as it can be detected in neonatal blood spots (Guthrie cards) retrospectively analyzed from affected children. Still, it takes a long time for full blown leukemia to develop (Wiemels, Cazzaniga et al. 1999) and this occurs only in a small percentage of children that are positive for this fusion (Mori, Colman et al. 2002). This indicates that the acquisition of the fusion gene is a pre-leukemic event and that additional genetic hits are required for the development of ALL.

There are reports showing that the *TEL-AML1* fusion can only be found in CD19+ but not CD19- cells. In contrast, another study showed that in pediatric B-ALL, leukemia specific aberrations can be found in the CD34+/CD38- fraction (George, Franklin et al. 2001) indicating the involvement of the HSC compartment. Recent results from Castor and colleagues (Castor, Nilsson et al. 2005) could nicely reconcile these contrasting findings; they observed that this CD34+/CD38- compartment can be divided into CD19+ and CD19- cells and that only the CD19+ fraction was positive for the *TEL-AML1* fusion. Importantly, this population is absent in normal individuals. Moreover, in these patients, the size of the CD34+/CD38-/CD19- fraction was unchanged compared to control and the myeloid cells in the patients did not harbor the *TEL-AML1* fusion indicating that the LSCs did not originate from HSCs in these cases, but from a CD19+ committed lymphoid population. These findings also highlight the importance of differentiating between 'cells of origin' and 'CSCs', which will be discussed in the following section.

B-ALL with the Philadelphia chromosome (Ph+ B-ALL) is another subset of ALL with a poor prognosis. These are usually characterized by either of two different commonly occurring breakpoints resulting in a BCR-ABL fusion protein of 210 kilodalton termed p210 BCR-ABL and another shorter form, the 190 kilodalton p190 BCR-ABL fusion protein. In the Castor et al. study, they analysed B-ALLs with both forms of *BCR-ABL* and found that the p210 form is expressed in cells of multiple lineages indicating its origin in a multipotent HSC. Furthermore, functional analysis showed that even though the HSCs harbored *BCR-ABL*, only CD19+ cells could induce leukemia reconstitution in mice and therefore potential LSC activity. This finding is very similar to the results reported in CML where preleukemic stem cells harbour the fusion gene and myeloid progenitors are candidate LSCs showing the highest leukemic activity. Interestingly in contrast to p210 positive B-ALL, in B-ALLs with the p190 form, the CD34+/CD38-/CD19- compartment was negative for the fusion gene and the CD19+ cells showed a high tumor propagating ability. These results suggested that the cell in which the *BCR-ABL* mutation first arose (*'cell of origin'*) seemed to be different in these two related subtypes of B-ALL (p210 BCR-ABL and p190 BCR-ABL_), even though the LSC in both cases could be a CD19+ cell. These data show that the LSC in lymphoid tumors seems to express B-lineage associated markers. The LSCs in other types of ALL such as T-ALL and in chronic lymphoid leukemia (CLL) remain to be identified and is likely to be the focus of investigation in coming years.

3. Cancer Stem Cell Concepts and Questions: Lessons from Leukemia

3.1. 'Cell of Origin' and the CSC

CSC candidates of various cancers have been identified and have been presented as the most therapeutically relevant targets for anti-cancer treatment. This approach, which relies mostly on the analysis of different tumor sub-populations for transplantability of the disease, identifies the cell with the highest tumorigenicity (CSC). However, an important point for the understanding of the disease is that the CSCs can differ from the cell in which the cancer predisposing mutation initially occurred, termed the *'cell of origin'*. The 'cell of origin' in cancer has been defined as a *'pre-CSC'* or a *'precancerous cell that gives rise to a cancer stem cell'* (Smith 2006). As discussed before, (see Section 2.2), it is suggested that t(8;21)$^+$ HSC are not leukemic, but some of their downstream progeny might achieve additional mutation(s) to become transformed into LSCs (Miyamoto, Weissman et al. 2000). The HSCs in this case would then be the *'cells of origin'* of the tumor or *'pre-LSCs'* and the LSCs would be the highly leukemogenic transformed progenitors. Similarly, in blast crisis CML (see Section 2.1) the cell of origin seems to be the HSCs, whereas the LSCs originate in the pool of committed myeloid cells (Figure 1).

Similarly, in *TEL-AML1* as well a p190 *BCR-ABL* positive B-ALLs (see Section 2.3), the disease seems to originate in B-cell progenitors which are also LSC candidates, thus demonstrating that in some instances the *'cell of origin'* and the LSC might be found in the same cell compartment, even though it cannot be ruled out that HSCs from these patients harbor yet undefined leukemia predisposing mutations before the known leukaemia-specific fusion gene confers leukemogenic potential leading to LSC formation.

In most malignancies the *'cell of origin'* is not known (Polyak and Hahn 2006). By definition, this cell, though it may or may not be able to propagate the tumor by itself, might feed a continuous supply of CSCs and therefore must be factored in for the design of a treatment strategy that aims at eliminating all the cells involved in the process of tumor maintenance. It is important to mention though, that the elimination of CSCs, but not the *'cell of origin'* might still be clinically effective and at least postpone disease relapse (Polyak and Hahn 2006). It is even conceivable that elimination of the CSCs with persistence of the *'cell of origin'* would cure a patient if the cell of origin has no leukemogenic potential. This would fit with observations in AML patients with e.g. the *AML1-ETO* fusion gene as many patients in persistent complete remission show the presence of *AM1-ETO* transcripts by PCR without experiencing a relapse of their disease.

3.2. CSCs: Are They Rare?

Another open question concerning CSCs is whether these cells are rare, like their normal counterparts or whether they can form a substantial proportion of tumors. Studies in multiple human tumors have shown that CSCs form a rare and phenotypically identifiable population (Bonnet and Dick 1997; Al-Hajj, Wicha et al. 2003; Singh, Hawkins et al. 2004; O'Brien, Pollett et al. 2007). However, all these studies have made use of the xenotransplantation of human cells in immunodeficient mice. It remains possible that the transplantation of cells in a foreign milieu favours the propagation of certain cells over others and underestimates the fraction of cells with tumorigenic potential. Therefore, the use of syngenic models of cancer should provide definitive evidence of whether there is a difference between the frequencies of CSCs in syngenic and xenogenic models. Importantly, Kroon et al., could show, in a syngenic mouse model of leukemia mediated by the *HoxA9* and *Meis1* proto-oncogenes, that the frequency of LSCs as high as 1:50 to 1:500 cells (Kroon, Krosl et al. 1998). In 2006, Somervaille and Cleary (Somervaille and Cleary 2006) demonstrated that colony forming cells which were frequent (20-30 %) were also leukemic stem cells in a mouse model of the *MLL-AF9* translocation as they could initiate leukemias and regenerate the tumor hierarchy. In both these cases, the frequencies of LSCs were much higher than the frequency of LSCs observed in human AML patients suggesting that xenotransplantation of human cancers underestimates LSC numbers. However, data from our own lab (Deshpande, Cusan et al. 2006) and unpublished observations) and from other labs (Neering, Bushnell et al. 2007) shows that in other syngenic murine leukemia models, the LSC fraction is comprised of a rare, phenotypically identifiable population. Recently, data from Kelly et al., (Kelly, Dakic et al. 2007) has shown a very high frequency of tumor propagating cells in syngenic models of B and T cell lymphoma as well as a myeloid leukemia model, although this particular study did not analyze these cells for the regeneration of the heterogeneity of the tumor, which is a key requirement for defining CSCs. These partly contradictory results might reflect the heterogeneity of AML or differences in the CSC pool even in the same tumor type in different individuals or at different stages of disease. There is some evidence for this: as discussed previously (see Section 2.1), in CML the LSC population not only seems to shift from the HSC to the GMP pool (change in identity of LSCs), there is also an expansion of the GMP/LSCs concomitant with disease progression (change in LSC pool size) (Jamieson, Weissman et al. 2004). These discrepancies could also be explained by the fact that different parameters have been used by different groups for defining CSCs. They underline the importance of evolving a consensus definition of the CSC in the scientific community, and some steps have been taken in this direction (Clarke, Dick et al. 2006).

4. Therapeutic Implications of Drug Resistant CSCs

Currently employed treatments for hematological malignancies include intense cytotoxic chemotherapy, radiation and allogenic bone marrow transplantation to induce immune reaction against the leukemia, while a few leukemias, notably CML are treated with specific therapies targeting deregulated molecular pathways or even the oncogenic molecules directly, such as the receptor tyrosine kinase pathway and the *BCR-ABL* fusion gene in CML. However, despite modern treatment approaches most leukemias relapse following these therapies and most patients succumb to the disease. The recurrence of the disease from therapy resistant CSCs is now believed, though not proven, to be one of the main reasons for relapse. In CML, it has been demonstrated that there are *BCR-ABL* positive LSCs that are quiescent and relatively refractory to imatinib, which is otherwise very effective in eliminating CML cells, reviewed in (Deininger, Buchdunger et al. 2005). Similarly non-cycling LSCs from human AML patients can be detected in serial transplantation experiments in mice (Hope, Jin et al. 2004) and these LSCs are resistant to *in vitro* treatment with 5-fluorouracil or tritiated thymidine which kills actively cycling cells (Terpstra, Ploemacher et al. 1996; Guan, Gerhard et al. 2003) suggesting that quiescent AML LSCs might escape killing by anti-proliferative agents currently used for treating cancer. Lastly, the size of the CSC pool might also determine prognosis and define the progression of the disease. For the development of LSC specific or at least associated therapies it is of utmost importance to define characteristics of LSCs which differ from the characteristics of normal hematopoietic stem cells.

5. Eradication of LSCs

Since LSCs share many features of normal HSCs, it is difficult to make a distinction between these cells, complicating efforts for the selective elimination of LSCs. Targeting LSCs with markers shared with HSCs would cause considerable toxicity to normal HSC. Therefore, it is important to characterize LSCs in great detail for understanding the differences between normal and leukemic stem cells. LSC specific therapies would typically entail the targeting of molecules specifically expressed by LSCs or the inhibition of pathways specifically activated in these cells. There has been some progress on both fronts in recent years, with considerable literature documenting LSC specific markers or pathways. It was shown that LSCs from human *de novo* AML can also express lineage markers such as CD123 (IL3Rα) and CD33 which are myeloid markers often expressed by leukemic blasts in certain types of AML (Jordan, Upchurch et al. 2000) (Sperr, Florian et al. 2005; van Rhenen, Moshaver et al. 2007). This data is consistent with the observation of lineage markers on LSCs in murine models of leukemia (Deshpande, Cusan et al. 2006; Somervaille and Cleary 2006). These results raise hopes for the selective targeting of these LSCs in the future by exploiting these markers. Drugs targeting the molecules expressed by human AML LSCs are currently being tested. Some examples are diphtheria toxin conjugated CD123 antibody (Hogge, Feuring-Buske et al. 2004) and the drug Gemtuzumab (Ozogamicin) which is a monoclonal antibody targeted against CD33 coupled with a cytotoxic agent (Tsimberidou, Giles et al. 2006). These epitopes are of interest, since an ideal candidate for therapy would be a molecule that is expressed on the surface of LSCs as well as the leukemic bulk but not on HSCs. Taussig et al., however, reported the expression of these marker also on normal HSCs challenging the notions of LSC specificity of these molecules (Taussig, Pearce et al. 2005). One of the interesting LSC specific markers in AML and CML is the adhesion molecule CD44. It was recently shown that the homing and engraftment of LSCs but not of normal HSCs could be impaired by blocking this marker, in separate studies on AML and CML models (Jin, Hope et al. 2006; Krause, Lazarides et al. 2006).

VLA-4 is an integrin which is expressed on the cell surface of subsets of AML is a mediator of the interactions of the leukemic cells with the bone marrow niche. AML patients in which the leukemic cells show a cell surface expression of this molecule have a higher relapse rate after chemotherapy than VLA-4 negative AMLs suggesting that VLA-4 positive LSCs are resistant to treatment. In mice the addition of anti-VLA4 antibody to other agents can effectively eliminate residual AML cells making it an attractive target for therapy in VLA-4 positive AMLs (Matsunaga, Takemoto et al. 2003).

A recent study showed that candidate LSCs of Ph+ ALL express markers of endothelial cells such as VE-cadherin, PECAM-1 and Flk-1 (Wang, O'Leary et al. 2007). These cells seemed to have lost dependence on cues from the bone marrow microenvironment for self-renewal and could use the BCR-ABL/VE-cadherin/beta-catenin pathway for bypassing the requirement of exogenous Wnt signaling. These results are similar to the results in CML where activated beta-catenin and *BCR-ABL* expression are crucial in the LSC formation and disease progression (Jamieson, Ailles et al. 2004). As discussed previously (see Section 2.1), Wnt signaling is abnormally activated in the GMP compartment in blast crisis CML and the self-renewal of these GMPs could be reversed by Axin, an inhibitor of the Wnt signaling pathway. This pathway is therefore an attractive therapeutic target for B-ALL as well as CML LSC eradication.

Leukemia studies in the mouse have shed light on overlapping pathways in LSCs and HSCs. However, it is possible that some pathways that are indispensable for LSC maintenance but redundant in HSCs (Stubbs and Armstrong 2007) Therefore the inhibition of such pathways would be an effective form of treatment, one such potential target being the tumor suppressor *Pten* (phosphatase and tensin homolog). Mice lacking this gene showed a progressive loss of stem cell maintenance and developed myeloproliferation followed by leukemia. Interestingly, the administration of the 'mammalian target of rapamycin' (mTOR) inhibitor Rapamycin to these mice could rescue HSC development and deplete AML LSCs indicating a differential activity of this factor in normal and tumor stem cells and identifying Rapamycin as a potential therapeutic agent for tumors with *Pten* mutations. (Yilmaz, Valdez et al. 2006; Zhang, Grindley et al. 2006). These data implicate the involvement of the PI3K/AKT/mTOR pathway in leukemia. Of note, both the AKT mTOR kinases are seen to be activated in human AML blasts and treatment with PI3K or mTOR inhibitors in combination with other chemotherapeutic agents can decrease LSC load in AML patient samples (Xu, Simpson et al. 2003; Xu, Thompson et al. 2005).

The plethora of data accumulating on the identification of LSCs in various subtypes of leukemia has intensified our search for LSC specific markers and pathways. Therapies that target these molecules, either alone or in combination with routinely used treatments could be of immense clinical benefit in these malignancies.

Conclusion

Growing appreciation of the involvement of stem cells and stem cell associated processes in malignant transformation has been an important advance in our understanding of cancer pathogenesis. As illustrated in the chapter using several examples, hematological malignancies have been particularly useful in elucidating key concepts of CSC biology. Many groups are currently focusing on ways and means of characterizing candidate CSCs in these malignancies and trying to learn more about differentially expressed surface epitopes or signal transduction pathways between normal and tumor stem cells. An understanding of the processes governing the formation and propagation of CSCs will have clear clinical implications for the future and will aid in the development of targeted therapies against cancer.

References

Al-Hajj, M., M. S. Wicha, et al. (2003). "Prospective identification of tumorigenic breast cancer cells." *Proc. Natl. Acad. Sci. USA* 100(7): 3983-8.

Bonnet, D. and J. E. Dick (1997). "Human acute myeloid leukemia is organized as a hierarchy that originates from a primitive hematopoietic cell." *Nat. Med.* 3(7): 730-7.

Bose, S., M. Deininger, et al. (1998). "The presence of typical and atypical BCR-ABL fusion genes in leukocytes of normal individuals: biologic significance and implications for the assessment of minimal residual disease." *Blood* 92(9): 3362-7.

Campbell, L. L. and K. Polyak (2007). "Breast tumor heterogeneity: cancer stem cells or clonal evolution?" *Cell Cycle* 6(19): 2332-8.

Castor, A., L. Nilsson, et al. (2005). "Distinct patterns of hematopoietic stem cell involvement in acute lymphoblastic leukemia." *Nat. Med.* 11(6): 630-7.

Chomel, J. C., F. Brizard, et al. (2000). "Persistence of BCR-ABL genomic rearrangement in chronic myeloid leukemia patients in complete and sustained cytogenetic remission after interferon-alpha therapy or allogeneic bone marrow transplantation." *Blood* 95(2): 404-8.

Clarke, M. F., J. E. Dick, et al. (2006). "Cancer Stem Cells--Perspectives on Current Status and Future Directions: AACR Workshop on Cancer Stem Cells." *Cancer Res.* 66(19): 9339-44.

Cobaleda, C., N. Gutierrez-Cianca, et al. (2000). "A primitive hematopoietic cell is the target for the leukemic transformation in human philadelphia-positive acute lymphoblastic leukemia." *Blood* 95(3): 1007-13.

Cox, C. V., R. S. Evely, et al. (2004). "Characterization of acute lymphoblastic leukemia progenitor cells." *Blood* 104(9): 2919-25.

Cox, C. V., H. M. Martin, et al. (2007). "Characterization of a progenitor cell population in childhood T-cell acute lymphoblastic leukemia." *Blood* 109(2): 674-82.

Cozzio, A., E. Passegue, et al. (2003). "Similar MLL-associated leukemias arising from self-renewing stem cells and short-lived myeloid progenitors." *Genes Dev.* 17(24): 3029-35.

Cuenco, G. M. and R. Ren (2001). "Cooperation of BCR-ABL and AML1/MDS1/EVI1 in blocking myeloid differentiation and rapid induction of an acute myelogenous leukemia." *Oncogene* 20(57): 8236-48.

Dalerba, P., R. W. Cho, et al. (2007). "Cancer stem cells: models and concepts." *Annu. Rev. Med.* 58: 267-84.

Daley, G. Q., R. A. Van Etten, et al. (1990). "Induction of chronic myelogenous leukemia in mice by the P210bcr/abl gene of the Philadelphia chromosome." *Science* 247(4944): 824-30.

Dash, A. B., I. R. Williams, et al. (2002). "A murine model of CML blast crisis induced by cooperation between BCR/ABL and NUP98/HOXA9." *Proc. Natl. Acad. Sci. USA* 99(11): 7622-7.

Deininger, M., E. Buchdunger, et al. (2005). "The development of imatinib as a therapeutic agent for chronic myeloid leukemia." *Blood* 105(7): 2640-53.

Deininger, M. W., J. M. Goldman, et al. (2000). "The molecular biology of chronic myeloid leukemia." *Blood* 96(10): 3343-56.

Deshpande, A. J. and C. Buske (2007). "Lymphoid progenitors as candidate cancer stem cells in AML: new perspectives." *Cell Cycle* 6(5): 543-5.

Deshpande, A. J., M. Cusan, et al. (2006). "Acute myeloid leukemia is propagated by a leukemic stem cell with lymphoid characteristics in a mouse model of CALM/AF10-positive leukemia." *Cancer Cell* 10(5): 363-74.

Fialkow, P. J. (1974). "The origin and development of human tumors studied with cell markers." *N. Engl. J. Med.* 291(1): 26-35.

Fialkow, P. J. (1979). "Clonal origin of human tumors." *Annu. Rev. Med.* 30: 135-43.

Fialkow, P. J., A. M. Denman, et al. (1978). "Chronic myelocytic leukemia. Origin of some lymphocytes from leukemic stem cells." *J. Clin. Invest* 62(4): 815-23.

George, A. A., J. Franklin, et al. (2001). "Detection of leukemic cells in the CD34(+)CD38(-) bone marrow progenitor population in children with acute lymphoblastic leukemia." *Blood* 97(12): 3925-30.

Golub, T. R., G. F. Barker, et al. (1995). "Fusion of the TEL gene on 12p13 to the AML1 gene on 21q22 in acute lymphoblastic leukemia." *Proc. Natl. Acad. Sci. USA* 92(11): 4917-21.

Guan, Y., B. Gerhard, et al. (2003). "Detection, isolation, and stimulation of quiescent primitive leukemic progenitor cells from patients with acute myeloid leukemia (AML)." *Blood* 101(8): 3142-9.

Haase, D., M. Feuring-Buske, et al. (1995). "Evidence for malignant transformation in acute myeloid leukemia at the level of early hematopoietic stem cells by cytogenetic analysis of CD34+ subpopulations." *Blood* 86(8): 2906-12.

Hogge, D. E., M. Feuring-Buske, et al. (2004). "The efficacy of diphtheria-growth factor fusion proteins is enhanced by co-administration of cytosine arabinoside in an immunodeficient mouse model of human acute myeloid leukemia." *Leuk. Res.* 28(11): 1221-6.

Hope, K. J., L. Jin, et al. (2004). "Acute myeloid leukemia originates from a hierarchy of leukemic stem cell classes that differ in self-renewal capacity." *Nat. Immunol.* 5(7): 738-43.

Huntly, B. J., H. Shigematsu, et al. (2004). "MOZ-TIF2, but not BCR-ABL, confers properties of leukemic stem cells to committed murine hematopoietic progenitors." *Cancer Cell* 6(6): 587-96.

Jaiswal, S., D. Traver, et al. (2003). "Expression of BCR/ABL and BCL-2 in myeloid progenitors leads to myeloid leukemias." *Proc. Natl. Acad. Sci. USA* 100(17): 10002-7.

Jamieson, C. H., L. E. Ailles, et al. (2004). "Granulocyte-macrophage progenitors as candidate leukemic stem cells in blast-crisis CML." *N. Engl. J. Med.* 351(7): 657-67.

Jamieson, C. H., I. L. Weissman, et al. (2004). "Chronic versus acute myelogenous leukemia: a question of self-renewal." *Cancer Cell* 6(6): 531-3.

Jin, L., K. J. Hope, et al. (2006). "Targeting of CD44 eradicates human acute myeloid leukemic stem cells." *Nat. Med.* 12(10): 1167-74.

Jordan, C. T., D. Upchurch, et al. (2000). "The interleukin-3 receptor alpha chain is a unique marker for human acute myelogenous leukemia stem cells." *Leukemia* 14(10): 1777-84.

Kelly, P. N., A. Dakic, et al. (2007). "Tumor growth need not be driven by rare cancer stem cells." *Science* 317(5836): 337.

Krause, D. S., K. Lazarides, et al. (2006). "Requirement for CD44 in homing and engraftment of BCR-ABL-expressing leukemic stem cells." *Nat. Med.* 12(10): 1175-80.

Krivtsov, A. V., D. Twomey, et al. (2006). "Transformation from committed progenitor to leukaemia stem cell initiated by MLL-AF9." *Nature* 442(7104): 818-22.

Kroon, E., J. Krosl, et al. (1998). "Hoxa9 transforms primary bone marrow cells through specific collaboration with Meis1a but not Pbx1b." *Embo J.* 17(13): 3714-25.

Lapidot, T., C. Sirard, et al. (1994). "A cell initiating human acute myeloid leukaemia after transplantation into SCID mice." *Nature* 367(6464): 645-8.

Li, C., D. G. Heidt, et al. (2007). "Identification of pancreatic cancer stem cells." *Cancer Res.* 67(3): 1030-7.

Li, S., R. L. Ilaria, Jr., et al. (1999). "The P190, P210, and P230 forms of the BCR/ABL oncogene induce a similar chronic myeloid leukemia-like syndrome in mice but have different lymphoid leukemogenic activity." *J. Exp. Med.* 189(9): 1399-412.

Matsunaga, T., N. Takemoto, et al. (2003). "Interaction between leukemic-cell VLA-4 and stromal fibronectin is a decisive factor for minimal residual disease of acute myelogenous leukemia." *Nat. Med.* 9(9): 1158-65.

Mayotte, N., D. C. Roy, et al. (2002). "Oncogenic interaction between BCR-ABL and NUP98-HOXA9 demonstrated by the use of an in vitro purging culture system." *Blood* 100(12): 4177-84.

Mehrotra, B., T. I. George, et al. (1995). "Cytogenetically aberrant cells in the stem cell compartment (CD34+lin-) in acute myeloid leukemia." *Blood* 86(3): 1139-47.

Melo, J. V. and D. J. Barnes (2007). "Chronic myeloid leukaemia as a model of disease evolution in human cancer." *Nat. Rev. Cancer* 7(6): 441-53.

Miyamoto, T., I. L. Weissman, et al. (2000). "AML1/ETO-expressing nonleukemic stem cells in acute myelogenous leukemia with 8;21 chromosomal translocation." *Proc. Natl. Acad. Sci. USA* 97(13): 7521-6.

Mori, H., S. M. Colman, et al. (2002). "Chromosome translocations and covert leukemic clones are generated during normal fetal development." *Proc. Natl. Acad. Sci. USA* 99(12): 8242-7.

Neering, S. J., T. Bushnell, et al. (2007). "Leukemia stem cells in a genetically defined murine model of blast-crisis CML." *Blood* 110(7): 2578-85.

O'Brien, C. A., A. Pollett, et al. (2007). "A human colon cancer cell capable of initiating tumour growth in immunodeficient mice." *Nature* 445(7123): 106-10.

Polyak, K. and W. C. Hahn (2006). "Roots and stems: stem cells in cancer." *Nat. Med.* 12(3): 296-300.

Quijano, C. A., D. Moore, 2nd, et al. (1997). "Cytogenetically aberrant cells are present in the CD34+CD33-38-19- marrow compartment in children with acute lymphoblastic leukemia." *Leukemia* 11(9): 1508-15.

Romana, S. P., H. Poirel, et al. (1995). "High frequency of t(12;21) in childhood B-lineage acute lymphoblastic leukemia." *Blood* 86(11): 4263-9.

Sell, S. (2004). "Stem cell origin of cancer and differentiation therapy." Crit. Rev. *Oncol. Hematol.* 51(1): 1-28.

Singh, S. K., C. Hawkins, et al. (2004). "Identification of human brain tumour initiating cells." *Nature* 432(7015): 396-401.

Smith, A. (2006). "A glossary for stem-cell biology." *Nature* 441(7097): 1060-1060.

Somervaille, T. C. and M. L. Cleary (2006). "Identification and characterization of leukemia stem cells in murine MLL-AF9 acute myeloid leukemia." *Cancer Cell* 10(4): 257-68.

Sperr, W. R., S. Florian, et al. (2005). "CD 33 as a target of therapy in acute myeloid leukemia: current status and future perspectives." *Leuk Lymphoma* 46(8): 1115-20.

Stubbs, M. C. and S. A. Armstrong (2007). "Therapeutic implications of leukemia stem cell development." *Clin. Cancer Res.* 13(12): 3439-42.

Takahashi, N., I. Miura, et al. (1998). "Lineage Involvement of Stem Cells Bearing the Philadelphia Chromosome in Chronic Myeloid Leukemia in the Chronic Phase as Shown by a Combination of Fluorescence-Activated Cell Sorting and Fluorescence In Situ Hybridization." *Blood* 92(12): 4758-4763.

Taussig, D. C., D. J. Pearce, et al. (2005). "Hematopoietic stem cells express multiple myeloid markers: implications for the origin and targeted therapy of acute myeloid leukemia." *Blood* 106(13): 4086-92.

Terpstra, W., R. E. Ploemacher, et al. (1996). "Fluorouracil selectively spares acute myeloid leukemia cells with long-term growth abilities in immunodeficient mice and in culture." *Blood* 88(6): 1944-50.

Tsimberidou, A. M., F. J. Giles, et al. (2006). "The role of gemtuzumab ozogamicin in acute leukaemia therapy." *Br. J. Haematol.* 132(4): 398-409.

Van Etten, R. A. (2001). "Models of chronic myeloid leukemia." *Curr. Oncol. Rep.* 3(3): 228-37.

van Rhenen, A., B. Moshaver, et al. (2007). "Aberrant marker expression patterns on the CD34+CD38- stem cell compartment in acute myeloid leukemia allows to distinguish the malignant from the normal stem cell compartment both at diagnosis and in remission." *Leukemia* 21(8): 1700-7.

Wang, L., H. O'Leary, et al. (2007). "Ph+/VE-cadherin+ identifies a stem cell like population of acute lymphoblastic leukemia sustained by bone marrow niche cells." *Blood* 110(9): 3334-44.

Wiemels, J. L., G. Cazzaniga, et al. (1999). "Prenatal origin of acute lymphoblastic leukaemia in children." *Lancet* 354(9189): 1499-503.

Xu, Q., S. E. Simpson, et al. (2003). "Survival of acute myeloid leukemia cells requires PI3 kinase activation." *Blood* 102(3): 972-80.

Xu, Q., J. E. Thompson, et al. (2005). "mTOR regulates cell survival after etoposide treatment in primary AML cells." *Blood* 106(13): 4261-8.

Yilmaz, O. H., R. Valdez, et al. (2006). "Pten dependence distinguishes haematopoietic stem cells from leukaemia-initiating cells." *Nature* 441(7092): 475-82.

Zhang, J., J. C. Grindley, et al. (2006). "PTEN maintains haematopoietic stem cells and acts in lineage choice and leukaemia prevention." *Nature* 441(7092): 518-22.

In: Cancer and Stem Cells
Eds: Thomas Dittmar and Kurt S. Zänker

ISBN 978-1-60456-478-5

Chapter 6

Stem Cells in Solid Tumors

Andres Matoso and Alexander Yu. Nikitin*
Department of Biomedical Sciences,
Cornell University, Ithaca, New York, 14853

Abstract

Emerging evidences suggest that the capacity of a neoplasm to grow and metastasize is dependent on a small subset of cells, so called cancer stem cells, that have such properties of normal stem cells as self-renewal, extensive proliferative capability, superior multidrug resistance and sustained telomerase expression. Although cancer stem cells of hematopoietic system have been relatively well characterized, their identification and characterization in solid cancers has begun relatively recently. Based on such parameters as cell surface markers and enhanced tumorigenic capacity, cancer stem cells have recently been isolated from a variety of solid tumor types, including those of the brain, the breast, the prostate, the colon, and the pancreas, in both humans and animal models. Importantly, biochemical pathways involved in self-renewal and maintenance of normal stem cells are frequently altered in solid cancers. Thus, it is likely that either normal stem cells represent a target of malignant transformation or more differentiated somatic cells re-acquire stem-cell like machinery during carcinogenesis. Understanding of the origin, biology and microenvironmental requirements of cancer stem cells and uncovering their differences from the normal stem cells may lead to finding new therapeutic targets that would selectively attack the most critical population of neoplastic cells and cure the disease.

Introduction

Solid organs and blood share the need to replenish their cell population in renovation cycles. Despite frequently short lifespans of their functional cellular components, these

* Correspondence: Alexander Yu. Nikitin, T2 014 VRT, Campus Rd., Ithaca, NY 14853. E-mail: an58@cornell.edu

organs maintain their cellular mass and normal architecture due to hierarchical cellular organization dependent on a small population of cells with the capacity to live for extended periods of time and maintain a high proliferative potential. Such cells are called stem cells for any given tissue. [reviewed in Blanpain et al., 2007; Eckfeldt et al., 2005; Morrison and Kimble, 2006].

The cancer stem cell model assumes that, similar to stem cells, only a very small subset of cells within the tumor population has the capacity to sustain neoplastic growth [Al-Hajj and Clarke, 2004; Pardal et al., 2003; Polyak and Hahn, 2006; Reya et al., 2001; Wicha et al., 2006]. This model originates from the "embryonal rest" theory formulated by Cohnheim and Durante over 150 years ago [reviewed in Sell, 2004].

The origin of cancer stem cells contemplates several possible scenarios. They can arise directly from somatic stem cells that have undergone malignant transformation, or from more differentiated cells that have acquired the machinery necessary for self-renewal (Figure 1). The first scenario is based on stem cell's ability to produce more stem cells, a property known as "self-renewal", as well as their ability to produce progeny cells that differentiate. Self-renewal and production of progeny cells are accomplished by symmetric and asymmetric division, respectively. A defective balance between these two modes of division has been proposed as the mechanism responsible for the initiation of cancer [reviewed in Al-Hajj and Clarke, 2004; Clevers, 2005; Morrison and Kimble, 2006; Nikitin et al., 2007; Polyak and Hahn, 2006; Wicha et al., 2006]. The second scenario has been proposed to occur if transit-amplifying or differentiated cells become less differentiated. In support of this possibility, a recent study by Takahashi et al. has shown that differentiated cells can be re-programmed to a pluripotent state by introducing just four factors, Oct3/4, Sox2, c-Myc, and Kfl4 [Takahashi and Yamanaka, 2006]. Alternatively, transit-amplifying or differentiated cells may acquire stem cell properties by cell fusion or horizontal gene transfer [Bjerkvig et al., 2005].

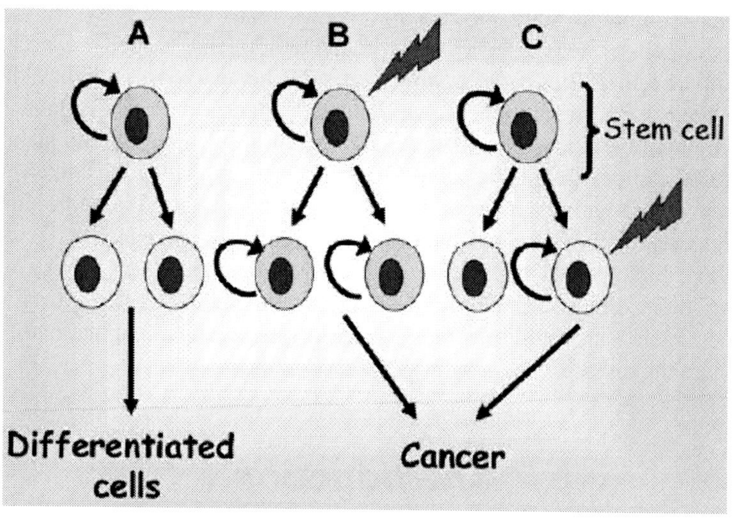

Figure 1. Schematic representation of cancer stem cell model. A. Tissues are organized in a hierarchical manner and contain somatic stem cells that have the capacity to self-renew and proliferate extensively. B. Model in which carcinogenic insult targets the somatic stem cell and its transformation results in uncontrolled self-renewal. C. Model in which the target for transformation is a more differentiated cell that has reacquired the capacity to self-renew.

Direct testing of cancer stem cells' existence has became possible with advances in stem cell technology. In fact, technologies such as refined cell sorting and transplantation assays made it possible to isolate different populations of cells and to demonstrate that phenotypically distinct populations of cancer cells were responsible for perpetuating the disease whereas others were not. Initial progress was limited to the hematopoietic system and led to identification of leukemia-initiating cellular subpopulation [Bonnet and Dick, 1997; Lapidot et al., 1994]. However, more recently, identification and characterization of stem cells in solid cancers has been pioneered by studies on breast cancer stem cells [Al-Hajj et al., 2003].

In this chapter, we summarize current knowledge on the properties and characteristics of solid cancer stem cells and their microenvironment, discuss molecular stem cell-related mechanisms frequently altered in cancer, and describe possible targets for new therapeutic approaches.

Cancer Stem Cells in Human Solid Tumors

Taking advantage of recently developed technology, investigators have demonstrated that only a minority of cells isolated from a human neoplasm have the ability to produce new clones or tumors when placed in cell culture or injected into immunocompromised mice, respectively (Table 1).

In 2003 Al-Hajj et al. first reported the isolation of cancer stem cells from a solid human tumor [Al-Hajj et al., 2003]. This study demonstrates that most human breast cancers have a small proportion of cells that have the capacity to form a new tumor when serially xenografted in NOD/SCID mice. With each passage tumors contained a stable ratio of $CD44^{+}$, $CD24^{-/low}$ $Lineage^{-}$ tumorigenic cancer cells and a phenotypically heterogeneous population of nontumorigenic cancer cells. These observations established that tumorigenic cells can generate both tumorigenic and nontumorigenic cells, thereby exhibiting properties of cancer stem cells.

Following a similar approach, cancer stem cells have also been isolated from brain tumors [Galli et al., 2004; Singh et al., 2003; Singh et al., 2004]. These studies were performed on glioblastoma multiforme and medulloblastoma. Intracerebral injections of $CD133^{+}$ cells reproduced the primary tumor, including the original phenotypic diversity [Singh et al., 2004]. In cell culture the $CD133^{+}$ subpopulations from these tumors could initiate clonally derived neurospheres and showed self-renewal, differentiation and proliferative characteristics similar of normal brain stem cells [Galli et al., 2004; Hemmati et al., 2003; Singh et al., 2004].

Two different studies have reported that prostate carcinoma cells expressing CD44 ($CD44^{+}$) are more proliferative, clonogenic, tumorigenic, and metastatic than the isogenic $CD44^{-}$ cells [Collins et al., 2005; Patrawala et al., 2006]. Additionally, these $CD44^{+}$ cancer cells show higher mRNA levels of several genes significant for stem cell biology, so called "stemness" genes, including Oct-3/4, Bmi-1, β-catenin and SMO [Patrawala et al., 2006].

Table 1. Isolation and characterization of human cancer stem cells

Organ	Markers	Isolated cells (%)	Self-renewal assay
Breast [Al-Hajj et al., 2003]	$CD44^{+}CD24^{-/low}$	11-35	Xenograft in NOD/SCID mice and serial transplantation
Brain [Singh et al., 2004]	$CD133^{+}$	5-30	Xenograft in NOD/SCID mouse brain and serial transplantation
Prostate [Collins et al., 2005]	$CD44^{+}/\alpha_2\beta_1^{hi}/CD133^{+}$	0.1	Colony-forming and long-term serial culture assays
Pancreas [Li et al., 2007]	$CD44^{+}$ $CD24^{+}ESA^{+}$	0.2-0.8	Subcutaneous midabdomen xenografts in NOD/SCID mice and serial transplantation
Colon [O'Brien et al., 2007; Ricci-Vitiani et al., 2007]	$CD133^{+}$	2.5±1.4	Subcutaneous and renal capsule transplantation in NOD/SCID mice

Epithelial ovarian cancer (EOC) is presumed to arise from the ovarian surface epithelium, but is marked with diverse histological subtypes [Nikitin and Hamilton, 2005; Scully, 1996]. This disease is known for its aggressive course and failure to respond to multiple chemotherapeutic treatments. Factors such as the variable differentiation potential and the failure of multidrug treatments suggest that EOC contains a population of cells with stem cell characteristics. Consistent with this possibility BCRP1 (ABCG2) protein, which is involved in the efflux of many drugs, is highly expressed in a Hoechst 33342-excluding side population of EOC cells that showed stem cells properties [Szotek et al., 2006].

Recently, a population of pancreatic cancer cells expressing $CD44^{+}$ $CD24^{+}ESA^{+}$ has been shown to have the ability to self-renew and produce differentiated progenies. These cells formed new tumors that were histologically indistinguishable from the original tumor after transplantation into NOD/SCID mice [Li et al., 2007]. Additionally, these cells expressed high levels of Sonic Hedgehog (Shh) which has previously been reported as abnormally expressed in pancreatic adenocarcinoma and pancreatic intraepithelial neoplasia [Thayer et al., 2003]. Notably, Shh pathway inhibition in pancreatic cancer has recently been shown to be effective against metastatic spread [Feldmann et al., 2007], giving a support to the concept of "migrating cancer stem cells" [Brabletz et al., 2005].

A prospective cancer stem cell population has also been identified in colon cancer. Renal capsule transplantation into NOD/SCID mice [O'Brien et al., 2007] or subcutaneous injection of colon cancer cells expressing CD133 [Ricci-Vitiani et al., 2007], identified a population of cells able to both renew themselves and differentiate, thereby allowing maintenance of tumor heterogeneity after several transplantation.

Taken together, the reported results strongly support the cancer stem cell hypothesis and its relevance to solid cancers. However, definitive demonstration that a single transplanted cell gives rise to all diverse subpopulations of neoplastic cells in any given tumor remains to be performed. Additionally, it should be noted that all animal experiments with human cancer cells involve transplantation into immunocompromised mice. Thus, the low frequency of tumor growth might instead reflect the small number of human cells that can adapt to the foreign environment [Kelly et al., 2007]. Experiments utilizing "humanized mice" with improved "human-like" microenvironment may be helpful to address this problem in the future. Use of immunocompetent mouse models of cancer represents another promising venue for cancer stem cell studies.

Stem Cells in Mouse Models of Cancer

In addition to circumventing problems with deficient immune response characteristic for xenograft models, genetically defined mouse models of human cancer allow assessment of the normal stem cell compartment, as well as sequential, stage by stage, evaluation of carcinogenesis. In spite of clear advantages for stem cells research, only a few models of solid cancer have been characterized so far in respect to cancer stem cells.

Recently, a regional pulmonary stem cell population, termed bronchioalveolar stem cells, was identified at the bronchioalveolar duct junction of the lung [Kim et al., 2005]. These cells were resistant to bronchiolar and alveolar damage in injury experiments, and proliferated during epithelial cell renewal in vivo. In clonal assays these cells exhibited self-renewal and were multipotent indicating their stem cell properties. Importantly, bronchioalveolar stem cells expanded in response to oncogenic *K-ras* both in culture and in precursors of lung tumors in situ. These data support the hypothesis that pulmonary stem cells may be a cell of origin in lung cancer.

The mouse prostate is another organ system suitable for addressing the role of stem cells in carcinogenesis [reviewed in Nikitin et al., 2007]. It has been reported that perturbation of the PTEN/AKT signaling pathway in Sca-1^+ mouse prostate cells with stem cell properties may lead to the initiation of carcinogenesis. Additionally, cancer progression is associated with a dramatic increase in Sca-1^+ cells [Xin et al., 2005]. Using prostate epithelium-specific conditional gene inactivation Wang et al. demonstrated that *Pten* loss is associated with increased basal cell density and concomitant expansion of a prostate stem/progenitor-like subpopulation [Wang et al., 2006]. Such expansion resulted in an increase in the transit-amplifying cell population and eventually led to cancer. However, the mechanism by which Pten controls prostate stem cell behavior remains unclear.

Due to its anatomic characteristics the mouse prostate is particularly well suited for morphological studies examining the relationship between cellular differentiation status and malignant transformation. Each prostate lobe is composed of a series of brunching ducts, where each duct consists of the proximal region attached to the urethra, the intermediate and distal regions [Sugimura et al., 1986]. Importantly, transit-amplifying cells and differentiated cells are located in the distal region, whereas prostate epithelial stem cells are concentrated in the proximal region of the duct [Burger et al., 2005; Lawson et al., 2007; Tsujimura et al.,

2002; Xin et al., 2005]. Our studies have demonstrated that conditional inactivation of *p53* and *Rb* in the prostatic epithelium results in aggressive metastatic carcinomas that arise only from the proximal region of prostatic duct [Zhou et al., 2007]. Intriguingly, these tumors express markers of luminal and neuroendocrine differentiation indicating that the cell of origin is at least bipotent [Zhou et al., 2006; Zhou et al., 2007]. The pattern of gene expression associated with p53 and Rb deficient prostate cancer is very similar to the one observed in human prostate carcinoma. Sixteen of the 18 genes most frequently altered in aggressive human prostate carcinoma are similarly affected in this mouse model. Among those, genes involved in stem cell regulation, Bmi-1, Ezh2 and Pim1, are up-regulated.

Currently characterized models suggest that populations of somatic stem or progenitor cells with pluripotent properties are especially susceptible to oncogenic transformation. These models are based on both the anatomic localization of cells with properties of stem cells and on cell surface markers. With rapid progress being made in identification and characterization of normal mouse stem cells in solid organs [reviewed in Blanpain et al., 2007; Eckfeldt et al., 2005], the explosion in the number of studies aimed at understanding the connection between normal stem cells and cancer is anticipated.

Linking Molecular Stem Cell Pathways to Cancer

Similarities in the biology of stem cells and cancer initiating cells such as the capacity for long-term self-renewal, the capability to develop into multiple lineages, the potential to proliferate extensively, the ability to develop multidrug resistance and the presence of sustained telomerase expression have given sustainability to the cancer stem cell hypothesis. Notably, many of the biochemical pathways known to be involved in regulation of stem cells are frequently altered in cancer.

Wnt/β-catenin signaling pathways have been shown to control a wide variety of cellular processes, including cellular specification, differentiation, migration and polarity. Deregulation of the Wnt/β-catenin pathway often results in the development of familial and/or sporadic epithelial cancers [Reya and Clevers, 2005]. The human *WNT* genes consist of about 20 members that encode cysteine-rich proteins that are secreted as glycoproteins. These glycoproteins bind and activate two classes of co-receptors, LDL related proteins (LRPs) and members of the Frizzled protein family. β-catenin is the major effector of the canonical Wnt pathway, and is located both in the intercellular membrane (adherens junctions) as well as the cytoplasm. The cytoplasmic pool of β-catenin is normally phosphorylated and targeted for ubiquitination-mediated degradation via a protein Axin scaffold. Axin scaffold consists of adenomatous poliposis coli (APC) protein, β-catenin and its GSK-3b kinase. When Wnt binds to its receptor Frizzled, the scaffold becomes inactive, and β-catenin accumulates in the cytoplasm. Stabilized β-catenin can then bind to TCF/LEF family of DNA-binding proteins, where it acts as a transcriptional co-factor activating target genes such as *FGF20*, *DKK1*, *WISP1*, *MYC*, and *CCND1* [Chamorro et al., 2005; He et al., 2006; He et al., 1998; Pennica et al., 1998; Tetsu and McCormick, 1999].

The importance of Wnt/β-catenin signaling in epithelial stem cells has been highlighted by mouse models expressing gain- or loss-of-function of this pathway. In a transgenic mouse model, expression of Wnt-1 in mammary epithelium expands a population of cells expressing progenitor cell markers keratin-6 and Sca-1. Notably, subsequent tumors express these markers and contain luminal and mioepithelial cells that share the same secondary mutations, suggesting that they come from a common progenitor cell [Li et al., 2003]. Ablation of β-catenin results in an absence of follicle morphogenesis in neonates [Huelsken et al., 2001], and a postnatal loss of the follicle stem cell niche [Lowry et al., 2005]. Similarly, overexpression of DKK1, a soluble inhibitor of Wnt ligands, results in the loss of intestinal crypts [Pinto et al., 2003], and a failure to develop hair follicles and mammary glands [Andl et al., 2002; Chu et al., 2004].

Genetic alterations that stabilize β-catenin are found in tumors in both mice and humans. The most frequent ones involve either APC, Axin, or the amino-terminus of β-catenin affecting the colon, liver, skin, stomach, ovaries, pancreas and prostate. Loss of APC occurs in 70-80% of human colorectal cancers, and mutations of β-catenin are present in half of the remaining cases [reviewed in Bienz and Clevers, 2000]. Similarly, loss of the wild-type allele of $APC^{Min/+}$ mice initiates adenoma formation [Moser et al., 1993; Oshima et al., 1995], and expression of a mutated form of β-catenin produces intestinal adenomas in mice [Romagnolo et al., 1999].

Additional evidence of the role of β-catenin both in self-renewal and cancer arises from the biology of the hair follicle. A constitutively active, oncogenic β-catenin transgene induces trichofolliculoma and pilomatricoma-like lesions of the hair follicle [Gat et al., 1998]. Trichofolliculoma can be also induced by a tamoximen-inducible transgenic system [Lo Celso et al., 2004]. Importantly, the most common pilomatricomas in humans carry activating mutations in β-catenin [Chan et al., 1999]. Furthermore, many human sebaceous tumors carry *LEF1* mutations, impairing LEF1 binding to β-catenin and transcriptional activation. Since it has been proposed that Wnt signaling transduced by LEF1 is required for early progenitors to enter into hair fate, it is likely that these progenitors are erroneously directed toward a sebocyte fate [Takeda et al., 2006].

The Notch signaling pathway has also been proposed to be involved in a wide range of human neoplasms [reviewed in Allenspach et al., 2002]. Notch is a transmembrane heterodimeric receptor, of which there are four distinct members (Notch1 to Notch4), that is activated by cell-membrane-associated ligands. Members differ in the number of EGF-like repeats in the extracellular domain and length of the intracellular domain [Maine et al., 1995]. The cell-membrane-associated ligands are categorized into three different subfamilies, where each subfamily contains several members. Notch ligands are collectively known as "DSL". When a Notch ligand binds to its receptor, the intracellular domain of the receptor is sequentially cleaved by metalloproteinases and γ-secretases. Released intracellular Notch translocates to the nucleus, where it can associate with DNA binding protein RBP-J to convert it into a transcriptional activator. Notch target genes belong to the Hes complex and consist of the b-HLH transcription factors Hes and Hey [Iso et al., 2003]. Like Wnt signaling, the physiologic effects of Notch include stem cell maintenance, specification of cell fate and regulation of differentiation [Artavanis-Tsakonas et al., 1999]. In mammals, Notch is expressed in different cell types. This suggests that Notch signaling participates not only in the interconnection among equivalent cells through lateral specification or inhibition, but also between different cell types. In the intestine, Notch signaling regulates cell fate determination in the crypt, as has been first demonstrated by a *Hes1* knockout mouse. Mice deficient for *Hes1* gene possess an increase in neuroendocrine cells, Paneth cells, and goblet cells, whereas they experienced a decreased population of eneterocytes [Jensen et al., 2000; Suzuki et al., 2005]. Conversely, knockout of *Math1* or gain-of-function mutations in *Notch* result in the opposite phenotype [Fre et al., 2005; Stanger et al., 2005; Yang et al., 2001]. Additionally, inhibition of γ-secretase [Searfoss et al., 2003] or conditional targeting of *RBP-J* in the mouse [van Es et al., 2005] results in expansion of the goblet cell population. Furthermore, blocking of γ-secretase promotes differentiation towards goblet cells in intestinal tumors of APC mutant mice [van Es et al., 2005]. Put together, evidence strongly suggests that Notch signaling plays a key role in intestinal development and fate determination, and may represent a potential therapeutic target in the treatment of intestinal cancer.

As in the intestine, Notch also plays an important role in proliferation and differentiation of the mammary gland epithelium. Notch4 overexpression leads to mammary gland tumors [Hu et al., 2006]. Additionally, ablation of RBP-J produces severe alveolar impairment during pregnancy [Buono et al., 2006].

Notch has been linked to the pathogenesis of small cell lung carcinoma (SCLC), an aggressive type of lung cancer with neuroendocrine (NE) differentiation [Borges et al., 1997; Sriuranpong et al., 2001]. Similar to intestine, skin and mammary gland, Notch signaling is involved in both normal pulmonary development and carcinogenesis. During development, Notch signaling controls pulmonary epithelial cell differentiation by activating HES. Activation of HES suppresses genes required for neuroendocrine (NE) differentiation, such as *ASH1* [Ito et al., 2000]. Mice deficient for ASH1 lack pulmonary neuroendocrine cells, while activated expression of ASH1 results in pulmonary hyperplasia and metaplasia [Borges et al., 1997; Ito et al., 2000; Linnoila et al., 2000]. However, these tumors do not express NE cell markers, meaning that ASH1 is not sufficient for NE differentiation. Conversely, when ASH1 is expressed associated to SV40 large T antigen the phenotype shown is lung adenocarcinoma with NE differentiation [Linnoila et al., 2000]. Notably, the downstream targets of large T antigen are p53 and Rb, which are frequently inactivated in human lung cancers [Kohno and Yokota, 1999].

Notch pathway has also been implicated in cervical cancer, since several reports have shown an elevated expression in cervical carcinoma cells. [Zagouras et al., 1995]. However, this observation has been challenged by one study that reports Notch1 downregulation in late stage HPV-infected tumors, and that Notch signaling counteracts HPV-induced transformation [Talora et al., 2002]. Normally a squamous epithelium covers the ectocervix, and a columnar epithelium covers the endocervical canal. The basal layer of the cervical epithelium contains a reserve cell precursor population that has the potential to undergo either squamous or columnar cell differentiation. In normal squamous ectocervix, only the spinosum layer has detectable Notch receptors, while in columnar endocervix, Notch1 and Notch2 are present in the reserve population of cells [Gray et al., 1999; Zagouras et al., 1995]. Although the definitive stem cell population of the cervix has not yet been identified, the basal epithelial cells of the endocervical-ectocervical junction are prone to metaplastic transformation. Furthemore, they express Notch1 and Notch2. These observations suggest that Notch may function as an important factor for cell fate decision in the squamous-columnar junction of the cervix; however, the relationship of Notch signaling to cervical carcinogenesis remains unclear.

The evidence discussed previously seems to clearly indicate that deregulation of the Notch pathway functions as an oncogene, promoting self-renewal and maintenance of epithelial stem cells; however, there is also evidence that implicates Notch as a tumor suppressor. For example, loss of Notch1 in adult cornea and epidermis results in epithelial hyperthickening and expansion of basal layers. The mechanism by which Notch1 acts as a tumor suppressor has been proposed to be through upregulation of p21 [Rangarajan et al., 2001]. In summary, the evidence presented above demonstrates the importance of the Notch signaling pathway in development and carcinogenesis. In particular, cell lineage determination appears to function as a key player in the oncogenic process.

Oct4 is a key regulator molecule essential for the formation and maintenance of the inner cell mass during mouse preimplantation development, and for self-renewal of pluripotent ES cells [Nichols et al., 1998; Scholer et al., 1990]. In the absence of Oct4, pluripotent cells revert to the throphoblast lineage both in vivo and in tissue culture. Additionally, over-expression of Oct4 in embryonic stem cells leads to differentiation towards endoderm lineage [Niwa et al., 2000]. This suggests that Oct4 is an important regulatory molecule in initial cell fate decisions during mammalian development.

In cancer, Oct4 has been found to be over expressed in seminoma and embryonal carcinoma of the testis [Jones et al., 2004], breast cancer [Ezeh et al., 2005], teratocarcinoma [Chambers and Smith, 2004] and dysgerminoma of the ovary [Cheng et al., 2004]. Its role in determination of pluripotency in early embryos, as well as its involvement in several human cancers, makes Oct4 an attractive factor to study in regards to potential applications in cancer therapeutic development.

Members of the *hedgehog* (*Hh*) gene family encode secreted proteins *Sonic*, *Indian* and *Desert* (*Shh*, *Ihh*, and *Dhh* respectively) that act as intercellular signals. These proteins have been implicated in many different processes in development, including cartilage differentiation, myotome and sclerotome specification, hair follicle development, limb morphogenesis and the specification of different neuronal cell types [Ingham, 1998; McMahon, 2000] .

Hh proteins enter the secretory pathway where they undergo an intramolecular cleavage and lipid modification reaction catalyzed by the carboxy-terminal portion of the precursor. The result is an amino-terminal peptide of 19 kDa esterified at its C terminus to a cholesterol molecule [Porter et al., 1996], which is responsible for all the signaling activities of the pathway. Response to Hh signal is controlled by two transmembrane proteins, the tumor suppressor Patched (Ptc) and the proto-oncogene Smoothened (Smo). Smo is a member of the seven-transmembrane receptor family, most closely related to the Frizzled family of Wnt receptors (see above). In the resting state, Ptc suppresses Smo activity. This suppression is released by Hh stimulation and transcriptional activation begins. One of the target genes is *Ptc* resulting in a negative feedback [Freeman, 2000]. Most of the regulatory functions of this pathway are carried by Gli1 and Gli2, which are activators, and Gli3, primarily a repressor [Park et al., 2000].

Hh pathway was first associated to human cancer after identification of *PTCH* as a tumor suppressor in Gorlin's syndrome, which is characterized by a increased risk of basal cell carcinoma (BCC), medulloblastoma and other tumors [Hahn et al., 1996; Johnson et al., 1996]. Medulloblastoma is thought to originate from cells of the external germinal layer (EGL) of the cerebellum [Kenney and Rowitch, 2000; Wechsler-Reya and Scott, 2001]. The Hh pathway has been suggested to maintain an undifferentiated subset of cells of the EGL that characteristically lack p27 experssion and are able to proliferate extensively. Consistently, mutations in the *PTCH* gene have been found in nodular medulloblastoma. These tumors have nests of cells expressing p27, surrounded by p27 negative proliferating cells [Schiffer et al., 1999]. The route by which Hh may regulate proliferation of medulloblastoma cells is through suppression of Rb function [Kenney and Rowitch, 2000]. Consistently, medulloblastoma also arises as a result of p53 and Rb deficiencies [Marino et al., 2000].

Disruption of pathways mediated by tumor suppressors p53 and Rb is so frequently associated with neoplasia that it has been viewed as the hallmark of cancer [Sherr and McCormick, 2002]. *Rb* is essential for cell cycle control and exerts diverse effects on cell proliferation, survival and differentiation. $p16^{ink4a}$ contributes to cell proliferation control by maintaining Rb in an inactive hypophosphorylated form, and growth suppression by p16 requires functional Rb [Lukas et al., 1995; Medema et al., 1995]. Inactivation of p16/Rb pathway, which can either result from inactivation of p16 or Rb, or from overexpression of cyclin D1 or Cdk4, is a common event in human carcinogenesis [Sherr, 1996, 2001], and it has been shown to be involved in the genesis of pancreatic carcinoma, melanoma, T cell acute lymphoblastic leukemia and breast cancer [Sherr and McCormick, 2002]. Furthermore, mice lacking p16 are highly susceptible to cancer induced by carcinogens [Krimpenfort et al., 2001; Sharpless et al., 2001]. Recent observations indicate that *Rb* and its pathway are involved in control of stem cell cycle progression, senescence and tissue homeostasis [Galderisi et al., 2006; Wenzel et al., 2007].

p53 is a transcriptional factor that regulates genes critical for cell cycle, apoptosis, senescence, and DNA repair, thus preventing genomic instability [reviewed in Lowe et al., 2004]. The main function of ARF/p53 pathway is to eliminate cells that have undergone malignant transformation that otherwise would result in cancer [Sherr and McCormick, 2002]. Transcriptional silencing of ARF is detected in certain types of human cancer, but p53 is defective in more than 50% of human malignancies [Levine, 1997]. Recently, *p53* has been shown to negatively regulate proliferation and survival of neural stem cells [Meletis et al., 2006], to mediate the onset of senescence of endothelial progenitor cells [Rosso et al., 2006] and to induce differentiation of embryonic stem cells [Lin et al., 2005; Qin et al., 2007].

Notably, p16/Rb and ARF/p53 pathways are extensively connected and may be coordinately regulated. One of such regulators is Bmi-1 (B lymphoma Mo-MLV insertion region), which executes at least a part of its functions by regulation of *p16* and $p14^{ARF}$, encoded by the *Ink4a* locus. Bmi-1 belongs to the Polycomb group of epigenetic chromatin modifiers and is implicated in repression of gene transcription [Valk-Lingbeek et al., 2004]. Bmi-1 has been shown to be required for maintenance and self-renewal of hematopoietic stem and progenitor cells in mice and is involved in control of cell proliferation, survival and differentiation [Park et al., 2003]. Deficiency of Bmi-1 results in over-expression of p16 and

Arf in mouse stem cells followed by a progressive loss of hematopoietic stem cells (HSCs) and in defects in the stem cell compartments of the nervous system [Aslanian et al., 2004; Molofsky et al., 2003; Park et al., 2003]. Even more, in the absence of Bmi-1, deficiency for p16/ARF partially rescues the stem cell defects, suggesting a role of p16/ARF as a mediator of Bmi-1 [Bruggeman et al., 2005; Molofsky et al., 2005; Molofsky et al., 2003]. In addition to its role in stem cell maintenance, Bmi-1 expression has been found to be altered in several human cancers [Raaphorst, 2005] and is highly expressed in leukemia stem cells [Lessard and Sauvageau, 2003].

As mentioned above, selective inactivation of p53 and Rb in the mouse prostate epithelium leads to metastatic prostate cancer. Importantly, cancer cells show a heterogeneous phenotype and arise from the prostate stem cell compartment thereby suggesting their possible origin from a pluripotent stem cell [Zhou et al., 2006; Zhou et al., 2007]. Further studies will address whether p53 and Rb alterations, individually or in combination, preferentially transform stem cells and if such transformation may determine aggressiveness of the neoplasia.

In an attempt to translate experimental evidence into clinical applications, a comparative mouse to human genomics approach identified an 11-gene signature that consistently displays a stem cell resembling profile. Importantly, this gene signature was present in distant metastases and primary tumors from a transgenic mouse model of prostate cancer and from cancer patients. Analyses of a set of 1,153 cancer patients diagnosed with 11 different types of cancer demonstrated that this 11-gene signature of primary tumors is a consistent powerful predictor of short term interval to disease recurrence, distant metastasis, and death after therapy in cancer patients [Glinsky et al., 2005]. It remains to be determined whether there is a causal relationship between activation of stem cell-resembling genes and malignant behavior of human cancer.

Taken together, there is a significant body of information on the pathways active in normal stem cells and their alterations cancer. This information provides an essential ground for further efforts towards the identification of potential therapeutic targets.

Stem Cell Niche and Cancer

The maintenance of stem cell properties is critically affected by the microenvironment called the niche [Li and Neaves, 2006; Moore and Lemischka, 2006]. The niche is composed of surrounding cells in a special location that functions to maintain the stem cells. The cells of the niche generate extrinsic factors that control stem cell number, proliferation and differentiation. It has been proposed that niche and its modifications may have an important role in cancer stem cell biology [reviewed inLi and Neaves, 2006; Yang and Wechsler-Reya, 2007].

Stem cell niche has particular properties depending on the organ site. For example, neural stem cells exist in vascular niches, into which endothelial cells secrete factors that regulate their functions [Palmer et al., 2000; Ramirez-Castillejo et al., 2006; Shen et al., 2004]. Interstingly, a recent study suggests that vascular niches in cerebral tumors are abnormal, and that they directly promote the generation of cancer stem cells, thereby contributing to tumor growth [Calabrese et al., 2007].

In skin, stem cells are located in the bulge of the hair follicle [Cotsarelis et al., 1990]. As aforementioned, Wnt signaling plays a role in promoting stem cells activation and expansion in the skin [Lowry et al., 2005; Silva-Vargas et al., 2005]. Notably, Wnt inhibitors have been found to be predominantly present in the stem cell niche, providing an environment of cell growth inhibition [Tumbar et al., 2004].

In the intestine, stem cells are located in between Paneth cells and proliferating progenitor cells [Potten et al., 1997; Radtke and Clevers, 2005], whereas Wnt inhibitors are predominantly expressed in intestine stem cells. Wnt is active in proliferating crypt cells, suggesting that the niche might play a role in controlling Wnt activation [Gregorieff et al., 2005; He et al., 2005].

As discussed above, conditional inactivation of *p53* and *Rb* in the mouse prostate epithelium leads to aggressive metastatic prostate cancer arising from the prostatic stem cell compartment located within the proximal region of the prostatic ducts [Zhou et al., 2006; Zhou et al., 2007]. However, in an ectopic transplantation assay, early mutant cells derived from either region of the prostatic ducts are capable of forming neoplasms within 3 months. Thus, microenvironment may play an essential role in controlling cancer progression in the context of specific prostatic compartments [Zhou et al., 2007].

There is now ample evidence to support the hypothesis that the microenvironment regulates carcinogenesis [reviewed in Bissell and Labarge, 2005]. However, the role of microenvironment in cancer stem cell biology only begins to be unraveled.

Anticancer Therapeutics Based on the Cancer Stem Cell Model

The idea that a small population of cancer stem cells with specific phenotypic and functional characteristics can sustain cancer growth has triggered a new direction in research of anticancer therapeutics. According to this concept, traditional therapies do not target cancer stem cells and therefore, after a period of remission, cancer relapses. The cancer stem cell model encourages a new therapeutic approach focused on the ability to target the stem cell subpopulation and their molecular pathways (Figure 2).

Several lines of investigations suggest that it might be possible to selectively strike cancer stem cells. Looking at mechanistic differences between normal and cancer stem cells, Yilmaz et al. [Yilmaz et al., 2006] addressed this issue by conditionally deleting the *Pten* in adult hematopoietic cells. Pten deficiency led to transplantable leukemia. *Pten* deletion also resulted in HSCs proliferation. However, this led to HSCs depletion via a cell-autonomous mechanism. In contrast to leukemia-initiating cells, HSCs were unable to maintain themselves without *Pten*. Treatment with rapamycin not only depleted leukemia-initiating cells, but also restored normal HSC function.

The cancer niche is also being studied as a possible target for cancer therapeutics. If the molecular interactions between the niche and normal or malignant stem cells are different, then it may become possible to develop agents that specifically block self-renewal signals transmitted by the niche of the cancer cell.

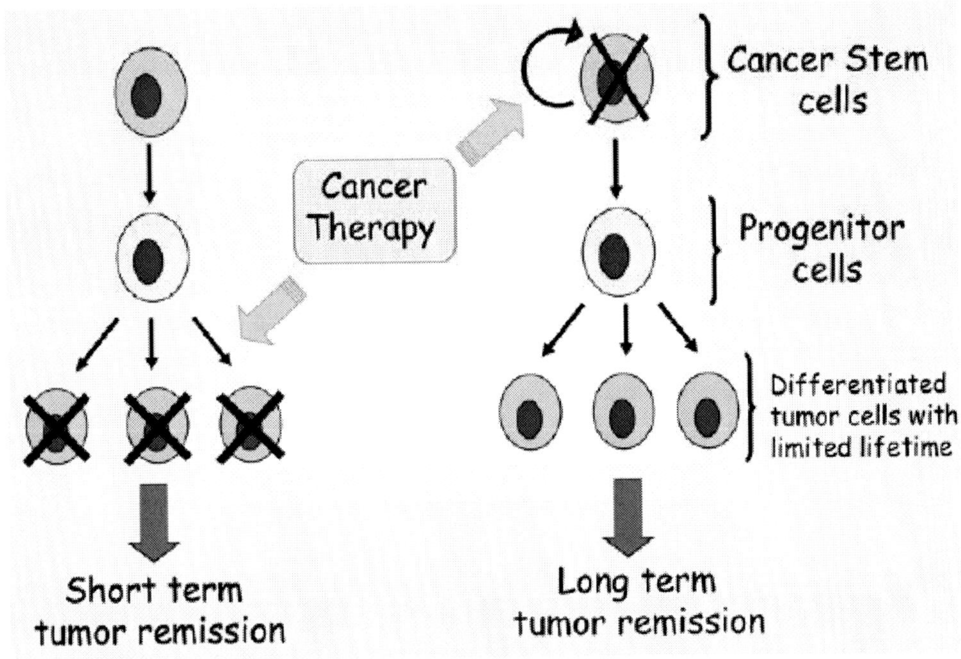

Figure 2. Schematic representation of different cancer therapy approaches. Traditional therapy usually targets rapidly dividing cells resulting in a short-term remission (left). Cancer therapy designed to target cancer stem cells would yield much longer remission and, hopefully, a permanent cure of the disease (right).

We have mentioned above that the Wnt signal favors cell proliferation, promotes cell growth and, therefore, has to be restricted in the adult stem cells to prevent tumorigenesis. The BMP signal generated from intestinal stem cell niche may serve as a "gatekeeper" to prevent abnormal activation of stem cells through suppression of Wnt/β-catenin activity [Reya et al., 2003]. Accordingly, mice bearing a mutant form of BMP have a significant increase in intestinal stem cell numbers. Furthermore, BMP signaling is able to inhibit β-catenin activity through regulation of PTEN activity [He et al., 2004]. Along this line of investigation, researchers have shown that BMPs, amongst which BMP4 elicits the strongest effect, trigger a significant reduction in the stem-like tumor initiated precursors of human glioblastomas [Piccirillo et al., 2006].

The design of new therapeutic strategies targeting the cancer stem cell population does not necessarily imply the design of expensive, sophisticated new drugs or agents. For example, a long known compound Parthenolide, has recently been shown to specifically combat cancer stem cells in acute (AML) and chronic myeloid leukemia (CML) [Guzman et al., 2005]. Parthenolide is a sesquiterpene lactone found to be the major active component in Feverfew (*Tanacetum parthenium*). This herbal medicine has been used to treat migraine and rheumatoid arthritis for centuries [Knight et al., 1995]. Additionally, in this study, it was demonstrated that parthenolide can induce robust apoptosis in primary human AML cells and blast crisis CML cells while sparing normal hematopoietic cells. Furthermore, analysis of progenitor cells using in vitro colony assays, as well as stem cells using NOD/SCID xenograft model, showed that parthenolide also preferentially targets AML progenitor and stem cell populations. Notably, in comparison to the standard chemotherapy drug cytosine arabinoside (Ara-C), parthenolide is much more specific to leukemia cells. Parthenolide-mediated apoptosis was also shown to be strongly associated with inhibition of nuclear factor kappa B, proapoptotic activation of p53, and increased reactive oxygen species.

The results of ongoing research aimed at targeting cancer stem cells are promising and continue to be built upon. Due to this, the way we treat cancer may soon be altered. Furthermore, with the development of new therapies, current parameters used to assess the therapeutic success must be reconsidered. Traditionally, a new treatment is considered successful when there is a dramatic decrease in the tumor load. A more comprehensive approach tying the therapeutic efficacy to eradication of the cancer stem cell population seems to be a reasonable new direction.

Conclusion

For many years cancer has been treated as a disease, where specific attention was paid to the behavior of bulky populations of neoplastic cells. The cancer stem cell concept provides a rationale for more selective targeting of a small population of cells responsible for cancer perpetuation. Recent studies have demonstrated the existence of stem cells in a variety of solid cancers and have paved the way to changing the manner in which we study and, hopefully, treat cancer.

Acknowledgements

We thank Melia G. Nafus for critical reading of the manuscript. This work was supported by NIH grants CA96823, CA112354 and RR17595 to AYN and by the Ovarian Cancer Research Fund Program of Excellence in Ovarian Cancer Research Postdoctoral Fellowship CUMC/POE02.06 to AM.

References

Al-Hajj, M., and Clarke, M.F. (2004). Self-renewal and solid tumor stem cells. *Oncogene 23*, 7274-7282.

Al-Hajj, M., Wicha, M.S., Benito-Hernandez, A., Morrison, S.J., and Clarke, M.F. (2003). Prospective identification of tumorigenic breast cancer cells. *Proc. Natl. Acad. Sci. USA 100*, 3983-3988.

Allenspach, E.J., Maillard, I., Aster, J.C., and Pear, W.S. (2002). Notch signaling in cancer. *Cancer Biol. Ther. 1*, 466-476.

Andl, T., Reddy, S.T., Gaddapara, T., and Millar, S.E. (2002). WNT signals are required for the initiation of hair follicle development. *Developmental Cell 2*, 643-653.

Artavanis-Tsakonas, S., Rand, M.D., and Lake, R.J. (1999). Notch signaling: cell fate control and signal integration in development. *Science 284*, 770-776.

Aslanian, A., Iaquinta, P.J., Verona, R., and Lees, J.A. (2004). Repression of the Arf tumor suppressor by E2F3 is required for normal cell cycle kinetics. *Genes Dev. 18*, 1413-1422.

Bienz, M., and Clevers, H. (2000). Linking colorectal cancer to Wnt signaling. *Cell 103*, 311-320.

Bissell, M.J., and Labarge, M.A. (2005). Context, tissue plasticity, and cancer: are tumor stem cells also regulated by the microenvironment? *Cancer Cell 7*, 17-23.

Bjerkvig, R., Tysnes, B.B., Aboody, K.S., Najbauer, J., and Terzis, A.J. (2005). Opinion: the origin of the cancer stem cell: current controversies and new insights. *Nature Rev. Cancer 5*, 899-904.

Blanpain, C., Horsley, V., and Fuchs, E. (2007). Epithelial Stem Cells: Turning over New Leaves. *Cell 128*, 445-458.

Bonnet, D., and Dick, J.E. (1997). Human acute myeloid leukemia is organized as a hierarchy that originates from a primitive hematopoietic cell. *Nature Med. 3*, 730-737.

Borges, M., Linnoila, R.I., van de Velde, H.J., Chen, H., Nelkin, B.D., Mabry, M., Baylin, S.B., and Ball, D.W. (1997). An achaete-scute homologue essential for neuroendocrine differentiation in the lung. *Nature 386*, 852-855.

Brabletz, T., Jung, A., Spaderna, S., Hlubek, F., and Kirchner, T. (2005). Opinion: migrating cancer stem cells - an integrated concept of malignant tumour progression. *Nature Rev. Cancer 5*, 744-749.

Bruggeman, S.W., Valk-Lingbeek, M.E., van der Stoop, P.P., Jacobs, J.J., Kieboom, K., Tanger, E., Hulsman, D., Leung, C., Arsenijevic, Y., Marino, S., *et al.* (2005). Ink4a and Arf differentially affect cell proliferation and neural stem cell self-renewal in Bmi1-deficient mice. *Genes Dev. 19*, 1438-1443.

Buono, K.D., Robinson, G.W., Martin, C., Shi, S., Stanley, P., Tanigaki, K., Honjo, T., and Hennighausen, L. (2006). The canonical Notch/RBP-J signaling pathway controls the balance of cell lineages in mammary epithelium during pregnancy. *Dev. Biol. 293*, 565-580.

Burger, P.E., Xiong, X., Coetzee, S., Salm, S.N., Moscatelli, D., Goto, K., and Wilson, E.L. (2005). Sca-1 expression identifies stem cells in the proximal region of prostatic ducts with high capacity to reconstitute prostatic tissue. *Proc. Natl. Acad. Sci. USA 102*, 7180-7185.

Calabrese, C., Poppleton, H., Kocak, M., Hogg, T.L., Fuller, C., Hamner, B., Oh, E.Y., Gaber, M.W., Finklestein, D., Allen, M., *et al.* (2007). A perivascular niche for brain tumor stem cells. *Cancer Cell 11*, 69-82.

Chambers, I., and Smith, A. (2004). Self-renewal of teratocarcinoma and embryonic stem cells. *Oncogene 23*, 7150-7160.

Chamorro, M.N., Schwartz, D.R., Vonica, A., Brivanlou, A.H., Cho, K.R., and Varmus, H.E. (2005). FGF-20 and DKK1 are transcriptional targets of beta-catenin and FGF-20 is implicated in cancer and development. *EMBO J. 24*, 73-84.

Chan, E.F., Gat, U., McNiff, J.M., and Fuchs, E. (1999). A common human skin tumour is caused by activating mutations in beta-catenin. *Nature Genet. 21*, 410-413.

Cheng, L., Thomas, A., Roth, L.M., Zheng, W., Michael, H., and Karim, F.W. (2004). OCT4: a novel biomarker for dysgerminoma of the ovary. *Am. J. Surg. Pathol. 28*, 1341-1346.

Chu, E.Y., Hens, J., Andl, T., Kairo, A., Yamaguchi, T.P., Brisken, C., Glick, A., Wysolmerski, J.J., and Millar, S.E. (2004). Canonical WNT signaling promotes mammary placode development and is essential for initiation of mammary gland morphogenesis. *Development 131*, 4819-4829.

Clevers, H. (2005). Stem cells, asymmetric division and cancer. *Nature Genet. 37*, 1027-1028.

Collins, A.T., Berry, P.A., Hyde, C., Stower, M.J., and Maitland, N.J. (2005). Prospective identification of tumorigenic prostate cancer stem cells. *Cancer Res. 65*, 10946-10951.

Cotsarelis, G., Sun, T.T., and Lavker, R.M. (1990). Label-retaining cells reside in the bulge area of pilosebaceous unit: implications for follicular stem cells, hair cycle, and skin carcinogenesis. *Cell 61*, 1329-1337.

Eckfeldt, C.E., Mendenhall, E.M., and Verfaillie, C.M. (2005). The molecular repertoire of the 'almighty' stem cell. *Nature Rev. Mol. Cell. Biol. 6*, 726-737.

Ezeh, U.I., Turek, P.J., Reijo, R.A., and Clark, A.T. (2005). Human embryonic stem cell genes OCT4, NANOG, STELLAR, and GDF3 are expressed in both seminoma and breast carcinoma. *Cancer 104*, 2255-2265.

Feldmann, G., Dhara, S., Fendrich, V., Bedja, D., Beaty, R., Mullendore, M., Karikari, C., Alvarez, H., Iacobuzio-Donahue, C., Jimeno, A., *et al.* (2007). Blockade of hedgehog signaling inhibits pancreatic cancer invasion and metastases: a new paradigm for combination therapy in solid cancers. *Cancer Res. 67*, 2187-2196.

Fre, S., Huyghe, M., Mourikis, P., Robine, S., Louvard, D., and Artavanis-Tsakonas, S. (2005). Notch signals control the fate of immature progenitor cells in the intestine. *Nature 435*, 964-968.

Freeman, M. (2000). Feedback control of intercellular signalling in development. *Nature 408*, 313-319.

Galderisi, U., Cipollaro, M., and Giordano, A. (2006). The retinoblastoma gene is involved in multiple aspects of stem cell biology. *Oncogene 25*, 5250-5256.

Galli, R., Binda, E., Orfanelli, U., Cipelletti, B., Gritti, A., De Vitis, S., Fiocco, R., Foroni, C., Dimeco, F., and Vescovi, A. (2004). Isolation and characterization of tumorigenic, stem-like neural precursors from human glioblastoma. *Cancer Res. 64*, 7011-7021.

Gat, U., DasGupta, R., Degenstein, L., and Fuchs, E. (1998). De Novo hair follicle morphogenesis and hair tumors in mice expressing a truncated beta-catenin in skin. *Cell 95*, 605-614.

Glinsky, G.V., Berezovska, O., and Glinskii, A.B. (2005). Microarray analysis identifies a death-from-cancer signature predicting therapy failure in patients with multiple types of cancer. *J. Clin. Invest. 115*, 1503-1521.

Gray, G.E., Mann, R.S., Mitsiadis, E., Henrique, D., Carcangiu, M.L., Banks, A., Leiman, J., Ward, D., Ish-Horowitz, D., and Artavanis-Tsakonas, S. (1999). Human ligands of the Notch receptor. *Am. J. Pathol. 154*, 785-794.

Gregorieff, A., Pinto, D., Begthel, H., Destree, O., Kielman, M., and Clevers, H. (2005). Expression pattern of Wnt signaling components in the adult intestine. *Gastroenterology 129*, 626-638.

Guzman, M.L., Rossi, R.M., Karnischky, L., Li, X., Peterson, D.R., Howard, D.S., and Jordan, C.T. (2005). The sesquiterpene lactone parthenolide induces apoptosis of human acute myelogenous leukemia stem and progenitor cells. *Blood 105*, 4163-4169.

Hahn, H., Wicking, C., Zaphiropoulous, P.G., Gailani, M.R., Shanley, S., Chidambaram, A., Vorechovsky, I., Holmberg, E., Unden, A.B., Gillies, S., *et al.* (1996). Mutations of the human homolog of Drosophila patched in the nevoid basal cell carcinoma syndrome. *Cell 85*, 841-851.

He, J., Sheng, T., Stelter, A.A., Li, C., Zhang, X., Sinha, M., Luxon, B.A., and Xie, J. (2006). Suppressing Wnt signaling by the hedgehog pathway through sFRP-1. *J. Biol. Chem. 281*, 35598-35602.

He, T.C., Sparks, A.B., Rago, C., Hermeking, H., Zawel, L., da Costa, L.T., Morin, P.J., Vogelstein, B., and Kinzler, K.W. (1998). Identification of c-MYC as a target of the APC pathway. *Science 281*, 1509-1512.

He, X.C., Zhang, J., and Li, L. (2005). Cellular and molecular regulation of hematopoietic and intestinal stem cell behavior. *Ann. N. Y. Acad. Sci. 1049*, 28-38.

He, X.C., Zhang, J., Tong, W.G., Tawfik, O., Ross, J., Scoville, D.H., Tian, Q., Zeng, X., He, X., Wiedemann, L.M., *et al.* (2004). BMP signaling inhibits intestinal stem cell self-renewal through suppression of Wnt-beta-catenin signaling. *Nature Genet. 36*, 1117-1121.

Hemmati, H.D., Nakano, I., Lazareff, J.A., Masterman-Smith, M., Geschwind, D.H., Bronner-Fraser, M., and Kornblum, H.I. (2003). Cancerous stem cells can arise from pediatric brain tumors. *Proc. Natl. Acad. Sci. USA 100*, 15178-15183.

Hu, C., Dievart, A., Lupien, M., Calvo, E., Tremblay, G., and Jolicoeur, P. (2006). Overexpression of activated murine Notch1 and Notch3 in transgenic mice blocks mammary gland development and induces mammary tumors. *Am. J. Pathol. 168*, 973-990.

Huelsken, J., Vogel, R., Erdmann, B., Cotsarelis, G., and Birchmeier, W. (2001). beta-Catenin controls hair follicle morphogenesis and stem cell differentiation in the skin. *Cell 105*, 533-545.

Ingham, P.W. (1998). Transducing Hedgehog: the story so far. *EMBO J. 17*, 3505-3511.

Iso, T., Kedes, L., and Hamamori, Y. (2003). HES and HERP families: multiple effectors of the Notch signaling pathway. *J. Cell. Physiol. 194*, 237-255.

Ito, T., Udaka, N., Yazawa, T., Okudela, K., Hayashi, H., Sudo, T., Guillemot, F., Kageyama, R., and Kitamura, H. (2000). Basic helix-loop-helix transcription factors regulate the neuroendocrine differentiation of fetal mouse pulmonary epithelium. *Development 127*, 3913-3921.

Jensen, J., Pedersen, E.E., Galante, P., Hald, J., Heller, R.S., Ishibashi, M., Kageyama, R., Guillemot, F., Serup, P., and Madsen, O.D. (2000). Control of endodermal endocrine development by Hes-1. *Nature Genet. 24*, 36-44.

Johnson, R.L., Rothman, A.L., Xie, J., Goodrich, L.V., Bare, J.W., Bonifas, J.M., Quinn, A.G., Myers, R.M., Cox, D.R., Epstein, E.H., Jr., *et al.* (1996). Human homolog of patched, a candidate gene for the basal cell nevus syndrome. *Science 272*, 1668-1671.

Jones, T.D., Ulbright, T.M., Eble, J.N., and Cheng, L. (2004). OCT4: A sensitive and specific biomarker for intratubular germ cell neoplasia of the testis. *Clin. Cancer Res. 10*, 8544-8547.

Kelly, P.N., Dakic, A., Adams, J.M., Nutt, S.L., and Strasser, A. (2007). Tumor growth need not be driven by rare cancer stem cells. *Science 317*, 337.

Kenney, A.M., and Rowitch, D.H. (2000). Sonic hedgehog promotes G(1) cyclin expression and sustained cell cycle progression in mammalian neuronal precursors. *Mol. Cell. Biol. 20*, 9055-9067.

Kim, C.F., Jackson, E.L., Woolfenden, A.E., Lawrence, S., Babar, I., Vogel, S., Crowley, D., Bronson, R.T., and Jacks, T. (2005). Identification of bronchioalveolar stem cells in normal lung and lung cancer. *Cell 121*, 823-835.

Knight, J.L., Gorai, P.A., Atwater, R.D., and Grothaus, L. (1995). Tibial polyethylene failure after primary porous-coated anatomic total knee arthroplasty. Aids to diagnosis and revision. *J. Arthroplasty 10*, 748-757.

Kohno, T., and Yokota, J. (1999). How many tumor suppressor genes are involved in human lung carcinogenesis? *Carcinogenesis 20*, 1403-1410.

Krimpenfort, P., Quon, K.C., Mooi, W.J., Loonstra, A., and Berns, A. (2001). Loss of p16Ink4a confers susceptibility to metastatic melanoma in mice. *Nature 413*, 83-86.

Lapidot, T., Sirard, C., Vormoor, J., Murdoch, B., Hoang, T., Caceres-Cortes, J., Minden, M., Paterson, B., Caligiuri, M.A., and Dick, J.E. (1994). A cell initiating human acute myeloid leukaemia after transplantation into SCID mice. *Nature 367*, 645-648.

Lawson, D.A., Xin, L., Lukacs, R.U., Cheng, D., and Witte, O.N. (2007). Isolation and functional characterization of murine prostate stem cells. *Proc. Natl. Acad. Sci. USA 104*, 181-186.

Lessard, J., and Sauvageau, G. (2003). Bmi-1 determines the proliferative capacity of normal and leukaemic stem cells. *Nature 423*, 255-260.

Levine, A.J. (1997). p53, the cellular gatekeeper for growth and division. *Cell 88*, 323-331.

Li, C., Heidt, D.G., Dalerba, P., Burant, C.F., Zhang, L., Adsay, V., Wicha, M., Clarke, M.F., and Simeone, D.M. (2007). Identification of pancreatic cancer stem cells. *Cancer Res. 67*, 1030-1037.

Li, L., and Neaves, W.B. (2006). Normal stem cells and cancer stem cells: the niche matters. *Cancer Res. 66*, 4553-4557.

Li, Y., Welm, B., Podsypanina, K., Huang, S., Chamorro, M., Zhang, X., Rowlands, T., Egeblad, M., Cowin, P., Werb, Z., *et al.* (2003). Evidence that transgenes encoding components of the Wnt signaling pathway preferentially induce mammary cancers from progenitor cells. *Proc. Natl. Acad. Sci. USA 100*, 15853-15858.

Lin, T., Chao, C., Saito, S., Mazur, S.J., Murphy, M.E., Appella, E., and Xu, Y. (2005). p53 induces differentiation of mouse embryonic stem cells by suppressing Nanog expression. *Nat. Cell Biol. 7*, 165-171.

Linnoila, R.I., Zhao, B., DeMayo, J.L., Nelkin, B.D., Baylin, S.B., DeMayo, F.J., and Ball, D.W. (2000). Constitutive achaete-scute homologue-1 promotes airway dysplasia and lung neuroendocrine tumors in transgenic mice. *Cancer Res. 60*, 4005-4009.

Lo Celso, C., Prowse, D.M., and Watt, F.M. (2004). Transient activation of beta-catenin signalling in adult mouse epidermis is sufficient to induce new hair follicles but continuous activation is required to maintain hair follicle tumours. *Development 131*, 1787-1799.

Lowe, S.W., Cepero, E., and Evan, G. (2004). Intrinsic tumour suppression. *Nature 432*, 307-315.

Lowry, W.E., Blanpain, C., Nowak, J.A., Guasch, G., Lewis, L., and Fuchs, E. (2005). Defining the impact of beta-catenin/Tcf transactivation on epithelial stem cells. *Genes Dev. 19*, 1596-1611.

Lukas, J., Parry, D., Aagaard, L., Mann, D.J., Bartkova, J., Strauss, M., Peters, G., and Bartek, J. (1995). Retinoblastoma-protein-dependent cell-cycle inhibition by the tumour suppressor p16. *Nature 375*, 503-506.

Maine, E.M., Lissemore, J.L., and Starmer, W.T. (1995). A phylogenetic analysis of vertebrate and invertebrate Notch-related genes. *Mol. Phylogenet. Evol. 4*, 139-149.

Marino, S., Vooijs, M., van Der Gulden, H., Jonkers, J., and Berns, A. (2000). Induction of medulloblastomas in p53-null mutant mice by somatic inactivation of Rb in the external granular layer cells of the cerebellum. *Genes Dev. 14*, 994-1004.

McMahon, A.P. (2000). More surprises in the Hedgehog signaling pathway. *Cell 100*, 185-188.

Medema, R.H., Herrera, R.E., Lam, F., and Weinberg, R.A. (1995). Growth suppression by p16ink4 requires functional retinoblastoma protein. *Proc. Natl. Acad. Sci. USA 92*, 6289-6293.

Meletis, K., Wirta, V., Hede, S.M., Nister, M., Lundeberg, J., and Frisen, J. (2006). p53 suppresses the self-renewal of adult neural stem cells. *Development 133*, 363-369.

Molofsky, A.V., He, S., Bydon, M., Morrison, S.J., and Pardal, R. (2005). Bmi-1 promotes neural stem cell self-renewal and neural development but not mouse growth and survival by repressing the p16Ink4a and p19Arf senescence pathways. *Genes Dev. 19*, 1432-1437.

Molofsky, A.V., Pardal, R., Iwashita, T., Park, I.K., Clarke, M.F., and Morrison, S.J. (2003). Bmi-1 dependence distinguishes neural stem cell self-renewal from progenitor proliferation. *Nature 425*, 962-967.

Moore, K.A., and Lemischka, I.R. (2006). Stem cells and their niches. *Science 311*, 1880-1885.

Morrison, S.J., and Kimble, J. (2006). Asymmetric and symmetric stem-cell divisions in development and cancer. *Nature 441*, 1068-1074.

Moser, A.R., Mattes, E.M., Dove, W.F., Lindstrom, M.J., Haag, J.D., and Gould, M.N. (1993). ApcMin, a mutation in the murine Apc gene, predisposes to mammary carcinomas and focal alveolar hyperplasias. *Proc. Natl. Acad. Sci. USA 90*, 8977-8981.

Nichols, J., Zevnik, B., Anastassiadis, K., Niwa, H., Klewe-Nebenius, D., Chambers, I., Scholer, H., and Smith, A. (1998). Formation of pluripotent stem cells in the mammalian embryo depends on the POU transcription factor Oct4. *Cell 95*, 379-391.

Nikitin, A.Y., and Hamilton, T.C. (2005). Modeling ovarian cancer in the mouse. In *Research Advances in Cancer*, R.M. Mohan, ed. (Kerala, Global Research Network), pp. 49-59.

Nikitin, A.Y., Matoso, A., and Roy-Burman, P. (2007). Prostate stem cells and cancer. *Histol. Histopathol. 22*, 1043-1049.

Niwa, H., Miyazaki, J., and Smith, A.G. (2000). Quantitative expression of Oct-3/4 defines differentiation, dedifferentiation or self-renewal of ES cells. *Nature Genet. 24*, 372-376.

O'Brien, C.A., Pollett, A., Gallinger, S., and Dick, J.E. (2007). A human colon cancer cell capable of initiating tumour growth in immunodeficient mice. *Nature 445*, 106-110.

Oshima, M., Oshima, H., Kitagawa, K., Kobayashi, M., Itakura, C., and Taketo, M. (1995). Loss of Apc heterozygosity and abnormal tissue building in nascent intestinal polyps in mice carrying a truncated Apc gene. *Proc. Natl. Acad. Sci. USA 92*, 4482-4486.

Palmer, T.D., Willhoite, A.R., and Gage, F.H. (2000). Vascular niche for adult hippocampal neurogenesis. *J. Comp. Neurol. 425*, 479-494.

Pardal, R., Clarke, M.F., and Morrison, S.J. (2003). Applying the principles of stem-cell biology to cancer. *Nature Rev. Cancer 3*, 895-902.

Park, H.L., Bai, C., Platt, K.A., Matise, M.P., Beeghly, A., Hui, C.C., Nakashima, M., and Joyner, A.L. (2000). Mouse Gli1 mutants are viable but have defects in SHH signaling in combination with a Gli2 mutation. *Development 127*, 1593-1605.

Park, I.K., Qian, D., Kiel, M., Becker, M.W., Pihalja, M., Weissman, I.L., Morrison, S.J., and Clarke, M.F. (2003). Bmi-1 is required for maintenance of adult self-renewing haematopoietic stem cells. *Nature 423*, 302-305.

Patrawala, L., Calhoun, T., Schneider-Broussard, R., Li, H., Bhatia, B., Tang, S., Reilly, J.G., Chandra, D., Zhou, J., Claypool, K., *et al.* (2006). Highly purified CD44+ prostate cancer cells from xenograft human tumors are enriched in tumorigenic and metastatic progenitor cells. *Oncogene 25*, 1696-1708.

Pennica, D., Swanson, T.A., Welsh, J.W., Roy, M.A., Lawrence, D.A., Lee, J., Brush, J., Taneyhill, L.A., Deuel, B., Lew, M., *et al.* (1998). WISP genes are members of the connective tissue growth factor family that are up-regulated in wnt-1-transformed cells and aberrantly expressed in human colon tumors. *Proc. Natl. Acad. Sci. USA 95*, 14717-14722.

Piccirillo, S.G., Reynolds, B.A., Zanetti, N., Lamorte, G., Binda, E., Broggi, G., Brem, H., Olivi, A., Dimeco, F., and Vescovi, A.L. (2006). Bone morphogenetic proteins inhibit the tumorigenic potential of human brain tumour-initiating cells. *Nature 444*, 761-765.

Pinto, D., Gregorieff, A., Begthel, H., and Clevers, H. (2003). Canonical Wnt signals are essential for homeostasis of the intestinal epithelium. *Genes Dev. 17*, 1709-1713.

Polyak, K., and Hahn, W.C. (2006). Roots and stems: stem cells in cancer. *Nature Med. 12*, 296-300.

Porter, J.A., Young, K.E., and Beachy, P.A. (1996). Cholesterol modification of hedgehog signaling proteins in animal development. *Science 274*, 255-259.

Potten, C.S., Booth, C., and Pritchard, D.M. (1997). The intestinal epithelial stem cell: the mucosal governor. *Int. J. Exp. Pathol. 78*, 219-243.

Qin, H., Yu, T., Qing, T., Liu, Y., Zhao, Y., Cai, J., Li, J., Song, Z., Qu, X., Zhou, P., *et al.* (2007). Regulation of apoptosis and differentiation by p53 in human embryonic stem cells. *J. Biol. Chem. 282*, 5842-5852.

Raaphorst, F.M. (2005). Deregulated expression of Polycomb-group oncogenes in human malignant lymphomas and epithelial tumors. *Hum. Mol. Genet. 14 Spec No 1*, R93-R100.

Radtke, F., and Clevers, H. (2005). Self-renewal and cancer of the gut: two sides of a coin. *Science 307*, 1904-1909.

Ramirez-Castillejo, C., Sanchez-Sanchez, F., Andreu-Agullo, C., Ferron, S.R., Aroca-Aguilar, J.D., Sanchez, P., Mira, H., Escribano, J., and Farinas, I. (2006). Pigment epithelium-derived factor is a niche signal for neural stem cell renewal. Nature. Neurosci. *9*, 331-339.

Rangarajan, A., Talora, C., Okuyama, R., Nicolas, M., Mammucari, C., Oh, H., Aster, J.C., Krishna, S., Metzger, D., Chambon, P., *et al.* (2001). Notch signaling is a direct determinant of keratinocyte growth arrest and entry into differentiation. *EMBO J. 20*, 3427-3436.

Reya, T., and Clevers, H. (2005). Wnt signalling in stem cells and cancer. *Nature 434*, 843-850.

Reya, T., Duncan, A.W., Ailles, L., Domen, J., Scherer, D.C., Willert, K., Hintz, L., Nusse, R., and Weissman, I.L. (2003). A role for Wnt signalling in self-renewal of haematopoietic stem cells. *Nature 423*, 409-414.

Reya, T., Morrison, S.J., Clarke, M.F., and Weissman, I.L. (2001). Stem cells, cancer, and cancer stem cells. *Nature 414*, 105-111.

Ricci-Vitiani, L., Lombardi, D.G., Pilozzi, E., Biffoni, M., Todaro, M., Peschle, C., and De Maria, R. (2007). Identification and expansion of human colon-cancer-initiating cells. *Nature 445*, 111-115.

Romagnolo, B., Berrebi, D., Saadi-Keddoucci, S., Porteu, A., Pichard, A.L., Peuchmaur, M., Vandewalle, A., Kahn, A., and Perret, C. (1999). Intestinal dysplasia and adenoma in transgenic mice after overexpression of an activated beta-catenin. *Cancer Res. 59*, 3875-3879.

Rosso, A., Balsamo, A., Gambino, R., Dentelli, P., Falcioni, R., Cassader, M., Pegoraro, L., Pagano, G., and Brizzi, M.F. (2006). p53 Mediates the accelerated onset of senescence of endothelial progenitor cells in diabetes. *J. Biol. Chem. 281*, 4339-4347.

Schiffer, D., Bortolotto, S., Bosone, I., Cancelli, I., Cavalla, P., Schiffer, P., and Piva, R. (1999). Cell-cycle inhibitor p27/Kip-1 expression in non-astrocytic and non-oligodendrocytic human nervous system tumors. *Neurosci. Lett. 264*, 29-32.

Scholer, H.R., Ruppert, S., Suzuki, N., Chowdhury, K., and Gruss, P. (1990). New type of POU domain in germ line-specific protein Oct-4. *Nature 344*, 435-439.

Scully, R.E., Young, R. H., and Clement, P. B. (1996). *Tumors of the ovaries, maldeveloped gonads, fallopian tube, and broad ligament.* (Washington, Armed Forces Institute of Pathology).

Searfoss, G.H., Jordan, W.H., Calligaro, D.O., Galbreath, E.J., Schirtzinger, L.M., Berridge, B.R., Gao, H., Higgins, M.A., May, P.C., and Ryan, T.P. (2003). Adipsin, a biomarker of gastrointestinal toxicity mediated by a functional gamma-secretase inhibitor. *J. Biol. Chem. 278*, 46107-46116.

Sell, S. (2004). Stem cell origin of cancer and differentiation therapy. *Crit. Rev. Oncol. Hematol. 51*, 1-28.

Sharpless, N.E., Bardeesy, N., Lee, K.H., Carrasco, D., Castrillon, D.H., Aguirre, A.J., Wu, E.A., Horner, J.W., and DePinho, R.A. (2001). Loss of p16Ink4a with retention of p19Arf predisposes mice to tumorigenesis. *Nature 413*, 86-91.

Shen, Q., Goderie, S.K., Jin, L., Karanth, N., Sun, Y., Abramova, N., Vincent, P., Pumiglia, K., and Temple, S. (2004). Endothelial cells stimulate self-renewal and expand neurogenesis of neural stem cells. *Science 304*, 1338-1340.

Sherr, C.J. (1996). Cancer cell cycles. *Science 274*, 1672-1677.

Sherr, C.J. (2001). The INK4a/ARF network in tumour suppression. *Nature Rev. Mol. Cell. Biol. 2*, 731-737.

Sherr, C.J., and McCormick, F. (2002). The RB and p53 pathways in cancer. *Cancer Cell 2*, 103-112.

Silva-Vargas, V., Lo Celso, C., Giangreco, A., Ofstad, T., Prowse, D.M., Braun, K.M., and Watt, F.M. (2005). Beta-catenin and Hedgehog signal strength can specify number and location of hair follicles in adult epidermis without recruitment of bulge stem cells. *Developmental Cell 9*, 121-131.

Singh, S.K., Clarke, I.D., Terasaki, M., Bonn, V.E., Hawkins, C., Squire, J., and Dirks, P.B. (2003). Identification of a cancer stem cell in human brain tumors. *Cancer Res. 63*, 5821-5828.

Singh, S.K., Hawkins, C., Clarke, I.D., Squire, J.A., Bayani, J., Hide, T., Henkelman, R.M., Cusimano, M.D., and Dirks, P.B. (2004). Identification of human brain tumour initiating cells. *Nature 432*, 396-401.

Sriuranpong, V., Borges, M.W., Ravi, R.K., Arnold, D.R., Nelkin, B.D., Baylin, S.B., and Ball, D.W. (2001). Notch signaling induces cell cycle arrest in small cell lung cancer cells. *Cancer Res. 61*, 3200-3205.

Stanger, B.Z., Datar, R., Murtaugh, L.C., and Melton, D.A. (2005). Direct regulation of intestinal fate by Notch. *Proc. Natl. Acad. Sci. USA 102*, 12443-12448.

Sugimura, Y., Cunha, G.R., and Donjacour, A.A. (1986). Morphogenesis of ductal networks in the mouse prostate. *Biol. Reprod. 34*, 961-971.

Suzuki, K., Fukui, H., Kayahara, T., Sawada, M., Seno, H., Hiai, H., Kageyama, R., Okano, H., and Chiba, T. (2005). Hes1-deficient mice show precocious differentiation of Paneth cells in the small intestine. *Biochem. Biophys. Res. Commun. 328*, 348-352.

Szotek, P.P., Pieretti-Vanmarcke, R., Masiakos, P.T., Dinulescu, D.M., Connolly, D., Foster, R., Dombkowski, D., Preffer, F., Maclaughlin, D.T., and Donahoe, P.K. (2006). Ovarian cancer side population defines cells with stem cell-like characteristics and Mullerian Inhibiting Substance responsiveness. *Proc. Natl. Acad. Sci. USA 103*, 11154-11159.

Takahashi, K., and Yamanaka, S. (2006). Induction of pluripotent stem cells from mouse embryonic and adult fibroblast cultures by defined factors. *Cell 126*, 663-676.

Takeda, H., Lyle, S., Lazar, A.J., Zouboulis, C.C., Smyth, I., and Watt, F.M. (2006). Human sebaceous tumors harbor inactivating mutations in LEF1. *Nature Med. 12*, 395-397.

Talora, C., Sgroi, D.C., Crum, C.P., and Dotto, G.P. (2002). Specific down-modulation of Notch1 signaling in cervical cancer cells is required for sustained HPV-E6/E7 expression and late steps of malignant transformation. *Genes Dev. 16*, 2252-2263.

Tetsu, O., and McCormick, F. (1999). Beta-catenin regulates expression of cyclin D1 in colon carcinoma cells. *Nature 398*, 422-426.

Thayer, S.P., di Magliano, M.P., Heiser, P.W., Nielsen, C.M., Roberts, D.J., Lauwers, G.Y., Qi, Y.P., Gysin, S., Fernandez-del Castillo, C., Yajnik, V., *et al.* (2003). Hedgehog is an early and late mediator of pancreatic cancer tumorigenesis. *Nature 425*, 851-856.

Tsujimura, A., Koikawa, Y., Salm, S., Takao, T., Coetzee, S., Moscatelli, D., Shapiro, E., Lepor, H., Sun, T.T., and Wilson, E.L. (2002). Proximal location of mouse prostate epithelial stem cells: a model of prostatic homeostasis. *J. Cell. Biol. 157*, 1257-1265.

Tumbar, T., Guasch, G., Greco, V., Blanpain, C., Lowry, W.E., Rendl, M., and Fuchs, E. (2004). Defining the epithelial stem cell niche in skin. *Science 303*, 359-363.

Valk-Lingbeek, M.E., Bruggeman, S.W., and van Lohuizen, M. (2004). Stem cells and cancer; the polycomb connection. *Cell 118*, 409-418.

van Es, J.H., van Gijn, M.E., Riccio, O., van den Born, M., Vooijs, M., Begthel, H., Cozijnsen, M., Robine, S., Winton, D.J., Radtke, F., *et al.* (2005). Notch/gamma-secretase inhibition turns proliferative cells in intestinal crypts and adenomas into goblet cells. *Nature 435*, 959-963.

Wang, S., Garcia, A.J., Wu, M., Lawson, D.A., Witte, O.N., and Wu, H. (2006). Pten deletion leads to the expansion of a prostatic stem/progenitor cell subpopulation and tumor initiation. *Proc. Natl. Acad. Sci. USA 103*, 1480-1485.

Wechsler-Reya, R., and Scott, M.P. (2001). The developmental biology of brain tumors. *Annu. Rev. Neurosci. 24*, 385-428.

Wenzel, P.L., Wu, L., de Bruin, A., Chong, J.L., Chen, W.Y., Dureska, G., Sites, E., Pan, T., Sharma, A., Huang, K., *et al.* (2007). Rb is critical in a mammalian tissue stem cell population. *Genes Dev. 21*, 85-97.

Wicha, M.S., Liu, S., and Dontu, G. (2006). Cancer stem cells: an old idea--a paradigm shift. *Cancer Res. 66*, 1883-1890.

Xin, L., Lawson, D.A., and Witte, O.N. (2005). The Sca-1 cell surface marker enriches for a prostate-regenerating cell subpopulation that can initiate prostate tumorigenesis. *Proc. Natl. Acad. Sci. USA 102*, 6942-6947.

Yang, Q., Bermingham, N.A., Finegold, M.J., and Zoghbi, H.Y. (2001). Requirement of Math1 for secretory cell lineage commitment in the mouse intestine. *Science 294*, 2155-2158.

Yang, Z.J., and Wechsler-Reya, R.J. (2007). Hit 'em where they live: targeting the cancer stem cell niche. *Cancer Cell 11*, 3-5.

Yilmaz, O.H., Valdez, R., Theisen, B.K., Guo, W., Ferguson, D.O., Wu, H., and Morrison, S.J. (2006). Pten dependence distinguishes haematopoietic stem cells from leukaemia-initiating cells. *Nature 441*, 475-482.

Zagouras, P., Stifani, S., Blaumueller, C.M., Carcangiu, M.L., and Artavanis-Tsakonas, S. (1995). Alterations in Notch signaling in neoplastic lesions of the human cervix. *Proc. Natl. Acad. Sci. USA 92*, 6414-6418.

Zhou, Z., Flesken-Nikitin, A., Corney, D.C., Wang, W., Goodrich, D.W., Roy-Burman, P., and Nikitin, A.Y. (2006). Synergy of p53 and Rb Deficiency in a Conditional Mouse Model for Metastatic Prostate Cancer. *Cancer Res. 66*, 7889-7898.

Zhou, Z., Flesken-Nikitin, A., and Nikitin, A.Y. (2007). Prostate cancer associated with p53 and Rb deficiency arises from the stem/progenitor cell-enriched proximal region of prostatic ducts. *Cancer Res. 67*, 5683-5690.

In: Cancer and Stem Cells
Eds: Thomas Dittmar and Kurt S. Zänker
ISBN 978-1-60456-478-5

Chapter 7

Cancer Stem Cells and Metastasis

Benjamin Tiede and Yibin Kang*
Department of Molecular Biology, Princeton University,
Washington Road, Princeton, NJ 08544, USA

Abstract

Recent insights regarding the function of cancer stem cells are particularly intriguing when considered in the context of the metastatic cascade. As evidence for the direct involvement of cancer stem cells in initiating the growth of metastatic lesions is scant, this chapter will focus on known events in malignant transformation that are likely to involve or affect cancer stem cells, which may give rise to primary tumors of varying degrees of malignancy and metastatic potentials. The role of cancer stem cells in the later steps of the metastasis cascade will also be discussed. Finally, this chapter will explore potential characteristics vulnerabilities of cancer stem cells involved in metastasis, and speculate on how these weaknesses may be exploited to generate novel therapeutic and diagnostic approaches.

Introduction

The cancer stem cell (CSC) hypothesis, although proposed many years ago, has undergone a renaissance in the past few years as evident by the isolation and characterization of CSCs responsible for initiating tumorigenesis of a variety of solid and hematopoietic malignancies [1]. Part of the excitement surrounding this field has hinged on the fact that CSCs have been shown to be responsible for driving the recurrence of chemoresistant tumors [2]. As such, research into CSC function has sought to identify critical CSC vulnerabilities in order to improve cancer treatment. Ironically though, most CSC studies have focused on the

* Author for correspondence: Yibin Kang, Ph.D. Department of Molecular Biology, Princeton University, Princeton, NJ 08544, USA, Phone: +1 609 258 8834; Fax: +1 609 258 2340; ykang@princeton.edu

role of CSCs during primary tumorigenesis, but not metastasis, which is responsible for 90% of cancer related fatalities [3]. Therefore, the primary goals of this chapter are to speculate on what portions of the metastatic cascade are mediated by CSCs, identify critical research needed to validate these claims, and finally discuss how cancer treatment can shift to focus on the role of CSCs in metastasis.

Before proceeding with investigating the role of CSCs in metastasis, it is important to operationally define two different types of CSCs that play a role in two distinct steps in the tumorigenesis/metastasis cascade. The first population of CSCs (herein referred to as primary tumor CSCs, or pCSCs) are those that have been extensively studied for their role in primary tumorigenesis, and may give rise to highly or lowly metastatic tumors depending on early oncogenic events that drive their formation. The other population of CSCs (dubbed metastatic CSCs or mCSCs) are tumor cells that break off from the primary tumor, travel to the distant sites of metastasis and are responsible for the initiation and the propagation of metastatic lesions.

Poor Prognosis, Primary Tumors and pCSCs

For many years, tumor progression was believed to be the end result of a series of Darwinian natural selections that repeatedly enriched for cells that were fit to survive in the primary tumor microenvironment. While this idea undoubtedly holds a great deal of credence, it did leave one conceptual gap unanswered; how could metastatic cells that are adapted to travel through the circulation and survive at foreign tissues or organs be selected for at the site of the primary tumor? It would seem to be the case that mutations that favor metastasis but do not confer an advantage in primary tumor growth would not be enriched for in the primary tumor. One possible reconciliation to this puzzle is that metastasis potential is actually endowed early during tumorigenesis whereby initial oncogenic events produce distinct classes of tumors with distinct degrees of malignancy [4]. This speculation is likely to hold true when evaluating tumors which consist of subtypes that have a high degree of cellular and molecular heterogeneity (such as breast cancer and leukemia), compared to more homogeneous tumors such as colon and pancreatic cancers [5]. As such, this chapter will primarily focus on evidence from breast cancer and leukemia.

The early predetermination of malignancy hypothesis is supported by numerous studies which provided evidence that different prognoses, including risk of recurrence and distant metastasis, can be detected by profiling the bulk of the primary tumor. The fact that these phenotypes are shared by many of the primary tumor cells suggests that these cells share a common ancestor that was transformed and then expanded into the bulk of the tumor, rather than the entire tumor undergoing the same deregulation independently. For example, genomic analysis of breast tumors indicated at least five different subtypes for breast cancer based on their distinct gene expression profiles: a basal epithelial-like group, an ERBB2-overexpressing group, a normal breast-like group, a luminal A and a luminal B group [6,7]. Survival analyses showed significantly different outcomes for the patients belonging to the various groups, including a poor prognosis for the basal-like, $ERBB2^{+}$ and luminal B subtypes [6]. Furthermore, it has been shown that expression profiling of primary tumor masses can identify poor prognosis signatures which can effectively predict metastasis formation [8, 9, 10, 11]. Finally, expression profiling of a range of mouse breast cancer models revealed both a common tumorigenesis signature shared by all tumor types, and unique signatures that depended on the initial oncogenic events that correlated with subsequent tumor malignancy phenotypes [12].

The fact that the bulk of the tumor mass expresses a gene signature that can predict metastasis behavior suggests that metastasis potential is endowed early in tumorigenesis so that most cells express the poor prognosis signature, rather than later in tumorigenesis where a few highly metastatic variants would break off from the primary tumor. However, it should be kept in mind that these possibilities are not mutually exclusive; proof that poor prognosis signatures exist in certain tumors does not rule out the possibility for rare metastasis variants to arise late in tumorigenesis. Genomic profiling of primary tumors or metastases by nature will not be able to detect rare, metastatic variants which would not be populous enough to influence total tumor RNA levels [13]. Nevertheless, identifying the precise origin and characterizing the early activity of pCSCs remains a critical avenue of research to be explored to help explain tumor progression and metastasis.

pCSC Origins and Metastasis

Connecting the observations about tumor poor prognosis signatures with the CSC theory of carcinogenesis, a number of questions arise concerning how the origin and propagation of pCSCs could possibly account for the tumor-wide poor prognosis signatures that are observed. For instance, it is unknown whether the same pCSC population can give rise to tumors of varying degrees of malignancy if challenged by different transformation events (see Figure 1). Factors such as genomic instability, oncogenic stress, and microenvironment interactions could potentially alter the same pCSC population to produce tumors of different phenotypes. Early evidence in a leukemia model indicates this is the case as pre-pCSCs from a dendritic cell like leukemia can differentiate into both benign and malignant cell types depending on a variety of factors including the injection site and the immune background of the host [14]. Future studies should seek to expand these observations by testing different oncogenic stresses on the same population of pCSCs or pre-pCSCs to determine the precise role of early oncogenic events, before the majority of the tumor is formed, in predisposing tumors to metastasize.

It is also feasible that similar oncogenic stresses challenging two distinct cell populations, for instance a normal adult stem cell and a committed progenitor, could produce tumors of varying degrees of malignancy (see Figure 2). Preliminary evidence supporting this notion has come from studies which have sought to define the origin of pCSCs, where it has been suggested that both normal stem cells and committed progenitors could serve as the target for transformation. It is believed that normal stem cells or committed progenitors, rather than mature cell types, are the target for transformation because many mutational events rely on DNA replication and cell division: events which are restricted to stem/progenitor cells [5, 15].

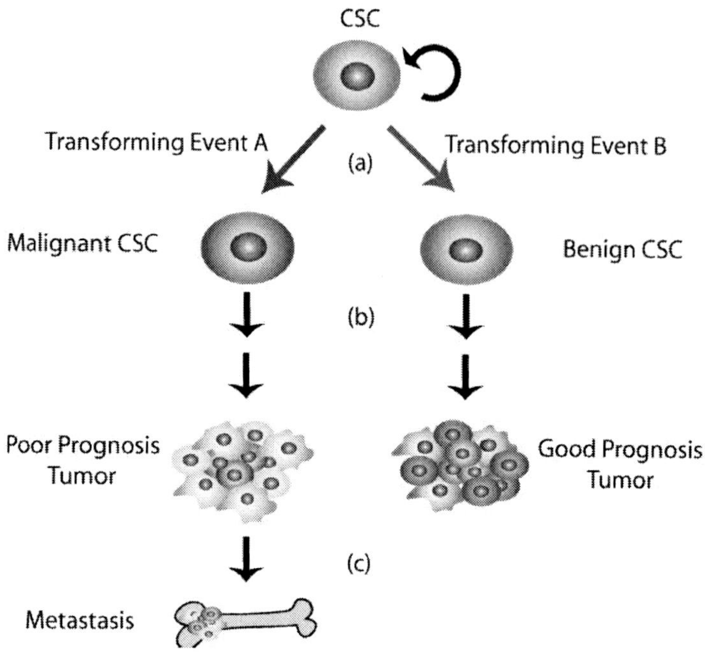

Figure 1. Single origin model of tumorigenesis. In this model, tumors of varying degrees of malignancy are the product of the same cellular origin because of different transformation events (a). These stresses result in the formation of distinct pCSCs (b) that divide and expand into good or poor prognosis tumors (c) that have a differential metastasis capacity.

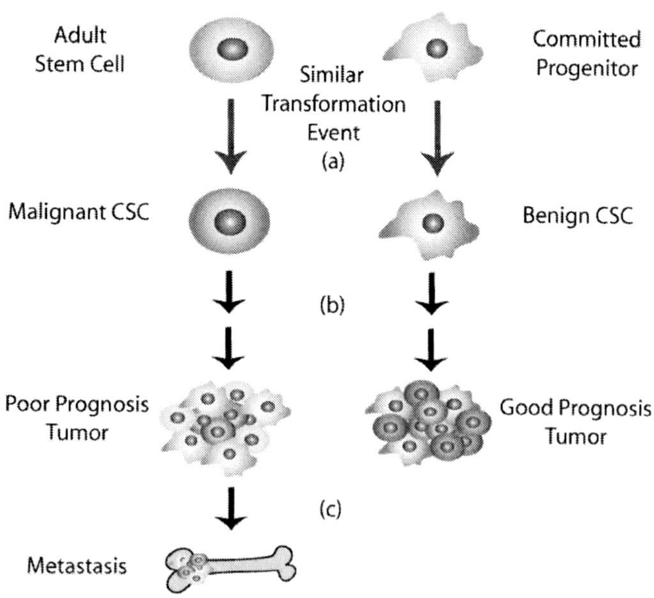

Figure 2. Multiple origin model of tumorigenesis. As opposed to Figure 1, in this scenario, differential metastasis ability is the result of a similar transformation event happening in different target populations (a, b). It is hypothesized, but not proven, that stresses initiated in normal adult stem cells will produce tumors that will metastasize more (c), because of their cellular plasticity and enhanced mobility.

The inherent self-renewal capacity and long lifespan of normal adult stem cells presumably allows for a greater window of opportunity for their transformation by oncogenic events that may occur over a long period of time. The fact that normal adult stem cells often share surface marker expression profiles with their cancerous counterparts suggests, but does not prove, that normal stem cells may be the origin of pCSCs [1]. For instance, it could be the case that transformed progenitors re-adopt a stem cell surface profile as part of their oncogenesis (there is a precedent for normal epithelial cells to re-adopt a stem cell phenotype in a Wnt-dependent fashion in the hair follicle [16]). Additionally, there is a ~6 fold expansion of mammary stem cells in pre-neoplastic mouse mammary glands in a breast cancer model [17], but again, this does not prove that the normal stem cells are the origin of pCSCs. What has been lacking in the field is the observation or induction of transformation of adult stem cells into pCSCs as opposed to retrospective analyses. Part of the reason why this has been difficult lies in the fact that outside of the hematopoietic system true, adult tissue-specific stem cells have been difficult to identify and isolate. In contrast, it has been much easier to identify committed progenitors because of the less stringent criteria needed to characterize and isolate them, and their relative abundance compared to tissue-specific stem cells.

The fact that committed progenitors are much more abundant than stem cells also suggests, based on probability, that they are more likely to be the target of oncogenic transformation. Given that committed progenitors are easier to isolate than true adult stem cells, it is not surprising that there is better evidence for committed progenitors serving as the origin of CSCs. For instance, committed myeloid progenitors have been shown to initiate leukemia development in mice when they are forced to overexpress Bcl-2 and BCR/ABL [18]. Furthermore, the 15:17 chromosome translocation associated with human acute promyelocytic leukemia (APL) is only found in committed progenitors, and not in hematopoietic stem cells [19]. Granulocyte-macrophage progenitors have also been shown to induce leukemia development, either when activating a self-renewal program through the upregulation of the Wnt/β-catenin pathway [20] or by the forced expression of the MLL-AF9 fusion protein [21]. Interestingly, expression profiling of the MLL-AF9 expressing cells revealed that they retained a progenitor gene expression profile, and not a hematopoietic stem cell profile. Similar evidence has also indicated that neural progenitors are likely to be the target of oncogenic transformations [22].

Given that there is evidence for both normal adult stem cells and committed progenitors to serve as the origin of CSCs, and knowing that there are many different paths to tumorigenesis, it is likely to be the case that both stem cells and committed progenitors can serve as the targets for transformation. In fact, it has been shown that EGFR activation, combined with the loss of Arf and Ink4a is sufficient to drive the formation of high grade malignant gliomas in both transformed astrocytes and neural stem cells [23]. What is not clear however is if CSCs derived from different cell types can produce tumors with varying degrees of malignancy. Preliminary evidence has indicated that the same oncogenic stress can induce the formation of tumors with differential metastasis ability if induced in different starting populations. Forced expression of SV-40 large T antigen, hTERT and H-ras-v12 in two distinct human mammary epithelial cell types, derived from the same origin but cultured in different conditions, resulted in tumors with completely different metastasis capacity [24].

Further characterization of the initial oncogenic events that drive CSC formation, particularly with respect to endowing the pCSCs with the ability to metastasize may help to identify clinically relevant prognostic indicators for future tumor malignancy. For instance, it may be possible to isolate pCSCs from a given tumor and determine if they express a unique signature, the figurative "root" of the poor prognosis signature, which would provide stronger prognostic value over sampling of the entire tumor. It also should be kept in mind that most experimental manipulations to decipher the origin of pCSCs typically (by design) test one experimental variable at a time (i.e. whether the challenging stem cells and progenitors with an oncogenic stress results in tumor formation). While this aids in analysis of data, it unfortunately leads to oversimplification of complex *in vivo* interactions.

For instance, it may be the case that an initial transformation event *in vivo* may happen in a stem cell population which results in a pre-neoplastic cell that after differentiating into a progenitor is subject to a second transformation event that leads to typical tumor growth. There is strong observational evidence in leukemia and comparatively weaker evidence from breast cancer studies to suggest this progressive tumorigenesis model happens *in vivo*. Hallmark fusion proteins associated with chronic myelogenous leukemia (CML) as well as acute myelogenous leukemia (AML) (BCR-ABL and AML1-ETO, respectively) can be detected in human hematopoietic stem cells, however these cells are not tumorigenic [20,25]. Instead, further mutations that are only seen in downstream progeny are required to fully initiate tumorigenesis. In breast cancer, it has been shown that tumorigenic $CD44^+$ CSCs are clonally related to and share many genomic alterations with $CD24^+$ cells, but that $CD24^+$ cells express unique mutations [26]. This observation was interpreted to mean that $CD24^+$ cells are the progeny of $CD44^+$ cells that have undergone and initial transformation event. Experimentally testing scenarios such as these (and not just making retroactive conclusions based on tumor heterogeneity) will require a new wave of innovative research design strategies.

Metastatic Cancer Stem Cells

In addition to playing significant roles early during the tumorigenesis process that ultimately affect metastasis propensity, CSCs also play a significant role after tumor formation, during the formation of the actual metastatic lesion. Just as pCSCs are required for the initiation of the primary tumor, mCSCs are likely to be required for the formation of metastatic lesions. It has been known that a single cell is capable of initiating metastasis [27]. Thus, given the high number of cells found circulating in the blood of cancer patients and the comparatively low metastasis incidence, it seems likely that only rare CSCs could initiate metastatic lesions. These CSCs, termed metastatic CSCs or mCSCs, are a distinct entity from the pCSCs that gave rise to the primary tumor (although they may share many of the same properties, such as expression of critical tumor propagation factors). mCSCs must also express proteins that endow them with the ability to survive in the blood or lymphatic system as well to adapt to the different environments at the future site of metastasis. For instance, it has been shown that pancreatic mCSCs are a contained in a subset of $CD133^+$ CSCs that also express CXCR4 [28], which is known to be important in homing/anchorage of metastatic cells. Just as pCSCs are rare within a primary tumor, and are the only cells that can induce formation of a new tumor, mCSCs may be the only cells that can break off from the primary tumor and form a metastatic lesion. This could explain the observation that many cancer cells can be detected in the blood of patients with primary tumors, but they all do not form metastasis [29]. Only when a mCSC colonizes a foreign tissue or organ will a metastatic lesion form.

Despite speculation of their existence, the direct identification of mCSCs has only been accomplished in one experimental system [28], but could be done by similar xenograft transplantation assays that are used to identify pCSCs. Instead of fractioning a primary tumor and testing different cell populations for their ability to form primary tumors in subcutaneous or orthotopic transplantation models, metastatic lesions or tumor cells collected from the circulation of tumor bearing subjects need to be collected, fractionated based on different cell surface profiles, and tested *in vivo* using experimental metastasis assays (see Figure 3a). These assays directly test the ability of cells to colonize the lung, bone, brain and other organs by injection into the blood circulation. If tumor cells were injected subcutaneously or orthotopically primary tumorigenesis would be a prerequisite of the cells in question, which may not be a property that mCSCs are endowed with. This approach understandably bypasses the initial intravasation step required for circulating tumor cells, but given the high numbers of circulating tumor cells that can be detected, this omission may not be a detrimental one. A complementary approach would involve isolating cells that initially lodge in the bone, lung or any metastatic site soon after injection in an experimental metastasis assay and testing to see if they have an enriched metastatic ability compared to the parental population that was initially injected (see Figure 3b). If this was the case, expression profiling could be used to identify relevant surface proteins that could be used to enrich for the mCSCs in the parental population which could then be characterized in subsequent testing.

It is interesting to note that in the identification of breast pCSCs, the majority of the tumor samples that were used to test pCSC function were pleural effusions, rather than primary tumors [30]. This could be the reason why the expression profiling of these cells identified a unique "invasiveness gene signature" that negatively correlated with metastasis free survival in breast and other cancer types [31]. Furthermore, cells with the breast CSC phenotype $CD44^+CD24^-$ [30] have been shown to be highly invasive *in vitro* [32], to overexpress motility and chemotaxis gene signatures [26], to be some of the first cells to metastasize to the bone in breast cancer patients [33], and when present in high numbers at the primary tumor to correlate clinically with distant metastasis [34]. These cells are also shown to contain a minority "side population", a group of cells known to have stem cell phenotypes and be chemoresistant [35]. These observations all suggest that breast pCSCs, in addition to forming primary tumors, may actually function as mCSCs as well.

Although the exact identity of mCSCs remains unknown, it is possible to study critical parts of the metastatic cascade that would affect their growth. For example, it has been shown that $CD133^+$ glioma CSCs are more adept at inducing angiogenesis, a critical early step in metastasis progression, during tumor formation compared to $CD133^-$ cells [36]. While this is clearly indicative of a role for CSCs in the early parts of the metastasis cascade, metastasis research relevant to the function of CSCs typically focuses on later steps in metastasis (i.e., determining tissue specificity, colonization and expansion).

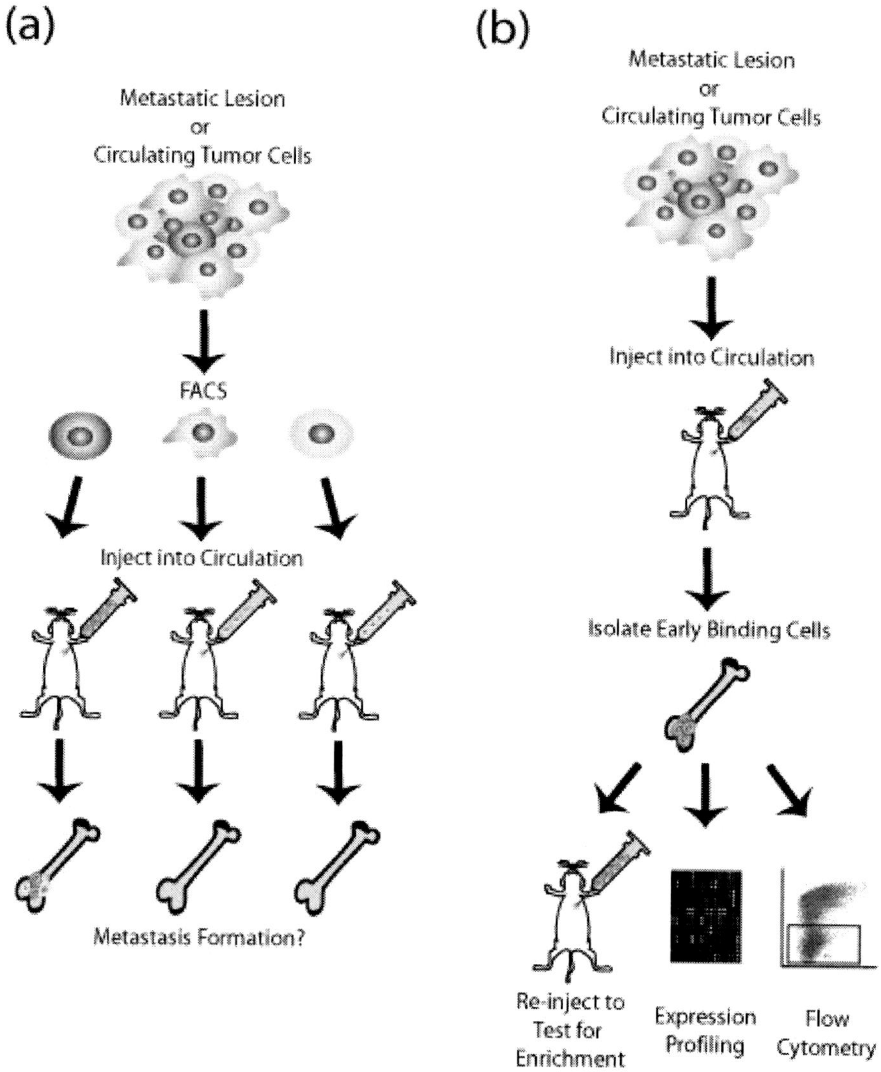

Figure 3. Two different strategies to prospectively identify mCSCs *in vivo*. In (a), a metastatic lesion or cancer cells isolated from the circulation of affected individuals are fractionated using FACS and then injected directly into the circulation of recipient mice. This allows for the direct determination of which cells are able to extravasate, colonize, and expand into a metastatic lesion, but requires the use of previously identified surface markers. As a complementary approach, (b) involves isolating similar tumor cells and injecting them directly into the circulation without fractionating them using FACS (labeling tumor cells with a drug selection marker or GFP would likely be critical before injecting). Soon after injection (~12hr to 2 days later), the cells which initially colonize the metastatic site are selected for, expanded in culture if needed, and reinjected to test for enriched tumorigenicity. These cells could be analyzed by expression profiling or flow cytometry to identify markers to enrich for these cells from other metastatic lesions to enable in further identification and characterization.

Just as pCSCs are thought to share properties with normal stem cells, so too is the case with mCSCs. Connecting these stipulations, one of the most relevant avenues of research related to mCSCs concerns the role of the supportive niche, or microenvironment that metastatic cells reside in.

The (PRE)-Metastatic Niche and mCSCs

From drosophila through vertebrates, the protection, growth, and differentiation of normal adults stem cells have been shown in a variety of systems to be regulated by nearby niche cells that provide both a physical location for stem cells to reside in as well as secreting molecules to regulate stem cell function (reviewed in [37]). Interestingly, signaling molecules, such as Wnts and TGFβ, found to be secreted at normal stem cell niches are factors known to be important in tumor growth and metastasis [38]. Additionally, if mCSCs are similar to normal stem cells in that they have a high degree of cellular plasticity, they are likely to be better then other tumor cells at surviving in a foreign niche that is different than the microenvironment at the site of the primary tumor. It is possible that when mCSCs engraft in a tissue they may kick out resident stem cells from their niche. For instance, it is known that osteolytic bone metastasis results in the activation of endosteal osteoclasts [39] which can promote the mobilization of endosteal hematopoietic progenitor cells in the bone marrow [40]. In addition to invading already established niches, metastatic cells have also been shown to induce niche formation prior to leaving the primary tumor site.

In a seminal report in 2005, it was shown that metastatic lung and melanoma cells secrete factors including vascular endothelial growth factor (VEGF) and placental growth factor (PlGF) which induce the recruitment of bone marrow derived cells to the future sites of metastasis (dubbed the pre-metastasis niche) [41]. Blocking these factors was sufficient to reduce tumor metastasis, and interestingly, treating mice with conditioned media from one tumor type was sufficient to redirect the tissue tropisms of the other type. This suggested that once the pre-metastasis niche was initiated, factors were secreted by cells in the niche back to the primary tumor to help recruit metastatic cells. Two possible candidates to mediate this effect are the S100 cytokines S100A8 and S100A9. These cytokines, expressed by myeloid cells, were shown to be upregulated in the pre-metastatic lungs of tumor bearing mice, and when blocked reduced metastasis to the lung [42]. The molecular basis of this effect seems to be the induction of the p38 Map kinase pathway which enhanced tumor cell migration and invasion [42]. Once located in the niche, it is speculated that mCSCs may enter a period of dormancy, similar to that of normal adult stem cells, whereby some re-activation signal may trigger their expansion into a full blown metastatic lesion (see Figure 4) [1]. However, at this point, this idea remains purely speculation and lacks experimental validation.

Other microenvironment factors known to be important during tumorigenesis and metastasis may specifically be important in the regulation of mCSC growth and expansion. For example, when secreted by stromal cells, growth regulators such as Bmp and its inhibitor GREMLIN-1, which are known to regulate normal stem cell proliferation, have been shown to regulate basal cell carcinoma primary tumor growth [43]. Whether this is true in metastasis, and specifically in the regulation of mCSC behavior, remains to be determined. A number of other heterotypic examples between tumor cells and their microenvironment known to play a role in metastasis, such as hypoxia and immune surveillance (reviewed in [44,45]), may also specifically affect mCSCs. However, without their precise identity known, direct studies to characterize these interactions remain far off. Once identified, tests could be designed to determine whether or not circulating cancer cells from a patient contain a population of mCSCs which would predict future metastasis.

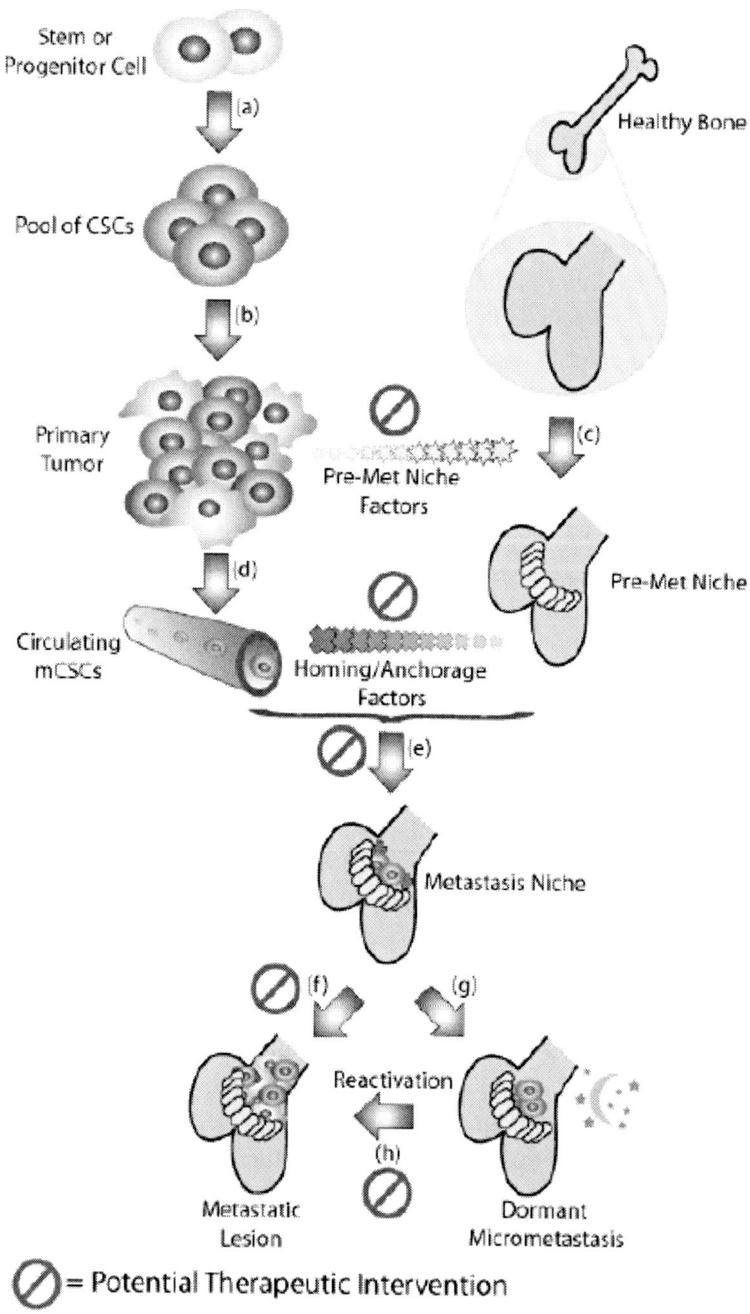

Figure 4. Critical stem cell-niche interactions in regulating metastasis (from [1]). Regardless of how it is derived (a), a pool of malignant pCSCs is formed which expands into a primary tumor (b). This primary tumor is capable of secreting pre-metastasis niche factors such as VEGF and PLGF (c) that induces the expression of homing and anchorage factors such as the S100 cytokines which guide circulating mCSCs (d). Once these mCSCs lodge in the niche (e), they can either proliferate into a metastatic lesion immediately (f) or enter into a period of dormancy (g) whereby reactivation signals induce their expansion (h). Ø = potential steps to target by therapeutic intervention.

As the mCSC population that initially lodges in a metastatic niche is likely very small, profiling the aforementioned niche responses to tumor metastasis may provide an easier means to detect early metastatic lesions. Further research into mCSC behavior, both reliant and independent of niche interactions hopefully will lead to the development of the most clinically effective cancer therapeutics to date.

Metastasis, CSCs and Chemotherapy

Much of the hype surrounding the CSC field has centered on the idea that by treating a small, typically chemoresistant population of cells responsible for initiating tumors, cancer treatment might finally deplete tumors of their lifeblood. However, the idea that these therapies might be designed to specifically ablate mCSCs has usually been little more than an afterthought. This fact should not be taken lightly as even if a CSC based therapy depletes all the tumor initiating cells from the primary tumor, mCSCs that have left the primary tumor and potentially have different molecular profiles than their primary tumor counterparts could be resistant to these therapies. It is also worth noting that many of these proposed therapies speculate on what the critical vulnerabilities of CSCs are, often times based on the known behavior of normal adult stem cells. However, before proceeding to discuss these approaches, it is important to think about the means of validating potential therapeutics, and about potential side effects of CSC based therapeutics.

The traditional standard of evaluating the effectiveness of a given anti-cancer drug is to determine the amount the drug can halt or shrink tumor growth. This is potentially problematic when considering CSC based therapeutics, since these cells are a minority population within a tumor. Treatment with CSC targeting agents in conjunction with traditional therapeutics may only result in a modest, if any, shrinking of the primary tumor compared to traditional drugs alone, but could have significant benefits when evaluating the recurrence- or metastasis-free survival. With respect to the potential side effects of CSC based therapy, there has been concern that if CSCs share properties with normal stem cells, then CSC based therapy may have deleterious side effects on these crucial cell types. This may not be much of a problem for breast cancer, where mastectomy is already an established acceptable treatment option but could be very serious for leukemia, where the normal stem cell and progenitor counterparts are essential for immune function. However, the increased proliferative potential of CSCs may provide a therapeutic window that could be exploited. This seems to be the case as leukemia initiating cells and normal hematopoietic stem cells have a differential dependence on the tumor suppressor PTEN [46].

Self-Renewal and Differentiation

Normal stem cells are known to possess the unique ability to self-renew to maintain a stem-cell pool and to differentiate into more committed progenitors. It is believed that either blocking CSC self-renewal ability or inducing differentiation may deplete these cells from the body. There are a variety of studies indicating this is the case in brain cancer. Treating glioblastoma derived neurospheres (cells dependent on stem cell function) with cyclopamine to block the Hedgehog pathway eliminated their ability to form new neurospheres. Additionally after cyclopamine treatment, glioblastoma cells were no longer able to form tumors *in vivo* [47]. Similar studies have demonstrated that using retinoic acid, a useful differentiation inducer in acute promyelocytic leukemia, also induces differentiation of glioblastoma cells [48]. Alternatively, using a γ-secretase inhibitor to block the Notch pathway resulted in differentiation of medulloblastoma cell lines, and a loss of colony- and tumor-forming ability. This effect appears to be due to a specific depletion of $CD133^+$ CSCs [49]. Despite these significant findings, it remains to be determined whether mCSCS can be targeted by similar strategies or if they require unique therapeutic targeting.

Metastasis Niche

One therapeutic strategy unique to mCSCs involves targeting the critical mCSC/niche interactions that affect homing, engraftment and growth of tumor cells. It has been shown that blocking the pre-metastasis niche initiation using VEGF or PIGF antibodies was sufficient to reduce metastasis [41]. However, after the niche is initiated, other factors may be useful drug targets in blocking the binding of mCSCs to the niche. One possible factor is CXCR4, which is critical for leukemia cells binding to their niche [50], is important in breast cancer metastasis [51], and has been shown to enrich for mCSCs in pancreatic cancer [28]. Another factor is CD44, which positively selects for breast pCSCs. Blocking CD44 in a acute myelogenous leukemia model resulted in a significant deficiency in engraftment, even when the leukemia CSCs were injected directly into the bone marrow, indicating a specific defect in binding not homing [52]. Similar conclusions were also drawn regarding the essential nature of CD44 in chronic myelogenous leukemia [53]. Once mCSCs are identified and characterized extensively, it will be interesting to note determine what other factors are supplied by the niche to maintain their growth, and if these are potential therapeutic targets.

Reactivation

It is speculated, but remains to be proven, that mCSCs reside in niches in a state of dormancy before expanding into a full blow metastatic lesion. If this is the case, identifying the critical reactivation factors will certainly be of great interest. These potential therapies could have an advantage over drugs that target the homing or seeding of mCSCs because by the time of tumor diagnosis, mCSCs may have already left the primary tumor, migrated and lodged in metastatic niches. However, developing these therapeutics will not happen in the near future since the dormancy model first needs to be validated and characterized before creating drugs.

CSC Clearance

Cell surface marker profiling of CSCs may be useful beyond teasing out tumor initiating populations from the bulk of the tumor mass; the markers identified may be useful in creating cell specific clearance therapies, such as DNA vaccines or oncolytic viruses. When $CD44^{+}CD24^{-/low}$ pleural effusion cells are infected with capsid modified oncolytic adenoviruses, their tumor initiating capacity is abrogated [35]. Furthermore, these viruses when administered after tumor formation were able to significantly deplete the $CD44^{+}/CD24^{-/low}$ population within tumors. Since the surface markers used to identify CSCs are also shared by normal, non tumor cells, specific targeting of the viruses to the CSC population is likely to be a major hurdle to overcome in this line of research.

Conclusion

The unprecedented excitement surrounding the CSC field is certainly grounded in significant theoretical and experimental evidence. This excitement is particularly warranted when considering the role of CSCs in metastasis, since metastasis is responsible for the overwhelming majority of cancer deaths coupled with the fact that CSCs have been shown to be chemoresistant [2, 3]. Characterizing the role of CSCs in metastasis involves two distinct portions of the metastatic cascade. First, the role of initial oncogenic events is important in deriving pCSCs that eventually produce tumors of varying degrees of malignancy. Understanding these events is likely to provide more prognostic, rather than therapeutic value. On the contrary, profiling the function of mCSCs, which are important for actually initiating and perpetuating metastatic lesion growth, may lead to novel therapeutic strategies. However, prudence dictates that scientists should acknowledge that while CSCs are a particularly intriguing line of research, at this juncture, we yet don't know if we will be successful in developing any new safe and effective therapeutics. Nevertheless, the future is filled with interesting avenues of research in the CSC field, many of which should shift to focus on the role of CSCs in metastasis and not just tumorigenesis. These studies may result in the development of the most powerful tools in prognostic and therapeutic oncology.

References

[1] Li F, Tiede B, Massague J, Kang Y (2006) Beyond tumorigenesis: cancer stem cells in metastasis. *Cell Res*.

[2] Bao S, Wu Q, McLendon RE, Hao Y, Shi Q, et al. (2006) Glioma stem cells promote radioresistance by preferential activation of the DNA damage response. *Nature* 444: 756-760.

[3] Jemal A, Siegel R, Ward E, Murray T, Xu J, et al. (2007) Cancer statistics, 2007. CA *Cancer J. Clin*. 57: 43-66.

[4] Bernards R, Weinberg RA (2002) A progression puzzle. *Nature* 418: 823.

[5] Stingl J, Caldas C (2007) Molecular heterogeneity of breast carcinomas and the cancer stem cell hypothesis. *Nat. Rev. Cancer*.

[6] Sorlie T, Perou CM, Tibshirani R, Aas T, Geisler S, et al. (2001) Gene expression patterns of breast carcinomas distinguish tumor subclasses with clinical implications. *Proc. Natl. Acad. Sci. USA* 98: 10869-10874.

[7] Perou CM, Jeffrey SS, van de Rijn M, Rees CA, Eisen MB, et al. (1999) Distinctive gene expression patterns in human mammary epithelial cells and breast cancers. *Proc. Natl. Acad. Sci. USA* 96: 9212-9217.

[8] van de Vijver MJ, He YD, van't Veer LJ, Dai H, Hart AA, et al. (2002) A gene-expression signature as a predictor of survival in breast cancer. *N. Engl. J. Med.* 347: 1999-2009.

[9] van 't Veer LJ, Dai H, van de Vijver MJ, He YD, Hart AA, et al. (2002) Gene expression profiling predicts clinical outcome of breast cancer. *Nature* 415: 530-536.

[10] Wang Y, Klijn JG, Zhang Y, Sieuwerts AM, Look MP, et al. (2005) Gene-expression profiles to predict distant metastasis of lymph-node-negative primary breast cancer. *Lancet* 365: 671-679.

[11] Ramaswamy S, Ross KN, Lander ES, Golub TR (2003) A molecular signature of metastasis in primary solid tumors. *Nat. Genet.* 33: 49-54.

[12] Desai KV, Xiao N, Wang W, Gangi L, Greene J, et al. (2002) Initiating oncogenic event determines gene-expression patterns of human breast cancer models. *Proc. Natl. Acad. Sci. USA* 99: 6967-6972.

[13] Hynes RO (2003) Metastatic potential: generic predisposition of the primary tumor or rare, metastatic variants-or both? *Cell* 113: 821-823.

[14] Chen L, Shen R, Ye Y, Pu XA, Liu X, et al. (2007) Precancerous stem cells have the potential for both benign and malignant differentiation. *PLoS ONE* 2: e293.

[15] Cairns J (2002) Somatic stem cells and the kinetics of mutagenesis and carcinogenesis. *Proc. Natl. Acad. Sci. USA* 99: 10567-10570.

[16] Ito M, Yang Z, Andl T, Cui C, Kim N, et al. (2007) Wnt-dependent de novo hair follicle regeneration in adult mouse skin after wounding. *Nature* 447: 316-320.

[17] Shackleton M, Vaillant F, Simpson KJ, Stingl J, Smyth GK, et al. (2006) Generation of a functional mammary gland from a single stem cell. *Nature* 439: 84-88.

[18] Jaiswal S, Traver D, Miyamoto T, Akashi K, Lagasse E, et al. (2003) Expression of BCR/ABL and BCL-2 in myeloid progenitors leads to myeloid leukemias. *Proc. Natl. Acad. Sci. USA* 100: 10002-10007.

[19] Turhan AG, Lemoine FM, Debert C, Bonnet ML, Baillou C, et al. (1995) Highly purified primitive hematopoietic stem cells are PML-RARA negative and generate nonclonal progenitors in acute promyelocytic leukemia. *Blood* 85: 2154-2161.

[20] Jamieson CH, Ailles LE, Dylla SJ, Muijtjens M, Jones C, et al. (2004) Granulocyte-macrophage progenitors as candidate leukemic stem cells in blast-crisis CML. *N. Engl. J. Med.* 351: 657-667.

[21] Krivtsov AV, Twomey D, Feng Z, Stubbs MC, Wang Y, et al. (2006) Transformation from committed progenitor to leukaemia stem cell initiated by MLL-AF9. *Nature*.

[22] Vescovi AL, Galli R, Reynolds BA (2006) Brain tumour stem cells. *Nat. Rev. Cancer* 6: 425-436.

[23] Bachoo RM, Maher EA, Ligon KL, Sharpless NE, Chan SS, et al. (2002) Epidermal growth factor receptor and Ink4a/Arf: convergent mechanisms governing terminal differentiation and transformation along the neural stem cell to astrocyte axis. *Cancer Cell* 1: 269-277.

[24] Ince TA, Richardson AL, Bell GW, Saitoh M, Godar S, et al. (2007) Transformation of Different Human Breast Epithelial Cell Types Leads to Distinct Tumor Phenotypes. *Cancer Cell* 12: 160-170.

[25] Blair A, Hogge DE, Ailles LE, Lansdorp PM, Sutherland HJ (1997) Lack of expression of Thy-1 (CD90) on acute myeloid leukemia cells with long-term proliferative ability in vitro and in vivo. *Blood* 89: 3104-3112.

[26] Shipitsin M, Campbell LL, Argani P, Weremowicz S, Bloushtain-Qimron N, et al. (2007) Molecular definition of breast tumor heterogeneity. *Cancer Cell* 11: 259-273.

[27] Fidler IJ, Talmadge JE (1986) Evidence that intravenously derived murine pulmonary melanoma metastases can originate from the expansion of a single tumor cell. *Cancer Res.* 46: 5167-5171.

[28] Hermann P, Huber S, Herrler T, Aicher A, Ellwart J, et al. (2007) Distinct Populations of Cancer Stem Cells Determine Tumor Growth and Metastatic Activity in Human Pancreatic Cancer. *Cell Stem Cell* 1: 313-323.

[29] Fidler IJ (2003) The pathogenesis of cancer metastasis: the 'seed and soil' hypothesis revisited. *Nat. Rev. Cancer* 3: 453-458.

[30] Al-Hajj M, Wicha MS, Benito-Hernandez A, Morrison SJ, Clarke MF (2003) Prospective identification of tumorigenic breast cancer cells. *Proc. Natl. Acad. Sci. USA* 100: 3983-3988.

[31] Liu R, Wang X, Chen GY, Dalerba P, Gurney A, et al. (2007) The prognostic role of a gene signature from tumorigenic breast-cancer cells. *N. Engl. J. Med.* 356: 217-226.

[32] Sheridan C, Kishimoto H, Fuchs RK, Mehrotra S, Bhat-Nakshatri P, et al. (2006) CD44+/CD24- breast cancer cells exhibit enhanced invasive properties: an early step necessary for metastasis. *Breast Cancer Res.* 8: R59.

[33] Balic M, Lin H, Young L, Hawes D, Giuliano A, et al. (2006) Most early disseminated cancer cells detected in bone marrow of breast cancer patients have a putative breast cancer stem cell phenotype. *Clin. Cancer Res.* 12: 5615-5621.

[34] Abraham BK, Fritz P, McClellan M, Hauptvogel P, Athelogou M, et al. (2005) Prevalence of CD44+/CD24-/low cells in breast cancer may not be associated with clinical outcome but may favor distant metastasis. *Clin. Cancer Res.* 11: 1154-1159.

[35] Eriksson M, Guse K, Bauerschmitz G, Virkkunen P, Tarkkanen M, et al. (2007) Oncolytic Adenoviruses Kill Breast Cancer Initiating CD44(+)CD24(-/Low) Cells. *Mol. Ther.*

[36] Bao S, Wu Q, Sathornsumetee S, Hao Y, Li Z, et al. (2006) Stem Cell-like Glioma Cells Promote Tumor Angiogenesis through Vascular Endothelial Growth Factor. *Cancer Res.* 66: 7843-7848.

[37] Moore KA, Lemischka IR (2006) Stem cells and their niches. Science 311: 1880-1885.

[38] Li L, Neaves WB (2006) Normal stem cells and cancer stem cells: the niche matters. *Cancer Res.* 66: 4553-4557.

[39] Guise TA, Mohammad KS, Clines G, Stebbins EG, Wong DH, et al. (2006) Basic mechanisms responsible for osteolytic and osteoblastic bone metastases. *Clin. Cancer Res.* 12: 6213s-6216s.

[40] Kollet O, Dar A, Shivtiel S, Kalinkovich A, Lapid K, et al. (2006) Osteoclasts degrade endosteal components and promote mobilization of hematopoietic progenitor cells. *Nat. Med.* 12: 657-664.

[41] Kaplan RN, Riba RD, Zacharoulis S, Bramley AH, Vincent L, et al. (2005) VEGFR1-positive haematopoietic bone marrow progenitors initiate the pre-metastatic niche. *Nature* 438: 820-827.

[42] Hiratsuka S, Watanabe A, Aburatani H, Maru Y (2006) Tumour-mediated upregulation of chemoattractants and recruitment of myeloid cells predetermines lung metastasis. *Nat. Cell Biol.* 8: 1369-1375.

[43] Sneddon JB, Zhen HH, Montgomery K, van de Rijn M, Tward AD, et al. (2006) Bone morphogenetic protein antagonist gremlin 1 is widely expressed by cancer-associated stromal cells and can promote tumor cell proliferation. *Proc. Natl. Acad. Sci. USA* 103: 14842-14847.

[44] Barnhart BC, Simon MC (2007) Metastasis and stem cell pathways. *Cancer Metastasis Rev.* 26: 261-271.

[45] Gupta GP, Massague J (2006) Cancer metastasis: building a framework. *Cell* 127: 679-695.

[46] Yilmaz OH, Valdez R, Theisen BK, Guo W, Ferguson DO, et al. (2006) Pten dependence distinguishes haematopoietic stem cells from leukaemia-initiating cells. *Nature* 441: 475-482.

[47] Bar EE, Chaudhry A, Lin A, Fan X, Schreck K, et al. (2007) Cyclopamine-Mediated Hedgehog Pathway Inhibition Depletes Stem-Like Cancer Cells in Glioblastoma. *Stem Cells*.

[48] Park DM, Li J, Okamoto H, Akeju O, Kim SH, et al. (2007) N-CoR pathway targeting induces glioblastoma derived cancer stem cell differentiation. *Cell Cycle* 6: 467-470.

[49] Fan X, Matsui W, Khaki L, Stearns D, Chun J, et al. (2006) Notch pathway inhibition depletes stem-like cells and blocks engraftment in embryonal brain tumors. *Cancer Res.* 66: 7445-7452.

[50] Tavor S, Petit I, Porozov S, Avigdor A, Dar A, et al. (2004) CXCR4 regulates migration and development of human acute myelogenous leukemia stem cells in transplanted NOD/SCID mice. *Cancer Res.* 64: 2817-2824.

[51] Kang Y, Siegel PM, Shu W, Drobnjak M, Kakonen SM, et al. (2003) A multigenic program mediating breast cancer metastasis to bone. *Cancer Cell* 3: 537-549.

[52] Jin L, Hope KJ, Zhai Q, Smadja-Joffe F, Dick JE (2006) Targeting of CD44 eradicates human acute myeloid leukemic stem cells. *Nat. Med.* 12: 1167-1174.

[53] Krause DS, Lazarides K, von Andrian UH, Van Etten RA (2006) Requirement for CD44 in homing and engraftment of BCR-ABL-expressing leukemic stem cells. *Nat. Med.* 12: 1175-1180.

In: Cancer and Stem Cells
Eds: Thomas Dittmar and Kurt S. Zänker

ISBN 978-1-60456-478-5

Chapter 8

Exercise, Stem Cells and Cancer

Emre Tunca, Karsten Krüger and Frank C. Mooren**
Department of Sports Medicine, Institute of Sports Sciences,
Justus-Liebig-University, Giessen, Germany

Introduction

In our modern industrialised world we are following a dangerous way, involving a gradually increasing caloric intake and a steady decline in physical activity. Physical inactivity has become an important risk factor for many chronic diseases such cardiovascular diseases, metabolic syndrome and also some types of malignant diseases. The sedentary lifestyle deprives the organism with exercise stimuli, which are necessary for metabolic homeostasis. This is indicated by a short look back into history of men. Our genetic background is still the same as in our historic ancestors, the nomadic hunter-gatherer, as convincing evidence shows that this ancient genome has remained essentially unchanged over the past 10,000 years and certainly not changed in the past 40-100 years. To ensure survival our ancestors had to cover great distances on their search for food. Therefore physical activity and exercise evolved as important factors for life and survival. These factors are still the most important natural stimuli to ensure a perfect harmony of physiological and biochemical processes fundamental to human life.

The following review should therefore give some information (1) about the role of exercise stimulus for stem cell mobilization and (2) what is currently known about exercise on tumour incidence and progression.

* Address for correspondence: Prof. Dr. Frank C. Mooren, Department of Sports Medicine, Justus-Liebig University Giessen, Kugelberg 62. 35394 Giessen. Tel: 49-641-9925210. Fax: 49-641-9925219. E-mail: frank-christoph.mooren@sport.uni-giessen.de

Exercise and Stem Cells

Regular physical exercise training is followed by structural adaptations in organs and tissues. For many years, it was believed that the responsible mechanisms for structural changes are either the mitotic activity of resident cells or the amplification and growth of available resources within the tissues. Today, accumulating evidence indicates that adaptation processes during exercise training are at least partially induced by resident and bone marrow derived stem cells with similar properties to those of embryonic stem cells (Ribatti et al. 2001). These stem cells have the potential to differentiate into mature cell types depending on specific activating signals. Stem cells are localized in "stem cell niches" in the bone marrow or within local tissues. Before activation they remain in an undifferentiated and quiescent state in the G0 phase of the cell cycle. Stem cell mobilization and activation is regulated by a variety of growth factors, enzymes, ligands and surface receptors. Stressful conditions such as exercise or exercise associated hypoxia induce a release of stem- cell-activating and -mobilizing factors which hamper the interactions between the cells and bone marrow stroma cells. These factors, including metallo-matrix proteases (MMP9), erythropoietin (EPO), granulocyte/monocyte colony-stimulating factor (GM-CSF), vascular endothelial growth factor (VEGF) and stromal-derived factor-1 (SDF-1) might be important mediators of the stress induced mobilization of stem cells into the circulation (Heissig et al. 2002).

Exercise and Endothelial Progenitor Cells

There is increasing evidence that the peripheral blood contains bone marrow derived premature cells which modulate cardiovascular function. Endothelial progenitor cells (EPCs), a subset of stem cells, have the potential to differentiate into mature endothelial cells. Therefore, EPCs might contribute to postnatal vessel-growth (Laufs et al. 2007).

Physical activity is associated with a reduction in cardiovascular events. Despite the wealth of evidence derived from epidemiological and interventional studies, there is limited understanding of the underlying molecular mechanisms. Notably, regular exercise training reduces vascular oxidative stress at least in part by increasing activity of endothelial nitric synthase (eNOS) and superoxide dismutase (SOD) and is able to restore dysregulated intracellular signalling pathways such as calcium signalling (Kojda et al. 2001, Fukai et al. 2000). Besides improving endothelial function, exercise training induces capillarization of the skeletal muscle and collateralization in patients with stenotic vascular diseases (Hu et al. 2003). For many years it was believed that the generation of new blood vessels in response to exercise training results from angiogenesis induced by local mitotic activity of endothelial cells. Recent studies provide evidence that invasion of stem and progenitor cells contribute to the growth of new blood capillaries (Custodis and Laufs, 2007).

Exercise regulates the activation and mobilization of EPCs, a specific subset of stem cells, which are involved in vasculogenesis, promoting vascular repair, inhibiting atherosclerosis, and increasing ventricular function after myocardial infarction (Dimmeler et al. 2001, Orlic et al. 2001, Assmus et al. 2002, Hill et al. 2003, Werner et al. 2003). Both, acute exercise and chronic training regimes regulate numbers of circulating EPCs.

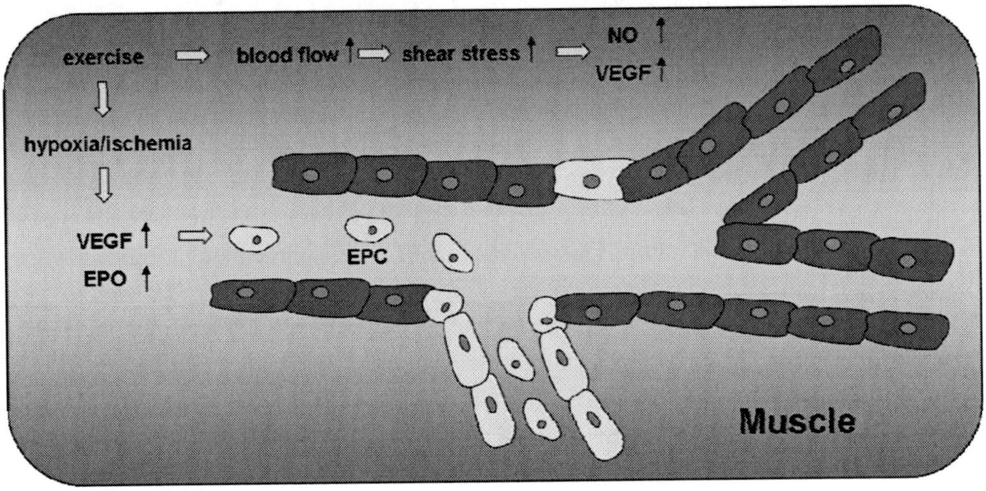

Figure 1. The effects of exercise on EPCs. Capillarization of the skeletal muscle is one important adaptation after endurance training. During acute exercise hypoxia and tissue-ischemia induces an upregulation vascular-endothelial growth factor (VEGF) and erythropoietin (EPO) which stimulates EPCs to proliferate and organize cell clusters. Furthermore, exercise-increased blood flow elevated blood flow which increases the production of nitric oxide (NO).

Likewise acute exercise has short term effects within hours on mobilization of EPCs into circulation. Adams et al. (2004) showed that the numbers of EPCs increased in patients with coronary artery disease 24h and 48h after exercise. Regarding acute exercise, the effects of the exercise mode seem to be an important determinant on EPC-mobilization. Laufs et al. (2005) investigated the effects of running of different duration and intensity on EPC numbers in the peripheral blood. Both, intensive running and moderate running for more than 30 minutes caused an increase of circulating progenitor cells, while running for 10 minutes failed. Simultaneously, Laufs et al. (2004) have shown that physical activity increased number of EPCs in the bone marrow, the blood and in the spleen of mice. This observation supports that exercise does not only mobilize stem cells from the bone marrow, but also stimulates production of cells in the bone marrow.

In addition, a 12-week regular endurance training increased the number of EPCs in the peripheral blood 2.9- fold. Furthermore, in coronary artery disease patients the number of EPCs in the peripheral blood was augmented significantly after 4 weeks of moderate endurance exercise (Laufs et al. 2004).

Exercise and Hematopoietic Stem Cells (HSCs)

Exercise is known to cause perturbations in peripheral leukocyte numbers. During exercise a leukocytosis occurs, which is mainly induced by a mobilization of granulocytes from the marginal pool and the bone marrow. Simultaneously lymphocyte numbers increase during exercise and fall under prexercise values after intensive exercise. One reason for the post-exercise decline of lymphocyte numbers is apoptosis (Mars et al. 1998, Mooren et al. 2002). An increased apoptosis might be a result of an enhanced cell turnover, and a regular loss of immunocompetent cells has to be compensated by an enhanced production of myeloid cells.

Even though these perturbations of leukocyte counts are well known, Bonsignore et al. (2002) were the first who investigated the influence of exercise on hematopoietic stem cells (HSCs). Both, acute exercise and regular exercise training influence HSC numbers in the peripheral blood. Acute exercise significantly increased HSCs into the circulation in the post-exercise period (Morici et al. 2005, Thijssen et al. 2006). This immediate mobilization seems to be age related, since the absolute increase of HSCs was attenuated in older men (Thijssen et al. 2006). In contrast, a half-marathon run and a marathon run reduced peripheral HSC-numbers at the following day, which might be a result of a delayed recruitment of cells into tissues (Bonsignore et al. 2002 Morici et al. 2005).

The influence of exercise on HSC –numbers in the blood seems to depend on the training status. Higher numbers of circulating stem cells were found in well trained athletes, while eight weeks of endurance training did not affect baseline numbers of circulating HSCs in untrained subjects (Bonsignore et al. 2002, Thijssen et al.2006). Chronically elevated HSC numbers in athletes might represent a hematopoietic adaptation to regular exercise training.

Potential Mechanisms for the Mobilization of EPCs and HSCs

Most studies also determined the potential factors which promote the mobilization of EPCs by exercise. One mechanism seems to be the exercise associated enhancement of shear stress which increases nitric oxide (NO) production. Aicher et al. (2003) have shown in mice that eNOS expression in bone marrow cells influences recruitment of EPCs. Furthermore, it was shown that voluntary-running induced enhancement of EPC numbers is related to the bioavailability of nitric oxide because upregulation was absent in eNOS-/- mice or in the presence of a nitric oxide synthase inhibitor (Laufs et al. 2004).

Another possible mediator of exercise-induced EPC mobilisation might be hypoxia, which leads to an enhanced production of several growth factors and hormones like VEGF and erythropoietin (Aicher et al. 2003). Furthermore, GM-CSF, G-CSF and chemokines like stromal-derived factor-1 (SDF-1) show increased levels after acute exercise. All these growth factors and cytokines are well known to induce progenitor cell mobilization (Laufs et al. 2004).

Exercise and Myogenic Satellite Cells

Physiological conditions such as exercise perturb the muscle's tensional and metabolic integrity. These perturbations of muscles homoeostasis is mechano-chemically transduced into molecular and cellular responses within the myofibres (Tidball 2005). These responses lead to specific structural changes that result in a task specific functional enhancement. In comparison to other organs, the skeletal muscle exhibits a remarkable capacity to adapt to physiologic stimuli such as exercise (Toigo and Boutellier 2006).

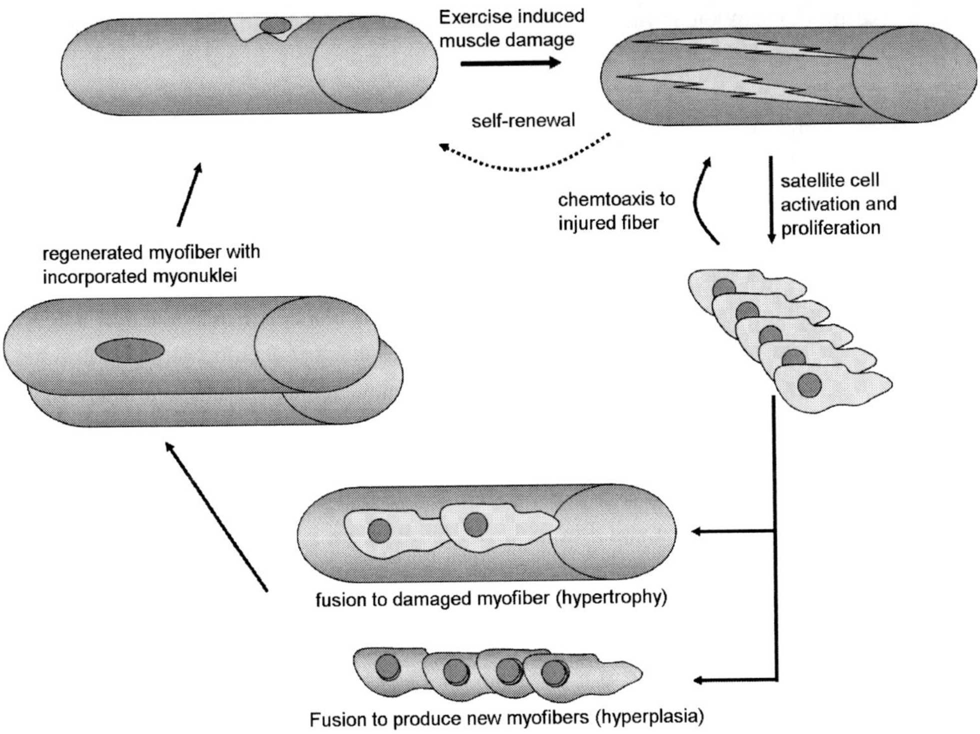

Figure 2. Mobilization of satellite cells after exercise-induced muscle damage. Exercise, especially resistance exercise and eccentric exercise, induces muscle damage, which initiates the activation and proliferation of satellite cells. Invading immune cells secrete variety of cytokines, which contribute to chemotaxis of satellite cells into the injured tissue. On the one hand, activated satellite cells fuse with existing fibers. On the other hand, the cells have the potential to fuse with each other and form completely new fibers.

Muscular adaptation to exercise depends on a specific stimulus resulting in the changes in the function and structure of muscle fibers. Adaptations to strength training were mainly attributed to hypertrophy of existent muscle, while endurance training resulting an enhanced capacity of metabolic and mitochondrial enzymes.

Structural and functional changes following strength or resistance training were - besides neuronal improvements - mainly referred to a change of muscle protein isoforms, improvement of enzyme activity and an increase of muscles cross sectional area. In addition, these adaptations can also be ascribed to the activation and differentiation of resident satellite cells. On the one hand, these cells have the ability to fuse to existing myofibers. On the other hand, activated satellite cells fuse and produce new myofibers resulting in adaptation by hyperplasia (Bischoff 1994).

The defining characteristic of quiescent satellite cells is that they are surrounded by the basal lamina and have a high nuclear-to-cytoplasmic ratio. Furthermore, they can be distinguished from myonuklei by more abundant heterochromatin (Schultz and McCormick, 1994). These morphological features are consistent with the finding that they are transcriptionally less active. Up to activation the cells rest in the G0 phase of the cell cycle. The quiescent cells do not express markers of terminal differentiation like the MyoD or MEF2 (Cornelison and Wold 1997). Instead they express a specific pattern of satellite cell markers like myocyte nuclear factor (MNF) and c-Met, the receptor for hepatocyte growth factor (HGF). Irintchev et al. (1994) identified M-cadherin, a calcium-dependent cell adhesion molecule, as a unique marker of the satellite cell pool. Activation of satellite cells occurs in response to various physical stressors like exercise. Exercise training is a physiological challenge that promotes an adaptational response of the muscle by satellite cell activation, proliferation, chemotaxis and fusion to existing fibers (Schultz and McCormick 1994). The migratory capacity of satellite cells is strongly dependent on the integrity of the basal lamina. Exercise, especially resistance and eccentric exercise, disturb the contact between the satellite cells and the basal lamina and change the integrity of the cell membrane (Schultz et al. 1985, Watt et al. 1991). Furthermore, exercise induced myotrauma initiates an inflammatory response resulting in an invasion of macrophages and neutrophils in the damaged muscle (Bischoff 1994, Vierck et al. 2000). Beside muscle infiltration and phagocytosis, the immune cells secrete a variety of cytokines that contribute to the regulation of satellite cells (Nathan 1987). Interestingly, in the presence of an enhanced immune response, there is an increase in satellite cell proliferation and differentiation (Lescaudron et al. 1999). Exercise-induced myotrauma results in a release of growth factors like insulin-like growth factor-1 (IGF-1), HGF and myogenic regulatory factors which further stimulate activation of satellite cells. Contrary, enhanced myostatin expression inhibits activation of satellite cells (McCroscery et al. 2003). Kadi and Thornell (1999) showed an increased expression of IGF-1 following muscle-damaging eccentric exercise. Resistance training reduced plasma-myostatine concentration at around 20 percent, which might contribute to an activation of satellite cells (Hellsten et al. 1990). Following activation the mitotic activity of the cells rises and the cytoplasmatic-to-nuclear ratio increases parallel to the number of intracellular organelles. Simultaneously activated satellite cells start to express myogenic markers like MyoD and myogenin. On the one hand activated satellite cells have the potential for self-renewal, which means they can substitute the original satellite cell pool. On the other hand, activated cells pass further differentiation. Fusing with existing muscle fibers might contribute to muscle-hypertrophy, while fusing with each other leads to a formation of completely new fibers (hyperplasia).

Exercise and Cancer

The first epidemiologic studies on the relationship between physical activity and cancer prevention were done in the thirties of the last century. In 1922 two studies were published independently analyzing among other things the cancer mortality rate among men with different occupations (Cherry 1922; Sivertsen and Dahlstrom 1922). It was reported that increasing physical activity decreased the cancer mortality rate lead to new aspects in cancer aetiology.

According to Courneya and Friedenreich (2001) the cancer experience can be divided into 2 experience periods. The first experience period is the pre-diagnosis period, which is subdivided into the 1) pre-screening and the 2) screening time periods. The second experience period is the post-diagnosis period. It is subdivided into 3) pre-treatment, 4) treatment, 5) post-treatment and 6) resumption time periods. Between both experience periods cancer will be diagnosed. For our intention, we will summarize the epidemiological studies into pre-diagnosis and post-diagnosis.

Considerable epidemiological studies investigated the link between physical activity and a reduced risk of several malignant diseases (pre-diagnosis period). Other studies examined the effect of physical activity on quality of life (QoL), the risk of recurrence and the length of the survival time (post-diagnosis period). Thereby the scientific evidence for the association between physical activity and cancer prevention is categorized in "convincing," "probable," "possible" and "insufficient" based on the definitions developed by the World Cancer Research Fund and American Institute for Cancer Research report on diet and cancer prevention (Potter JD. Food 1997) (Table 1).

The most common types for analytical epidemiological studies concerning the association between physical activity and cancer risk are the cohort type and the case-control type. The cohort study type is a longitudinal study, in which individuals are analysed over the time concerning one ore more expositions (e.g. physical activity). For the evaluation exposed and non-exposed individuals are compared to measure the incidence and/or the mortality rate. There are two different types of a cohort study. One is the retrospective study, in which datas concerning the expositions are taken from the past and the incidence and/or mortality are analysed subsequently. Another type is the prospective cohort study, in which datas are taken at the beginning of the study and the cohort is analysed for the following time over several years (follow-up). In case-control studies diseased individuals are recruited and compared to non-diseased individuals concerning different risk factors. Case-control studies are most suitable for rare diseases. In contrast to cohort studies, it is impossible to analyse an incidence of a disease when using a case-control study.

Table 1. Description of levels of evidence (descriptions from the World Cancer Research Fund/American Institute for Cancer Research) (Potter J.D., 1997)

Level of evidence	Description
Convincing	Epidemiological studies show consistent associations, with little or no evidence to the contrary. There should be a substantial number of acceptable studies (more than 20), preferably including prospective designs, conducted in different population groups and controlled for possible confounding factors. Exposure data should refer to the time preceding the occurrence of cancer. Dose-response relationships should be supportive of a causal relationship. Associations should be biologically plausible. Laboratory evidence is usually supportive.
Probable	Epidemiological studies showing associations are either not so consistent, with a number of studies not supporting the association, or the number or type of studies is not extensive enough to make a more definite judgment. Mechanistic and laboratory evidence is usually supportive.
Possible	Epidemiological studies are generally supportive, but are limited in quantity, quality or consistency. There may or may not be supportive mechanistic or laboratory evidence. Alternatively, there are few or no epidemiological data, but strongly supportive evidence from other disciplines.
Insufficient	There are only a few studies, which are generally consistent, but really do no more than hint at a possible relationship. Often, more well-designed research is needed.

Physical Activity during Cancer Pre-Diagnosis Period

Nearly 200 epidemiological studies have been performed up to date about the relation of physical activity and the incidence of various malignant diseases. Most convincing epidemiologic evidence has been shown for a relation between physical activity and the prevention of colon cancer for both men and women. Interestingly, studies on the influence of physical activity on the prevention from rectal cancer revealed no association.

Friedenreich and Orenstein (2002) reported that 43 of the 51 conducted studies on colon and colorectal cancer revealed an association between physical activity and cancer risk reduction among the most physically active male and female participants. This reduction averaged between 40%-50%, elevating up to 70% when comparing people of the highest activity level with those of the lowest activity level. Samad, Taylor, Marshall, and Chapman (2005) recently published a meta analysis in which they analysed the results of 47 studies investigating the association between physical activity and the risk of colorectal cancer. Nineteen of the 47 analysed studies were cohort studies and 28 were case-control studies. Forty of the analysed studies revealed a reduction of risk in cancer in males and only 18 showed an association between physical activity and risk reduction in females. The analysed cohort studies revealed that risk reduction of colon cancer in physically active male was associated with any type of physical activity. Both occupational and recreational activity revealed a risk reducing effect on colon cancer. In contrast, women with high levels of occupational activity showed no risk reducing effect on colon cancer. Only women, who were active at high levels in their recreation time had a lowered risk to suffer from colon cancer. The analysed case-control studies revealed, however, a reduced risk for both sexes independently from the type of activity.

A very recently done study used the California Teachers cohort, a prospective cohort of female teachers and administrators residing in California, ages 22 to 84 years at baseline and with no prior history of colon cancer (Mai et al. 2007). The study demonstrated that lifetime recreational physical activity had a reducing effect on colon cancer risk among postmenopausal women who had never used hormone therapy. In contrast, recreational physical activity had no additional effect on women who underwent a hormone therapy and had therefore lower risk of colon cancer.

There is a negative correlation between physical activity and the incidence of breast cancer, which is classified as convincing. However, the situation is not as consistent as that found for colon cancer. This might be attributed to the fact, that many different aspects have to be considered such as hormone receptor status, age at diagnosis (premenopausal vs. postmenopausal), body mass index etc. Monninkhof et al. (2007) evaluated 19 cohort studies and 29 case control studies of 76 identified potentially relevant studies, published between 1994 and 2006, and concluded that there is evidence that physical activity has a decreasing effect on breast cancer risk. They also concluded from their evaluation that stronger benefit occurred among postmenopausal women than among premenopausal women. Three of the analysed cohort studies, which measured total activity, showed different results. One found an association between physical activity and risk reduction, one found no association, and the third one found a risk increase with evidence for a dose-response effect. Analysing the cohort studies revealed that 8 of the 17 studies on leisure time activity showed a reduced risk, whereas the remaining 9 found no association. Concerning the case-control studies assessing total activity, 4 of 6 studies revealed a decrease risk in breast cancer ranging from 21% to 52%. Monninkhof et al. also report that 14 of the 28 case-control studies, publishing data on leisure time activity and breast cancer risk, observed a risk reduction in breast cancer ranging from 23% to 65%. A dose-response relationship was found in 9 of 14 studies, which observed a risk reduction.

The prospective study by McTiernan et al. (2003), which included 74171 women, revealed the importance of body mass index. They found a reduced cancer risk with increasing levels of physical activity. However, this effect was not observed in women with a BMI of greater than 28,5.

Prostate cancer is another most commonly occurring cancer type worldwide. The evidence for an association between physical activity and its prevention is only classified as probable, because data of those studies were less consistent than that for colon and breast cancer. Currently, there are about 36 studies, which investigated the relationship between physical activity and prostate cancer risk (Friedenreich and Thune 2001; Friedenreich and Orenstein 2002; Lee 2003). Eighteen of the 36 studies found a risk reduction averaging from 10% to 30% for men, who were most physically active. Nine studies reported of no association between physical activity and prostate cancer risk. In contrast, 4 studies found an increasing risk. A recent study by Patel et al. (2005) pointed to the role of tumour grading as an important factor whether a tumour might be sensitive to an exercise stimulus or not. The authors could demonstrate among men enclosed in the American Cancer Society Cancer Prevention Study II Nutrition Cohort, that recreational physical activity was not effective in preventing the number of tumour cases. However, physical activity more than 35 metabolic equivalent task-hours per week lowered the risk of an aggressive prostate cancer.

Evidences for an association between physical activity and prevention from other cancer types were classified as possible (lung, endometrium) and insufficient (e.g. testis, ovary, kidney, pancreas, thyroid, and melanoma) (for details see: Friedenreich and Orenstein 2002; American Institute for Cancer Research Report on Physical Activity and Cancer 2005).

Finally, one study aimed to describe the association between leisure-time physical activity and incidence of cancer in the general population of Danish adult men and women (Schnohr et al. 2005). The six most frequent cancer types of both sexes were included in that analysis and incident cases were recorded during a follow-up period of 14 years. The authors concluded that there were no, or only weakly, inverse associations between physical activity in leisure-time and incidence of cancer. The only exception was for cancer of the ovary.

Together, it can be concluded that there is accumulating evidence for a positive effect of physical activity on cancer incidence, especially for colon and breast cancer. There are still contradictory results of the effect of physical activity on cancer prevention. However, it has to be admitted that only a minority of studies found an increased cancer risk with increasing physical activity levels (Polednak 1976; West et al. 1991; Pukkala et al. 1993; Dorgan et al. 1994; Cerhan et al. 1997; Sung et al. 1999). Methodological considerations seem to be the major problems for the inconsistencies. As reviewed by Friedenreich and Orenstein (2002) and commented by McTiernan et al. (1999) there are several aspects influencing research findings: a) Accurately/completely assessment of physical activity (e.g. type, frequency, duration, intensity, and activity levels the entire lifetime); b) Subgroup effects (racial and ethnic background, sex, age, energy intake, weight, body mass index, and level of athletic fitness); c) Confounding (Association of physical activity with other risk factors, like smoking, alcohol, weight maintenance, etc.); d) Type of studies (conduction of controlled clinical trials to examine specific biological mechanisms). Taken together, analysing the association between physical activity and cancer prevention should always consider the different variables mentioned above to get a detailed insight into the mechanisms.

Physical Activity during Cancer Post-Diagnosis

Although the mortality rates for various cancers are still high, the 5-year relative survival rate of all sites of cancers is at present 66% (American Cancer Society. Cancer Facts and Figures 2006). For some site-specific cancers the 5-year relative survival rate has improved markedly since the 1970s (prostate, breast, colon, rectum, and leukaemia).

The common modes of cancer therapy are surgery, radiation therapy, and systemic therapy. Systemic therapy can be subdivided into chemotherapy, hormone therapy and immunotherapy (biologic). The above mentioned therapies are given alone or to improve the therapy in combination. Beside their therapeutically effect, all this interventions have many side effect (see Table 2). These side effects have additionally effects on life of cancer survivors. For example, it is referred that fatigue is influencing life, respectively QoL, long time after the last cancer therapy. Consequently, cancer therapy with all its side effects has an intensive negative impact on mind, physiology and sociology of cancer survivors.

These facts (higher survival rate and side effects) has generated large interest and forced research effort to improve quality of life (QoL), to reduce the risk of recurrence, to extend survival and to reduce mortality, respectively.

Recently published reviews have evaluated studies on the association between physical activity/exercise during and after a cancer therapy (Courneya 2003; McTiernan 2004; Stevinson, Lawlor , Fox 2004; Galvao, Newton 2005; Humpel, Iverson 2005; Schmitz et al. 2005, Pinto, Trunzo 2005; McNeely et al. 2006; Kirshbaum 2006). It seems that physical activity/exercise has consistently beneficial effects on physiological and psychological aspects of cancer patients, e.g. QoL-improvement, fatigue, cardio-respiratory fitness, depression.

Table 2. Examples of side effects of various cancer therapies

Mode of therapy	Side effect
Surgery	Pain, infection, diarrhoea, loss of function, etc.
Radiotherapy	Pain, fatigue, diarrhoea, cardiomyopathy, etc.
Chemotherapy	Fatigue, anaemia, neutropenia, thrombocytopenia, etc.
Hormone therapy	Loss of muscle substance, fatigue, osteoporosis, etc.
Immunotherapy	Similar to chemotherapy

Recently published studies analyzed the influence of physical activity on recurrence and cancer-specific and overall mortality by prospective, observational studies on patients with stage III colon cancer and stage I to II colorectal cancer (Meyerhardt et al. 2006; Meyerhardt et al. 2006). They concluded that physical activity appears to reduce the risk of recurrence, cancer specific and overall mortality.

Other recently published studies analyzed the association between physical activity and survival rate or QoL in breast cancer patients (Holmes et al. 2005; Milne et al. 2007). Holmes et al. found that physical activity after a breast cancer diagnosis at any category of activity higher than the reference category of less than 3 metabolic equivalent task-hours per week lowered the risk of death from this disease. The maximal benefit occurred among women who performed moderate intensive physical activity with little evidence of increased benefit for vigorous exercise. Milne et al. analyzed the association between physical activity/weight loss and QoL and concluded from their results that physically active and healthy weight breast cancer survivors experienced a better QoL. The only variable that decreased the association between physical activity and QoL was age. They found that QoL was higher for women under age 65 who were physically active. In contrast, women over 65 who were also physically active experienced no change in their QoL. They recommend that patients after successful breast cancer therapy should undergo any exercise or weight loss interventions as early as possible in order to maintain QoL.

Recently performed studies on association between physical activity and QoL concerning different cancer types (endometrial, bladder, head and neck, and ovarian) concluded all that physical activity has a beneficial effect on QoL (Courneya et al. 2005; Rogers et al. 2006; Karvinen et al. 2007; Stevinson et al. 2007). Some of these studies, however, pointed to the fact that among cancer survivors only a few met public health physical activity guidelines. In contrast, it has to mention that most training guidelines for cancer patients and survivors, which are available in the literature, are not supported by experimental evidence. Humpel and Iverson (2005) demonstrated in their recent review that there is no direct specific evidence about which type, frequency, duration or intensity of exercise is most effective in cancer therapy and rehabilitation.

Physical Activity, Cancer and Murine Tumour Models

Animal tumour models, especially murine animals, are of high interest for understanding the various aspects of carcinogenesis, tumour progression, metastasis, and tumour angiogenesis. Especially they are a useful approach to investigate the underlying mechanisms how exercise might affect tumour initiation und development. These models include implanted, transplanted, and spontaneous, carcinogen (chemical, radiation) induced and genetically engineered tumours (Hoffmann-Goetz 2003; Heijstek, Kranenburg, Borel Rinkes 2005; Ottewell, Coleman, Holen 2006; Frese and Tuveson 2007).

Orthotopic implantation/injection means the implantation/injection of tumour cells into the same organ, respectively tissue, as their site of origin. This is of great advantage, because the tumour cells are embedded at a site of physiological similarity. Orthotopic transplantation can be used with human (xenogeneic) or animal (allogeneic) tumour cells and allows the analysis of the tumour growth and metastasis *in vivo* (Kobaek-Larsen et al. 2000; Bornmann et al. 2007). To date, to our knowledge there is no published study using an orthotopic model to analyse the association between exercise and tumour. The reason for this minor interest in orthotopic tumour models to analyse exercise-tumour interactions could be explained by the fact that immunodeficient mice are used. Those animals do not reject orthotopic implants, respectively transplants, of xenogeneic or allogeneic tumour cells, but are unable to respond in a normal immunological manner, because of their compromised cellular and humoral immunity. To solve this problem, syngeneic animals/models can be used. Those animals are without the limit of a compromised immune system. Syngeneic animals are genetically identical by inbreeding of many generations and therefore tolerate tumour transplants with the same genetic background. In contrast to orthotopic models, syngeneic models are limited to animal tumour cells and the insights are therefore less transferable to human situations. Genetic tumour models concern transgenic or knock-out murine animals. Genetically predisposed animals enable the analysis of gene-environment interactions, e.g. exercise, and other factors such as gender, age. The most frequently used tumour model in research on exercise and cancer are the carcinogen induced tumours, especially chemically induced, e.g. azoxymethane (AOM), dimethylhydrazine (DMH), and N-methy-N-nitrosourea (NMU). Incidence, organ-specific site of tumour formation and type of tumour depend on several aspects, in particular route, time, dose, duration and frequency of administration, and age, sex and genetic background (strain).

A number of studies analyzed the influence of exercise on several aspects of cancer development using chemically induced, allogeneic and syngeneic tumour models (Baracos 1989; Thompson et al. 1995; Zielinski et al. 2004; Murphy et al. 2004). All studies reported consistently an inhibitory effect of exercise on tumour growth, while the results lack clarity about the exercise intensity needed. The exercise protocols used included swimming and running on a treadmill at low (~35% VO_{2max}) and high (~80%-100% VO_{2max}) intensities, particularly until exhaustion. Some results suggested that exercise has to be performed at high intensities to achieve an inhibitory effect on tumour growth and metastasis. In contrast, the study of Westerlind et al. (2003) analyzed the effect of moderate exercise training on mammary tumour development in adolescent rats using a chemically induced tumour model. They reported that moderate exercise training was also effective to increase tumour latency and to delay tumour growth.

Davis et al. (1998) used a syngeneic tumour model in order to determine whether an acute bout of exercise is able to affect pulmonary metastasis. Furthermore they addressed the effect of exercise intensity by comparing moderate intensity (~ 55%-65% of maximal performance) against exhaustive exercise. The mean exercise intensity during exhaustive trial was estimated to be around 75% of maximal performance and lead to a decreased number of tumour metastasis compared to both control sedentary conditions and to short-time exercise conditions at moderate intensity.

Some studies used genetic predisposed mice. In detail a mutation in the *adenomatous polyposis coli* (*Apc*) gene was investigated, which results in the production of multiple intestine adenomas (Colbert et al. 2000; Mehl et al. 2005; Moser, Pitot, and Dove 1990). In these studies heterozygous mice of both sexes for the *Apc* gene were used. Both studies used nearly the same exercise treadmill protocol with a moderate intensity estimated to be 55%-65% of maximal oxygen uptake (VO_{2max}) (Taylor 1987), while Mehl et al. used also a voluntary free wheel exercise approach. In this model mice have 24 hours access to a wheel, which serves as a model for enhanced physical activity. Colbert et al. reported a sex-specific effect of exercise on polyp number, which was observed only in male mice, but was not statistical significant. Similarly, Mehl et al. observed that treadmill exercise had a significantly reducing effect on polyp number and size in male mice. However, free wheel running had no effect.

Other recently published studies used UVB-light to induce tumour models using SKH-1 mice (Michna et al. 2006; Lu et al. 2006). Both studies used voluntary free wheel running as an exercise model and found that exercise decreased UVB-light induced tumours and carcinogenesis, respectively.

A recently published study analysed for the first time whether exercise modulates the antitumor efficacy of a chemotherapeutic agent (Doxorubicin) on breast cancer (Jones et al. 2005). Athymic nu/nu female mice were subcutaneously (s.c.) implanted with human MDA-MB-231 breast carcinoma xenografts. The used exercise protocol was a progressive treadmill running, in which the intensity corresponded at last to 70% to 75% of murine maximal oxygen uptake (VO_{2max}). They reported that tumour growth delay was significantly prolonged in the doxorubicin-only and exercise + doxorubicin groups compared with exercise-only and control groups. But, exercise in combination with the chemotherapeutic agent had no additional effect on tumour dormancy compared to doxorubicin-only. As they discussed, a number of differences limit the extrapolation on human situation, e.g. using of immature and athymic mice and s.c. implantation rather than orthotopic.

In summary, the results of the animal studies support the view of an anti-cancerous effect of exercise and physical activity. However, it seems noteworthy to analyze more systematically and in more detail the different parameters (intensity, frequency, duration) of exercise and their effect on cancer development, especially for different cancer types. As mentioned above, minor differences in exercise protocols can lead to partially different results. Beside these more descriptive approaches more studies are desirable which try to understand the underlying biological mechanisms of the exercise effects.

Perspectives

The above chapter tried to summarize what is currently known about the effects of exercise on stem cells on the one hand and on cancer development on the other hand. About the effects of exercise on cancer stem cells we can only speculate at the moment because as far as we know there are no studies available on this topic. However, two aspects of exercise seemed worth to be highlighted – the role of exercise in cell turnover and in inflammation. There is growing evidence that the maturation arrest of tissue-based stem cells is closely linked to the development of not only teratocarcinomas and haematological malignancies, but also carcinomas. In the pathophysiological cascade chronic inflammation seems to be a major mechanism for the promotion of certain tumours, such as primary liver tumours or gastric cancer. A milieu rich of inflammatory cells and their secreted mediators appears therefore critical for tumour progression in some cases (Alison et al. 2007). Interestingly, exercise has profound anti-inflammatory effects as indicated by both cross-sectional and longitudinal studies. Serum levels of inflammatory mediators such as TNF-alpha and C-reactive protein are inversely correlated with the levels of physical activity and fitness (Ford 2002). Until now the anti-inflammatory role of exercise has been studied primarily with regard to chronic vascular diseases and insulin resistance. Whether this effect may be operative during tumour progression as well remains to be shown.

Finally, the exercise stimulus seems to have profound effects on cell turnover as indicated by enhanced proliferation and apoptosis rates. Unfortunately, this has been shown so far only for immune cells and not for other cell types. Lymphocytes of trained athletes showed greater proliferation rates than lymphocytes of sedentary controls (Nieman et al. 1993). In breast cancer patients the mitogen-induced proliferation of lymphocytes was enhanced after a 6-week training programme compared to sedentary controls (Hutnick et al. 2005). In addition, we could show that lymphocyte basal apoptosis rates of high-performance athletes were enhanced in comparison to less well trained runners (Mooren et al. 2004). These preliminary data suggest that exercise might stimulate cell turnover which is crucial for adult tissue regenerative capacity. Enhanced cell turnover, however, should result in a reduced maturation time giving potential carcinogenic agents only limited time to induce genetic alterations which are a necessary prerequisite for the maturation arrest. However, this is only one possible hypothesis which needs much more experimental evidence. Together, our reviewed data suggest impressively that exercise and physical activity are an important and necessary stimulus with crucial consequences also for stem cell mobilization and development of malignant diseases.

References

Adams V, Lenk K, Linke A, Lenz D, Erbs S, Sandri M, Tarnok A, Gielen S, Emmrich F, Schuler G, Hambrecht R. 2004. Increase of circulating endothelial progenitor cells in patients with coronary artery disease after exercise-induced ischemia. *Arterioscler Thromb. Vasc. Biol.* 24(4):684-90.

Aicher A, Heeschen C, Mildner-Rihm C, Urbich C, Ihling C, Technau-Ihling K, Zeiher AM, Dimmeler S. 2003. Essential role of endothelial nitric oxide synthase for mobilization of stem and progenitor cells. *Nat. Med.*9(11):1370-6. Epub 2003 Oct 12.

Alison MR, Murphy G, Leedham S. 2007. Stem cells and cancer: a deadly mix. *Cell Tissue Res.* 16; [Epub ahead of print].

Assmus B, Schächinger V, Teupe C, Britten M, Lehmann R, Döbert N, Grünwald F, Aicher A, Urbich C, Martin H, Hoelzer D, Dimmeler S, Zeiher AM. 2002. Transplantation of Progenitor Cells and Regeneration Enhancement in Acute Myocardial Infarction (TOPCARE-AMI). *Circulation.* 10;106(24):3009-17.

Baracos V.E. 1989. Exercise inhibits progressive growth of the Morris hepatoma 7777 in male and female rats. *Can. J. Physiol. Pharmacol.* 67:864-870.

Bischoff R, Heintz C.Enhancement of skeletal muscle regeneration. *Dev. Dyn.* 1994 Sep;201(1):41-54.

Bonsignore MR, Morici G, Santoro A, Pagano M, Cascio L, Bonanno A, Abate P, Mirabella F, Profita M, Insalaco G, Gioia M, Vignola AM, Majolino I, Testa U, Hogg JC. 2002. Circulating hematopoietic progenitor cells in runners. *J. Appl. Physiol.* 93(5):1691-7.

Bornmann C., Graeser R., Esser N., Ziroli V., Jantscheff P., Keck T., Unger C., Hopt U.T., Adam U., Schaechtele C., Massing U., von Dobschuetz E. 2007. A new liposomal formulation of Gemcitabine is active in an orthotopic mouse model of pancreatic cancer accessible to bioluminescence imaging. *Cancer Chemother Pharmacol.* in press.

Cerhan J.R., Torner J.C., Lynch C.F., Rubenstein L.M., Lemke J.H., Cohen M.B., Lubaroff D.M., and Wallace R.B. 1997. Association of smoking, body mass, and physical activity with risk of prostate cancer in the Iowa 65+ Rural Health Study (United States). *Cancer Causes Control.* 8:229-238.

Cherry T. 1922. A theory of cancer. *Med. J. Aust.* 1:425-438.

Colbert L.H., Davis J.M., Essig D.A., Ghaffar A., and Mayer E.P. 2000. Exercise and tumor development in a mouse predisposed to multiple intestinal adenomas. *Med. Sci. Sports Exerc.* 32:1704-1708.

Cornelison DD, Wold BJ. 1997. Single-cell analysis of regulatory gene expression in quiescent and activated mouse skeletal muscle satellite cells. *Dev. Biol.* 15;191(2):270-83.

Courneya K.S. 2003. Exercise in Cancer Survivors: An Overview of Research. *Med. Sci. Sports Exerc.* 35:1846-1852.

Courneya K.S., Friedenreich C.M. 2001. Framework PEACE: an organizational model for examining physical exercise across the cancer experience. *Ann. Behav. Med.* 23:263-72.

Courneya K.S., Karvinen K.H., Campbell K.L., Pearcey R.G., Dundas G., Capstick V., Tonkin K.S. 2005. Associations among exercise, body weight, and quality of life in a population-based sample of endometrial cancer survivors. *Gynecologic Oncology.* 97:422-430.

Custodis F, Laufs U. Physical exercise and endothelial progenitor cells. 2007. *J. Cardiopulm. Rehabil. Prev.* 27(2):74-5.

Davis J.M., Kohut M.L., Jackson D.A., Colbert L.H., Mayer E.P., and Ghaffar A. 1998. Exercise effects on lung tumor metastases and in vitro alveolar macrophage antitumor cytotoxicity. *Am. J. Physiol.* 43:R1454-R1459.

Dimmeler S, Aicher A, Vasa M, Mildner-Rihm C, Adler K, Tiemann M, Rutten H, Fichtlscherer S, Martin H, Zeiher AM.2001. HMG-CoA reductase inhibitors (statins) increase endothelial progenitor cells via the PI 3-kinase/Akt pathway. *J. Clin. Invest.* 108(3):391-7.

Dorgan J.F., Brown C., Barrett M., Splansky G.L., Kreger B.E., D'Agostino R.B., Albanes D., and Schatzkin A. 1994. Physical activity and risk of breast cancer in the Framingham Heart Study. *Am. J. Epidemiol.* 139:662-669.

Ford ES. 2002. Does exercise reduce inflammation? Physical activity and C-reactive protein among U.S. adults. *Epidemiology.* 13(5):561-8.

Frese K.K. and Tuveson D.A. 2007. Maximizing mouse cancer models. *Nature Reviews Cancer.* 7:645-658.

Friedenreich C.M. and Orenstein M.R. 2002. Physical Activity and Cancer Prevention: Etiologic Evidence and Biological Mechanisms. *J. Nutr.* 132:3456S-3464S.

Friedenreich C.M., and Thune I. 2001. A review of physical activity and prostate cancer. *Cancer Causes Control.* 12:461-475.

Fukai T, Siegfried MR, Ushio-Fukai M, Cheng Y, Kojda G, Harrison DG. 2000. Regulation of the vascular extracellular superoxide dismutase by nitric oxide and exercise training. *J. Clin. Invest* 105(11):1631-9.

Galvao D.A., Newton R.U. 2005. Review of exercise intervention studies in cancer patients. *J. Clin. Oncol.* 23:899-909.

Heijstek M.W., Kranenburg O., Borel Rinkes I.H.M. 2005. Mouse Models of Colorectal Cancer and Liver Metastases. *Dig. Surg.* 22:16-25.

Heissig, B., K. Hattori, S. Dias, et al. 2002. Recruitment of stem and progenitor cells from the bone marrow niche requires MMP-9 mediated release of kit-ligand. *Cell* 109: 625-637.

Hellsten Y, Richter EA, Kiens B, Bangsbo J. 1999. AMP deamination and purine exchange in human skeletal muscle during and after intense exercise. *J. Physiol.* 1;520 Pt 3:909.

Hoffman-Goetz L. 2003. Physical Activity and Cancer Prevention: Animal-Tumor Models. *Med. Sci. Sport Exerc.* 35:1828-1833.

Holmes M.D., Chen W.Y., Feskanich D., Kroenke C.H., Colditz G.A. 2005. Physical Activity and Survival After Breast Cancer Diagnosis. *JAMA.* 293:2479-2486.

Hu Y, Davison F, Zhang Z, Xu Q. 2003. Endothelial replacement and angiogenesis in arteriosclerotic lesions of allografts are contributed by circulating progenitor cells. *Circulation.* 23;108(25):3122-7.

Humpel N., Iverson D.C. 2005. Review and critique of the quality of exercise recommendations for cancer patients and survivors. *Support Care Cancer.*13:493-502.

Hutnick NA, Williams NI, Kraemer WJ, Orsega-Smith E, Dixon RH, Bleznak AD, Mastro AM. 2005. Exercise and lymphocyte activation following chemotherapy for breast cancer. *Med. Sci. Sports Exerc.* 37(11):1827-35.

Ikebuchi K, Ihle JN, Hirai Y, Wong GG, Clark SC, Ogawa M. 2007. Synergistic factors for stem cell proliferation: further studies of the target stem cells and the mechanism of stimulation by interleukin-1, interleukin-6, and granulocyte colony-stimulating factor. *Blood.* 72(6):2007-14.

Irintchev A, Zeschnigk M, Starzinski-Powitz A, Wernig A. 1994. Expression pattern of M-cadherin in normal, denervated, and regenerating mouse muscles. *Dev. Dyn.* 199(4):326-37.

Jones L.W., Eves N.D., Courneya K.S., Chiu B.K., Baracos V.E., Hanson J., Johnson L., and Mackey J.R. 2005. Effects of exercise training on antitumor efficacy of doxorubicin in MDA-MB-231 breast cancer xenografts. *Clin. Cancer Res.* 11:6695-6698.

Kadi F, Thornell LE. 1999. Training affects myosin heavy chain phenotype in the trapezius muscle of women. *Histochem. Cell Biol.* 112(1):73-8.

Karvinen K.H., Courneya C.S., North S., and Venner P. 2007. Associations between exercise and quality of life in bladder cancer survivors: a population-based study. *Cancer Epidemiol. Biomarkers Prev.* 16:984-990.

Kirshbaum M.N. 2006. A review of the benefits of whole body exercise during and after treatment for breast cancer. *Journal of Clinical Nursing.* 16:104-121.

Kobaek-Larsen M., Thorup I., Diederichsen A., Fenger C., and Hoitinga M.R. 2000. Review of colorectal cancer and its metastases in rodent models: comparative aspects with those in humans. *Comp. Med.* 50:16-26.

Kojda G, Cheng YC, Burchfield J, Harrison DG. 2001. Dysfunctional regulation of endothelial nitric oxide synthase (eNOS) expression in response to exercise in mice lacking one eNOS gene. *Circulation*. 12;103(23):2839-44.

Kraemer WJ, Ratamess NA, French DN. 2002. Resistance training for health and performance. *Curr. Sports Med. Rep*. 1(3):165-71.

Laufs U, Urhausen A, Werner N, Scharhag J, Heitz A, Kissner G, Böhm M, Kindermann W, Nickenig G.. 2005. Running exercise of different duration and intensity: effect on endothelial progenitor cells in healthy subjects. *Eur. J. Cardiovasc. Prev. Rehabil.* 12(4):407-14.

Laufs U, Werner N, Link A, Endres M, Wassmann S, Jurgens K, Miche E, Bohm M, Nickenig G. 2004. Physical training increases endothelial progenitor cells, inhibits neointima formation, and enhances angiogenesis. *Circulation*. 109(2):220-6. Epub 2003 Dec 22.

Lee I-Min. 2003. *Physical Activity and Cancer prevention – Data from Epidemiological Studies*. 35:1823-1827.

Lescaudron L, Peltékian E, Fontaine-Pérus J, Paulin D, Zampieri M, Garcia L, Parrish E. 1999. Blood borne macrophages are essential for the triggering of muscle regeneration following muscle transplant. *Neuromuscul. Disord.* 9(2):72-80.

Lu Y.-P., Lou Y.-R., Nolan B., Peng Q.-Y., Xie J.-G., Wagner G.C., and Conney A.H. 2006. Stimulatory effect of voluntary exercise or fat removal (partial lipectomy) on apoptosis in the skin of UVB light-irradiated mice. *PNAS*. 103:16301-16306.

Mai P.L., Sullivan-Halley J., Ursin G., Stram D.O., Deapen D., Villaluna D., Horn-Ross P.L., Clarke C.A., Reynolds P., Ross R.K., West D.W., Anton-Culver H., Ziogas A., and Bernstein L. 2007. Physical Activity and Colon Cancer Risk among Women in the California Teachers Study. *Cancer Epidemiol. Biomarkers Prev*. 16:517-525.

Mars M, Govender S, Weston A, Naicker V, Chuturgoon A. 1998. High intensity exercise: a cause of lymphocyte apoptosis? *Biochem. Biophys. Res. Commun*. 19;249(2):366-70.

McNeely M.L., Campbell K.L., Rowe B.H., Klassen T.P., Mackey J.R., Courneya K.S. 2006. Effects of exercise on breast cancer patients and survivors: a systematic review and meta-analysis. *CMAJ*. 175:34-41.

McTiernan A. 2004. Physical activity after cancer: physiologic outcomes. *Cancer Invest*. 22:68-81.

McTiernan A., Kooperberg C., White E. et al. 2003. Recreational physical activity and the risk of breast cancer in postmenopausal women. The Women's Health Initiative Cohort Study. *JAMA*. 290:1331-1336.

McTiernan A., Schwartz R.S., Potter J., and Bowen D. 1999. Exercise Clinical Trials in Cancer Prevention Research: A Call to Action. *Cancer EpidemiolBiomarkers Prev*. 8:201-207.

Mehl K.A., Davis J.M., Clements J.M., Berger F.G., Pena M.M., and Carson J.A. 2005. Decreased intestinal polyp multiplicity is related to exercise mode and gender in ApcMin/+ mice. *J. Appl. Physiol*. 98:2219-2225.

Meyerhardt J.A., Giovannucci E.L., Holmes M.D., Chan A.T., Chan J.A., Colditz G.A., and Fuchs C.S. 2006. Physical Activity and Survival After Colorectal Cancer Diagnosis. *J. Clin. Oncol*. 24:3527-3534.

Meyerhardt J.A., Heseltine D., Niedzwiecki D., Hollis D., Saltz L.B., Mayer R.J., Thomas J., Nelson H., Whittom R., Hantel A., Schilsky R.L., and Fuchs C.S. 2006. Impact of Physical Activity on Cancer Recurrence and Survival in Patients With Stage III Colon Cancer: Findings From CALGB 89803. *J. Clin. Oncol.* 24:3535-3541.

Michna L., Wagner G.C., Lou Y.-R., Xie J.G., Peng Q.-Y., Lin Y., Carlson K., Shih W.J., Conney A.H., and Lu Y.-P. 2006. Inhibitory effects of voluntary running wheel exercise on UVB-induced skin carcinogenesis in SKH-1 mice. *Carcinogenesis.* 27:2108-2115.

Milne H.M., Gordon S., Guilfoyle A., Wallman K.E., and Courneya K.S. 2007. Association between physical activity and quality of life among Western Australian breast cancer survivors. *Psycho-Oncology.* in press.

Monninkhof E.M., Ellias S.G., Vlems F.A., van der Tweel I., Jantine Schuit A., Voskuil D.W., and van Leeuwen F.E. 2007. Physical Activity and Breast Cancer: A Systematic Review. *Epidemiology.* 18:137-157.

Mooren FC, Blöming D, Lechtermann A, Lerch MM, Völker K. 2002. Lymphocyte apoptosis after exhaustive and moderate exercise. *J. Appl. Physiol.* 93(1):147-53.

Mooren FC, Lechtermann A, Völker K. 2004. Exercise-induced apoptosis of lymphocytes depends on training status. *Med. Sci. Sports Exerc.* 36(9):1476-83.

Morici G, Zangla D, Santoro A, Pelosi E, Petrucci E, Gioia M, Bonanno A, Profita M, Bellia V, Testa U, Bonsignore MR. 2005. Supramaximal exercise mobilizes haematopoietic progenitors and reticulocytes in athletes. *Am. J. Physiol. Regul. Integr. Comp. Physiol.* 2005 Jul 14.

Moser A.R., Pitot H.C., and Dove W.F. 1990. A dominant mutation that predisposes to multiple intestinal neoplasia in the mouse. *Science.* 247:322-324.

Murphy E.A., Davis J.M., Brown A.S., Carmichael M.D., Mayer E.P., and Ghaffar A. 2004. Effects of moderate exerfcise and oat β-glucan on lung tumor metastases and macrophage antitumor cytotoxicity. *J. Appl. Physiol.* 97:955-959.

Nieman DC, Henson DA, Gusewitch G, Warren BJ, Dotson RC, Butterworth DE, Nehlsen-Cannarella SL. 1993. Physical activity and immune function in elderly women. *Med. Sci. Sports Exerc.* 25(7):823-31.

Nickenig G. 2005. Running exercise of different duration and intensity: effect on endothelial progenitor cells in healthy subjects. *Eur. J. Cardiovasc Prev. Rehabil.* 12(4):407-414.

Ottewell P.D., Coleman R.E., Hilen I. 2006. From genetic abnormality to metastases: murine models of breast cancer and their use in the development of anticancer therapies. 96:101-13.

Patel A.V., Rodriguez C., Jacobs E.J., Solomon L., Thun M.J., and Calle E.E. 2005. Recreational Physical Activity and Risk of Prostate Cancer in a Large Cohort of U.S. Men. *Cancer Epidemiol. Biomarkers Prev.* 14:275-279.

Pinto B.M., Trunzo J.J. 2005. Health Behaviour during and after a Cancer Diagnosis. *Cancer.* 104(11 Suppl):2614-23.

Polednak A.P. 1976. College athletics, body size, and cancer mortality. *Cancer.* 38:382-387.

Pukkala E., Poskiparta M., Apter D., and Vihko V. 1993. Life-long physical activity and cancer risk among Finish female teachers. *Eur. J. Cancer Prev.* 2:369-376.

Rehman J, Li J, Parvathaneni L, Karlsson G, Panchal VR, Temm CJ, Mahenthiran J, March KL.2004. Exercise acutely increases circulating endothelial progenitor cells and monocyte-/macrophage-derived angiogenic cells. *J. Am. Coll Cardiol.* 16;43(12):2314-8.

Rogers L.Q., Courneya K.S., Robbins K.T., Malone J., Seiz A., Koch L., Rao K., Nagarkar M. 2006. Physical activity and quality of life in head and neck cancer survivors. *Support Care Cancer.* 14:1012-1019.

Samad A.K.A., Taylor R.S., Marshall T., and Chapman M.A.S. 2005. A meta-analysis of the association of physical activity with reduced risk of colorectal cancer. *Colorectal Dis.* 7:204-213.

Sandri M, Adams V, Gielen S, Linke A, Lenk K, Krankel N, Lenz D, Erbs S, Scheinert D, Mohr FW, Schuler G, Hambrecht R. 2005. Effects of exercise and ischemia on mobilization and functional activation of blood-derived progenitor cells in patients with ischemic syndromes: results of 3 randomized studies. *Circulation.* 28;111(25):3391-9. Epub 2005 Jun 13.

Schmitz K.H., Holtzman J., Courneya K.S., Masse L.C., Duval S., and Kane R. 2005. Controlled Physical Activity Trials in Cancer Survivors: A Systematic Review and Meta-analysis. *Cancer Epidemiol. Biomarkers Prev.* 14:1588-1595.

Schnohr P., Gronbaek M., Petersen L., Hein H.O. and Sorensen T. IA. 2005. Physical activity in leisure-time and risk of cancer: 14-year follow-up of 28,000 Danish men and women. *Scandinavian Journal of Public Health.* 33:244-249.

Schultz E, Jaryszak DL. 1985. Effects of skeletal muscle regeneration on the proliferation potential of satellite cells. *Mech. Ageing Dev.* 30(1):63-72.

Schultz E, McCormick KM. 1994. Skeletal muscle satellite cells. *Rev. Physiol. Biochem. Pharmacol.* 123:213-57. Review.

Sivertsen I. and Dahlstrom A.W. 1922. The relation of muscular activity to carcinoma: a prelimanary report. *J. Cancer Res.* 6:365-378.

Steiner S, Niessner A, Ziegler S, Richter B, Seidinger D, Pleiner J, Penka M, Wolzt M, Huber K, Wojta J, Minar E and Kopp CW. 2005. Endurance training increases the number of endothelial progenitor cells in patients with cardiovascular risk and coronary artery disease. *Atherosclerosis* 181: 305-310.

Stevinson C., Faught W., Steed H., Tonkin K., Ladha A.B., Vallance J.K., Capstick V., Hepansky A., Courneya K.S. 2007. Associations between physical activity and quality of life in ovarian cancer survivors. *Gynecologic Oncology.* 106:244-250.

Stevinson C., Lawlor D.A. and Fox K.R. 2004. Exercise interventions for cancer patients: systematic review of controlled trials. *Cancer Causes and Control.* 15:1035-1056.

Sung J.F., Lin R.S., Pu Y.S., Chen Y.C., Chang H.C., and Lai M.K. 1999. Risk factors for prostate carcinoma in Taiwan: a case-control study in a Chinese population. *Cancer.* 86:484-491.

Taylor C.R. 1987. Structural and functional limits to oxidative metabolism: insights from scaling. *Annu. Rev. Physiol.* 49:135-146.

Thijssen DH, Vos JB, Verseyden C, van Zonneveld AJ, Smits P, Sweep FC, Hopman MT, de Boer HC. 2006. Haematopoietic stem cells and endothelial progenitor cells in healthy men: effect of aging and training. *Aging Cell.* 5(6):495-503.

Thompson H.J., Westerlind K.C., Snedden J.R., Briggs S., Singh M. 1995. Inhibition of mammary carcinogenesis by treadmill exercise. *J. Natl. Cancer Inst.* 87:453-455.

Tidball JG. 2005. Inflammatory processes in muscle injury and repair. *Am. J. Physiol. Regul. Integr. Comp. Physiol.* 288(2):R345-53. Review.

Toigo M, Boutellier U. 2006. New fundamental resistance exercise determinants of molecular and cellular muscle adaptations. *Eur. J. Appl. Physiol.* 97(6):643-63.

Werner N, Wassmann S, Ahlers P, Schiegl T, Kosiol S, Link A, Walenta K, Nickenig G. 2007. Endothelial progenitor cells correlate with endothelial function in patients with coronary artery disease. *Basic Res. Cardiol.* 102(6):565-71.

West D.W., Slattery M.L., Robison L.M., French T.K., and Mahoney A.W. 1991. Adult dietary intake and prostate cancer risk in Utah: a case-control study with special emphasis on aggressive tumors. *Cancer Causes Control.* 2:85-94.

Westerlind K.C., McCarty H.L., Schultheiss P.C., Story R., Reed A.H., Baier M.L., and Strange R. 2003. Moderate exercise training slows mammary tumor growth in adolescent rats. *European Journal of Cancer Prevention.* 12:281-287.

Zielinski M.R., Muenchow M., Wallig M.A., Horn P.L., and Woods J.A. 2004. Exercise delays allogeneic tumor growth and reduces intratumoral inflammation and vascularization. *J. Appl. Physiol.* 96:2249-2256.

In: Cancer and Stem Cells
Eds: Thomas Dittmar and Kurt S. Zänker
ISBN 978-1-60456-478-5

Chapter 9

Human Adult Stem Cells as Targets for Cancer Stem Cells: Evolution; Oct-4 Gene and Cell-to-Cell Communication

James E. Trosko *

Center for Integrative Toxicology, National Food Safety Toxicology Center
Dept. Pediatrics and Human Development, College of Human Medicine,
Michigan State University, East Lansing, Michigan

Abstract

To examine the factors involving human carcinogenesis in order to design new strategies for prevention and treatment, a new approach from the current reductionalistic molecular oncological view will have to be made. In addition, this view must take into account both biological and cultural evolutionary factors that interact with the biology of the pathogenesis of cancer. An integrated hypothesis that links many incomplete hypotheses, such as the stem cell or de-differentiation theories of cancer, the multi-stage, multi-mechanism or "initiation/promotion/progression" theory, the mutation and epigenetic theories of carcinogenesis, and the "cancer stem cells" hypothesis, has been outlined. The emergence of somatic and germ-line stem cells during the biological evolution of the multi-cellular organism created new functions to regulate, homeostatically, phenotypes such as growth control, differentiation, apoptosis, senescence and adaptive functions of terminally differentiated cells. The evidence supporting the stem cells as target cells for the initiation process was reviewed. The biological consequence of the initiation of an adult stem cell appears to be the inhibition of asymmetric cell division, or the blockage of "mortalization" of a normal "immortal" stem cell, not the "immortalization" of a normal, "mortal" cell. Promotion, functionally, is the clonal expansion of initiated stem cells by both mitogenesis and the inhibition of apoptosis. These promoting conditions occur during wound healing, compensatory

* E-Mail: james.trosko@ht.msu.edu

hyperplasia after cell death, chronic inflammation, growth factors and by many dietary and environmental, non-mutagenic chemicals. All of these promoting conditions inhibit cell-cell communication either by disruption of gap junctions in progenitor cells or by interfering with secreted negative growth regulator-receptor signalling in cells not having functional gap junctions, thereby releasing initiated stem cells from mitotic inhibition. Tumor promoters are characterized by threshold levels, exposing the initiated cells for regular and long periods of time in the absence of anti-promoters and having species, gender, cell-type specificities. The normal stem cell appears to give rise to the initiated stem cell which ultimately can accrue all the phenotypes of an invasive, metastatic "cancer stem cell". As the tumor grows, some of these cancer stem cells can partially differentiate to become cancer "non-stem cells". Finally, to understand how cultural evolution affects the human cancer patterns, domestication of certain animals helped to change dietary habits which can influence the carcinogenic process. These dietary factors can influence the adult stem cells in utero and postnatally, so as to either increase or decrease the risk to cancer by altering the stem cell pools and by increasing or decreasing the promotion of the initiated stem cells.

"Nothing in biology makes sense except in the light of evolution."
T. Dobzansky [1]

Introduction: The Complexicity of a Complicated Disease; The Interaction of Biological and Cultural Evolutionary Factors

The use of this quote by Theodosius Dobzhansky was done with a specific intent, namely, that in any attempt to understand carcinogenesis in human beings, outside the process of both biological and cultural evolution, will always come up with incomplete explanations. This review will attempt to provide some newer insights to this extremely complex disease. It should also be stated up front that "cancer" is not a single disease but multiple diseases that share several phenotypes or "hallmarks of cancer" [2]. Indeed, each cancer will be characterized by different phenotypes and genotypes within the tumor itself, due to both genetic and epigenetic instability as the tumor progresses.

Given this reality, one might wonder if any meaningful prevention and treatment strategies can be developed, not only for specific types of cancer (e.g., lung, prostate, colon), but, also, for different individuals with the same diagnosed cancer that shares the same 6 "hallmarks of cancer". This brings to mind a story of Albert Einstein' remark to a reporter who heard him gave a public lecture on his new theory of relativity. After his talk, this young reporter asked, "Professor Einstein, now that you physicists understand the workings of the universe, don't you think it's *complicated?* Einstein looked at the reporter and responded by saying, "Young man, if you *know nothing* of the universe, it is, indeed, *very complicated!* However, when you *begin to understand* it, it is *merely complex!*"

The goal of this overview *Commentary* is to try to integrate a number of well-known hypotheses of carcinogenesis (e.g., the stem cell versus the de-differentiation hypotheses, the multi-stage, multi-mechanism or "initiation, promotion, progression hypothesis; mutation versus epigenetic theories; oncogene- tumor suppression gene hypothesis of carcinogenesis). The attempt will, hopefully, demonstrate that this complicated carcinogenic process is "merely" complex. However, even with this incomplete understanding, new improved strategies can be made to prevent and treat the various cancers. Hopefully, unlike the old Indian fable of the six blind men who tried to describe the whole elephant, from which they only touched one part, medical science will at least try to integrate the different parts from various individual views in order to get a more realistic view of carcinogenesis.

No One Appendage Describes an Elephant, Nor Does Only One Thing Cause Cancer!

From early Greek observations to *Percival Pott's* observation on the relationship of soot to scrotal cancers in chimney sweepers and to the recent "discovery" of "cancer stem cells" [3], fundamental observations for hundreds of years have been made that give some insight into the factors influencing this whole animal/human biological process. However, the embryologists, pathologists, physiologists, biochemists, and molecular biologists saw cancers within the prisms of their reductionalistic training. The explosion of reductionalistic data being produced today, unfortunately, has no integrated framework on to which these data can be meaningfully interpreted. Because of the "success" of modern molecular oncology, with the discovery of oncogenes and tumor suppressor genes, many of the old observations and insights concerning the whole animal process of carcinogenesis have been ignored. The very idea that understanding the sequence of the human DNA will give us the "answer" to why we get cancer and how we can "cure" it, sounds much like the old fable of the 6 blind man.

In the field of embryology, Markert saw cancer as some developmental process that had been interfered with ("Cancer as a disease of differentiation") [4]. The following quote from one of his papers describes, beautifully, his perspective that has much relevance to our current understanding [5].

> "Cells interact and communicate during embryonic development and through inductive stimuli mutually direct the divergent courses of their differentiation. Very little cell differentiation is truly autonomous in vertebrate organisms. The myriad cell phenotypes present in mammals, for example, must reflect a corresponding complexity in the timing, nature, and amount of inductive interactions. Whatever the nature of inductive stimuli may be, they emerge as a consequence of specific sequential interactions of cells during embryonic development.
>
> The first embryonic cells, blastomeres, of mice and other mammals are all totipotent. During cleavage and early morphologenesis these cells come to occupy different positions in the three-dimensional embryo. Some cells are on the outside, some inside. The different environments of these cells cause the cells to express different patterns of metabolism in accordance with their own developing programs of gene function. These patterns of metabolism create new chemical environments for nearby cells and these changed environments induce yet new programs of gene function in responding cells. Thus a progressive series of reciprocal interactions is established between the cellular environment and the genome of each cell. These interactions drive the cell along a specific path of differentiation until a stable equilibrium is reached in the adult.

> Thereafter little change occurs in the specialized cells and they become remarkably refractory to changes in the environment. They seem stably locked into the terminal patterns of gene function characteristic of adult cells. The genome seems no longer responsible to the signals that were effective earlier in development.
> Of course, changes can occur in adult cells that lead to renewed cell proliferation and altered differentiation as seen in neoplasms, both benign and malignant, but such changes are very rare indeed when one considers the number of cells potentially available for neoplastic transformation. Possibly, mutations in regulatory DNA of dividing adult cells can occasionally lead to new and highly effective programs gene function that we recognize as neoplastic or malignant. However, most genetic changes in adult cells can probably lead to cell death since random changes in patterns of gene activity are not likely to be beneficial."

Pierce, also, saw carcinogenesis as a defect in the differentiation of stem cells ("Cancer as a stem cell disease) [6]. After examining many hundreds of Morris hepatomas, Van R. Potter proposed the concept of "oncogeny as partially blocked ontogeny" [7]. It should be noted that while these scientists did not have individual stem cells on which to study the process of carcinogenesis, the concept of stem cells was sufficient to explain both the processes of development and carcinogenesis. It should be noted that the operational definition of an embryonic stem cell of today is that they will form teratomas when placed back into an adult animal. Ironically, both embryologists and stem cell researchers use this observation of the cancer field as a criterion of stemness.

When it was shown that all the cells within a tumor were clonally- derived, it provided even more experimental evidence of the role of stem cells and differentiation in carcinogenesis. It might seem a bit conflicting that, while all the cells within a tumor are genotyically and phenotypically unique [8], they were all derivatives of a single stem cell. The concept of genomic and epigenomic instability of the carcinogenic process was created to explain this apparent dilemma [9, 10]. It must be pointed out, however, the idea that genomic and epigenomic stability is the "cause" of cancer has to be tempered with the possibility that these might be the consequence of a cell becoming a cancer cell, rather that the instability being the "cause" of cancer". Regardless of the ultimate resolution of this academic problem, this heterogeneity has been, and will continue to be, a major problem for prevention and treatment of cancer. That this is the case, for each tumor and each cell within that tumor, a different intracellular physiology, generated by different gene expressions and genetic abnormalities, poses a problem for treatment strategies.

From Single Cell Organisms to Multi-Cellular Organisms: Cancer as the "Faustian Bargain" We Paid for Our Survival

Until relatively recently, both the public and scientists wondered why the germ theory could not explain cancer as a disease. Even though clues that environmental agents, such as chimney soot, were associated with scrotal cancers by Percival Pott, it was difficult to put together a meaningful scientific hypothesis at that time. Although the clue that genetic factors might play a role came when Boveri [11] noticed abnormalities in chromosomes in cancer cells, until more direct evidence, such as the lack of the ability to repair ultraviolet light-induced DNA lesions in a cancer prone skin cancer syndrome, xeroderma pigmentosum [12], did a new perspective emerge. The role of the inability to repair UV-induced DNA lesions was associated with the production of mutations [13. 14] and the molecular basis of specific UV mutations in the p53 tumor suppressor gene of skin cancer cells [15]. The new paradigm was generated, "cancers as mutagen" [16], that took hold and from that time until just recently, carcinogenesis research became very reductionalistic with the new focus on the specific genes in cells, when mutated, "proto-oncogenes" and "tumor suppressor" were thought to provide the ultimate understanding of the carcinogenic process.

There is no doubt today, that the production of mutations does play a role in the complex carcinogenic process, as evidenced by (a)the inherited germ line mutations that led to cancer predispositions, such as the xeroderma pigmentosum, retinoblastoma, Down's, Fanconi's anemia, etc [17]; (b) agents associated with the induction of cancer inducing mutations in various short term in vitro assays; (c) mutations found in the oncogenes or tumor suppressor genes of cancer cells; and (d) DNA lesions found in cells of the cancer prone organs treated with various carcinogens. However, as will be discussed later, this view was too narrow, for it now has been shown that epigenetic alterations in the nuclear genome (*defined here as the alteration in the expression of the genome at the transcriptional, translational or posttranslational levels*) could also give raise to a component of the carcinogenic process.

However, to continue the focus on the role of evolution and cancer, one must realize that without mutations (as well as epigenetic changes) in the genome, that first living single cell organism would not have survived as a species. Clearly, if that early organism did not form any new genetic sequences, when the environment changes, as it inevitably has changed, and will continue to change, the genes that coded for those proteins and enzymes would be useless in the new challenging environment. The species could not survive in new harsh environments. Therefore, without the ability to protect DNA from having DNA lesions and from repairing, perfectly, the DNA lesions being formed by the errors of DNA repair or by errors of DNA replication, mutations could be generated in a population .In such cases, possibly one of those mutations could code for a protein that allows the organism to survive and reproduce, and, thus, saving the species. However, we must view the two extremes in mutation production. No mutations clearly lead to species failure in a changing environment. Too many mutations would also complicate survival. This is especially true in a multi-cellular organism.

Therefore, obviously, during the course of evolution, a balance was made between (a) protecting the DNA from any external damage that might lead to mutations and the perfect repair and replicating of DNA (which would lead to the extinction of the species) and (b) the lack of excessive DNA protection and the excessive production of errors of DNA repair and replication (which would also lead to the extinction of the species). While single cell organisms survive by unrestricted or immortalized ability to reproduce, in a population that is large enough, the population will have a few individuals that had accrued a mutation that allowed it to survive and reproduce when its sibs could not. Only temperature, nutrient depletion, pH changes and radiation would have environmental limiting influence on these single cell organisms' ability to proliferate.

When during the course of biological evolution that the first multi-cellular organism appeared, several new phenotypes had to accompany this new society of cells. Clearly, the aggregation of cells into a closed system would not have survived environmental changes had there not been some evolutionary advantage. One advantage would have been the appearance of specialized cells within the closed system that would enhance the survivability of the group as a whole. The appearance of the ability to form these specialized cells or *to differentiate* from a very primitive state to a very high "differentiated" cell, which could perform "higher order" functions, such as touch, sight, thermal regulation, muscle movement, etc., added to the single cell organism's ability to proliferate in, basically, an uncontrolled manner.

However, if a social colony of cells, which could form cooperating, but specialized functions, had no growth control, the colony would, in effect, become a tumor. Therefore, a second new phenotype had to be a new form of *growth control* in a closed system. In a society of single cell organisms, there are methods of "communicating" with each other via secreted factors. During the transition from the single cell to the multi-cell organism, this communication mechanism was not lost, but it was supplemented by the appearance of the gap junction, a membrane-associated protein channel that allows direct transfer of ions and small regulatory substrates to be transferred between the coupled cells [18]. Today, twenty connexion genes, those coding the proteins that are assembled into hexamers that comprise the hemi-channel of the cell which couples with the neighboring hemi-channel, are evolutionarily conserved, thus implying their importance in the survival of the metazoan [19]. These different connexion genes appear to serve the function of providing differential signalling mechanisms to regulate various cellular functions, including allowing for differential differentiation within an organism [20]. Equally important, these new means of communication between neighboring cells in direct contact with each other seem to be involved in growth control via "contact inhibition" [21].

Another new phenotype also appeared during this transition in evolution. It was the function of *programmed cell death* or *apoptosis*. If, in fact, a multi-cellular organism was to be successful in maintaining its species, it could also "improve" its ability to survive by changing its phenotype to add new survival functions, such as the transition from an insect larva to a flying butterfly. However to make this extraordinary advance, those specialized cells of the larva had to give way to new cells that would be needed for pigmentation, flight muscles, wings and other new sensory organs. This could only happen if whole battery of genes in those cells, needed for the larval function, is replaced with new differentiated cells having new battery of genes expressed for the new functions of a flying butterfly. The original fertilized egg of that butterfly had both sets of genes but they were expressed only when needed for that particular stage of development.

Equally important during this transition of the single to multi-cell organism was the "Faustian" bargain. That is, in return for higher order functions that differentiation of highly specials cells could give to the species' survival, was the "mortality" or senescence of the whole organism. Clearly, if *all* the cells of the multi-cellular organism senesced or became mortal, the species would not survive. With the appearance of the ability to form specialized *"immortal" germ cells,* the "Faustian" bargain, then, excluded the germ cells from the curse of "mortality". Moreover, if the multi-cell organ was to have additional adaptive functions, such as continued growth of the non-germ line cells, tissue replacement of damaged or diseased tissue, and for extended life span, not only was the germ-line cells privileged with the characteristic of "immortality", but also, some somatic or non-germ cells were selected that had this feature. These germ line and somatic "immortal cells" are the so-called adult "stem" cells.

If we now view these new phenotypes that emerged during multi-cellular development, and if we view what happens in a multi celled organism when it has a cancer, we note that cancers (a) no longer have growth control; (b) can not terminally differentiate; (c) do not apoptose normally; and (d) have the ability to be immortal. In effect, they have "de-evolved" to a single-cell organism-like state. It is interesting to note that the appearance of the connexion gene appeared early in the evolution of the multi-cellular organism [22]. It is also interesting that cancer cells have no functional gap junctional intercellular communication [23], either because the connexion genes were never expressed or that they were expressed but rendered non-functional by activated oncogenes or mutations [24]. Whether this association of the loss of function of the gap junction with the loss of growth control, differentiation, abnormal apoptosis and the appearance of immortality in the cancer cell was just coincidence or causal, has to be resolved.

Stem Cells, Cell Communication and Development

During the development of a human being from a single fertilized egg, the zygote or "toti-potent" stem cell, approximately 100 trillion cells are produced. In order that development of the embryo, fetus, neonate, adolescent , mature and geriatric individual be normal, a very delicate orchestration of communication processes (extra-, intra, and gap junctional inter-cellular communication mechanisms) must be integrated, in order that the hierarchy of different cell types (embryonic, pluri-potent, multi-potent, bi-polar stem cells; progenitor stems, and terminally-differentiated cells) be done in a sequential, concatenated manner to allow the total genome to be specifically regulated in each cell type (Figure 1).

Genes for "stemness", such as Oct-4, nanog, Sox-2 [25], must be expressed in the embryonic and adult stem cells (multi-potent, bi-polar). Other genes must be expressed in order that specific differentiation genes might be regulated during development, growth and in cell replacement in tissues, and during wound-healing. Gap junctions genes, the 20 connexin genes [19], do seem to be required for the specific differentiation of cells within and between tissues of different organs [20]. Temporal expressions of genes are needed for the normal process of apoptosis or programmed cell death and even for removal of damaged cells [26]. For cells in solid tissues, gap junction function seems to be required for apoptosis to occur [27].

This extremely complex communication between the adult stem cells in their niches [28], their committed progenitor or "transit" cells [29], and the terminally- differentiated daughter cells must exist. Since it seems that the early blastocyte cells do not have function gap junctions [30], and that several adult human stem cells also do nor express their connexion genes or have functional gap junctional intercellular communication (GJIC) [31], communication between the stem cells and the surrounding committed progenitor cells, that do seem to have gap junctions, and the terminally differentiated cells, that might or might not have gap junctions during their whole life time, must be mediated by secreted factors [32-33]. The progenitor cells, both epithelial, endothelial, and fibroblasts, do have contact-inhibitory means to regulate proliferation [34]. Gap junctions have been associated with growth control [35], differentiation [36] and apoptosis [27].

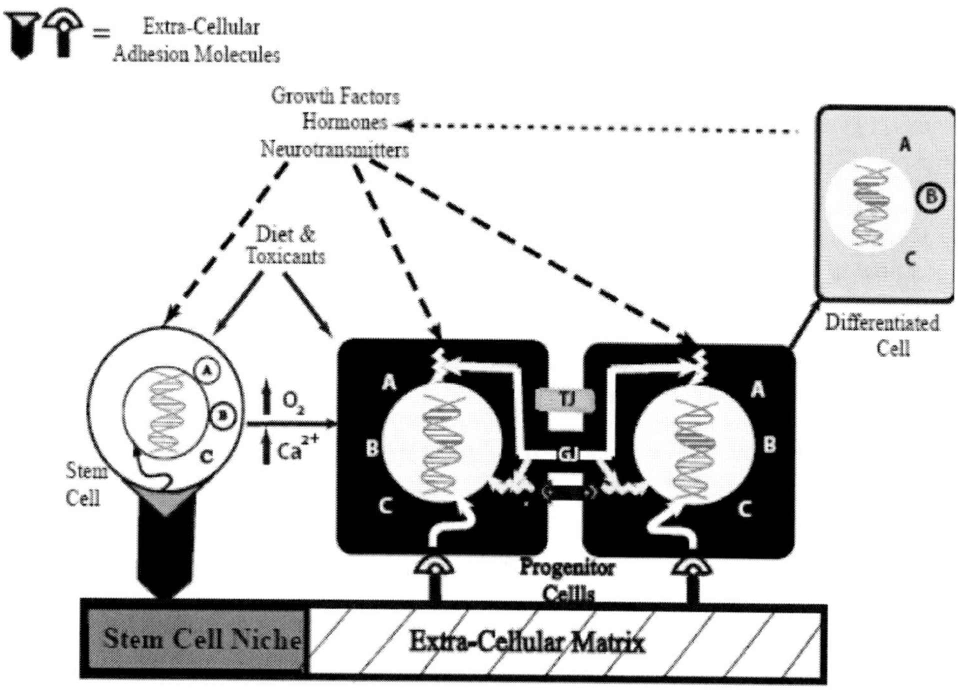

Figure 1. Gap junctions in cellular homeostasis. Extracellular signals, such as growth factors, toxicants, extra-cellular matrices and cell adhesion molecules that vary for each cell type (adult stem cell, progenitor and terminally-differentiated), interact with membrane receptors, which then activate intracellular signal transduction pathways that induce the transcription of genes (A,B,C) through activated transcription factors. These specific intracellular pathways operate under cascading systems that cross communicate with each other in controlling the expression of genes that direct the proliferation, differentiation and apoptosis of cells within a tissue. These multiple intracellular signalling check points are further modulated by intercellular signals traversing gap junctions, thereby maintaining the homeostatic state of a tissue. Abnormal interruption of these integrated signalling pathways by food-related and environmental toxicants results in diseased states, such as the tumor promotion phase of carcinogenesis, teratogenesis during early development, atherogenesis, immunotoxicity, reproductive- and neuro-toxicities.

The stem cell is defined as a cell that has the ability to divide either symmetrically to form two identical daughter stem cells (if it divides to commit both daughter to terminal differentiation, that would be the end of that stem cell's contribution to the organism's life) or asymmetrically to form one daughter cell (a progenitor) that is now committed to form a lineage of differentiated .cells and one daughter that remains capable of self-renewal or stemness. To view stem cells, in this light, is to realize that a stem cell is naturally an "immortal" cell and it becomes "mortal" when it is induced to form a terminally-differentiated or "mortal" cell. Therefore, this decision point in a multi-cellular organism's evolutionary advance over single cell organism, namely, the control of symmetric versus asymmetric cell division will be of critical importance during normal development and during carcinogenesis.

Exactly how a stem cell determines whether it should divide symmetrically or asymmetrically is not currently known. However, from a conceptual standpoint, the stem cell must receive a number of signalling mechanisms. The first is signalling the stem cell receives from its anchored niche-substrate extra-cellular molecules. In the case of non-anchored stem cells, extra-cellular secreted signalling ions and molecules probably provide the same signal. Together with the secreted factors such as a hormone, growth factor, cytokine, chemokine, or ions, such as calcium, that might trigger some specific intra-cellular signalling, , the net-effect of these signals would be result of the "cross-talk" of these extra- cellar signalling triggered intra-cellular signal pathways. Together with an important environmental factor, oxygen [37], the net effect of the interactive signals determine which genes are going to be transcribed and which existing proteins will be posttranslationally-modified for activity, inaction or ubquitization. That will lead to the molecular decision mechanism for symmetric or asymmetric cell division.

Conceptually, one model that might help to explain how the role of gap junctions might come into play in this process of symmetric and asymmetrical stem cell division. In Figure2, it is speculated that, depending on the mix of signals a stem cell gets in its niche, the stem cell anchored to the niche extra-cellar matrix might form a mitotic division plane that is parallel to the plane of the stem cell niche extra-cellular matrix. In this case, the new daughter that is still attached to the niche extra-cellular matrix will continue to receive the same signal as did its stem cell mother.

On the other hand, because the other daughter is not attached to the extra-cellular niche matrix and does not communicate directly via gap junctions to its sister cell (a stem cell), its new mix of signals coul d induce the expression of connexin genes and form functional gap junctions. This cell is now a progenitor cell and is growth inhibited every time it is stimulated to proliferate by these gap junctions and it can differentiate via these gap junctions.

On the other hand, if the mix of signals the anchored stem cell gets triggers genes that cause the mitotic division plane to be vertical to the stem cell niche plane, then both new daughter cells would still be anchored to the same extra-cellular matrix molecule that helped to determine stemness. Since neither sister stem cell has gap junctions, they do not differentiate.

The Stem Cell or De-Differentiation Hypothesis of Carcinogenesis

One of the oldest theories of cancer is that a cancer cell started as a stem cell but was blocked in its ability to terminally differentiate or to become "mortal". That is the essence of Markert's quote and led to his view that cancer was a disease of differentiation [4]. In addition, the views of Pierce ("Cancer as a stem cell disease") [6], Potter's concept of "oncogeny as partially blocked ontogeny" [7], together with the experimental demonstrations of the clonal origin of all the cells within a tumor [37-38] and the immortally of tumor cells, contribute to a hypothesis that the normal immortal stem cell was the target cell for the ultimate cancer cell.

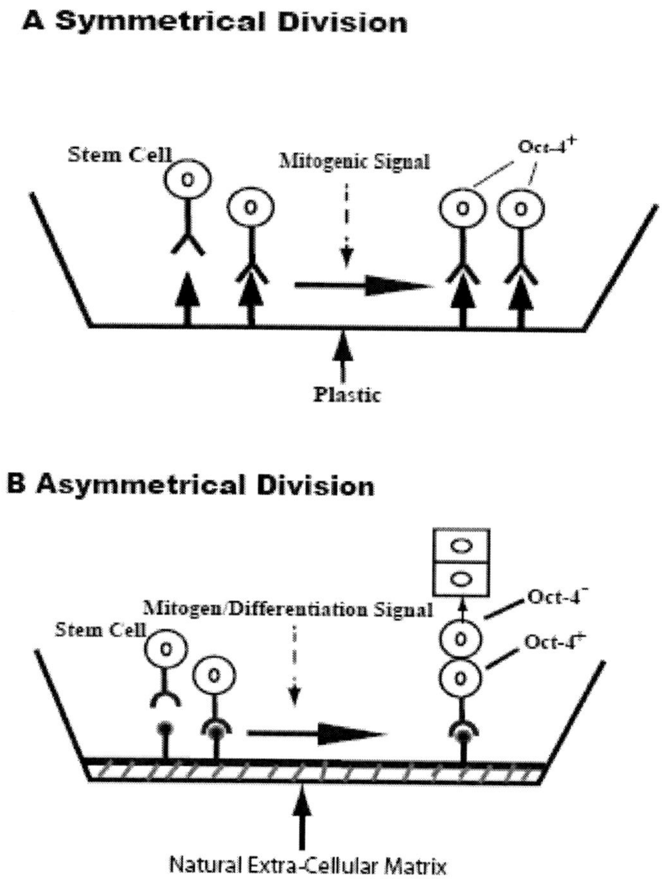

Figure 2. These diagrams illustrate two possible means by which stem cells (Oct-4+) decide to divide by symmetrical or asymmetrical division. In panel A, if a stem cell binds to a specific extracellular matrix, as symbolized by attaching to a coated plastic dish, the signal received combines with signals in the medium (growth factors, Ca++, nutrients, oxygen, etc.) to stimulate genes and gene products to bring about the division plane to be perpendicular to the attachment plane. As a result, both daughter cells continue to have identical signalling as did the maternal stem cell (symmerical cell division or expansion of the stem cell population). In panel B, the stem cell binds to a different substrate molecule, as represented by a natural extra-cellular molecule, such as laminin or collagen type 4. In this case, the signal this substrate molecule induces a different intracellular signal that interacts with the same signals from the medium, Ca++, oxygen, etc. to stimulate different genes and gene products to cause a division plane within the stem cell to be formed parallel to the attachment plane. In this case, the daughter cell on the bottom will mimic the same intracellular signalling as its maternal stem cell. Important to note that if these stem cells do not have functional gap junctional intercellular communication, then these signals are not transmitted to the other daughter cell because that daughter cell does not interact with the substrate signal. As a result, these daughter cells receive a different set of combined signals that trigger a commitment to become a progenitor and ultimately terminally differentiated progeny.

Yet this hypothesis has not gone unchallenged, as there are those who feel any cell, save those terminally-differentiated cells with no nuclei (red blood cells or lens cells), can de-differentiate to the "embryonic-stem" cell state and then progress to the carcinogenic process. In more modern terms, this "de-differentiation" might be re-named, "re-programmed" [39]. In deed, with some evidence being presented, adult differentiated mouse fibroblasts have been interpreted to be re-programmed after being genetically modified to over express copies of the Oct-4 gene [40-42]. Yet, these data also can be challenged in that the original adult mouse skin fibroblast culture probably contained some normal adult skin stem cells expressing Oct-4. The transfected recovered cells might have been a transfected normal skin adult stem cell. More experiments will be needed to resolve this possibility.

The de-differentiation hypothesis does challenge the basic tenet in science, namely, *Ocham's Razor*. Whenever multiple hypotheses are offered to explain an observation, one should first stick with the simplest explanation for it is the easiest to disprove. In the case of the de-differentiation hypothesis, one needs to re-program the genome , such that, at least those genes that limited the life span of the progenitor or terminally differentiate cell would need to be repressed and the stemness or Oct.4 gene be expressed. Basically, while in principle, this is logical, it does add another step in an otherwise, already complex carcinogenic process.

Probably another concept that has to be considered, in the context of the stem cell theory, is the current paradigm in the cancer field, namely, that the first step in the carcinogenic process must be the induction of "immortalization" in a normal, "mortal" cell [43]. In this paradigm, cancer is thought to arise from a normal, mortal cell, such as a primary culture of mammalian tissue. Since these primary cells, primarily fibroblasts, were characterized as having a finite life span in vitro, the "Hayflick limit" [44], any induced neoplastic cell derived from this population was assumed to be "mortal". Therefore, the first step in the carcinogenic process was to induce "immortality" in a mortal, normal cell. This allowed the immortalized cell to live long enough to accrue additional genetic and epigenetic changes needed for complete neoplastic transformation. However, if the target cell for carcinogenesis is the stem cell, then one can see the current paradigm is exactly backwards. If the stem cell, which is naturally "immortal" until it is induced to differentiate or to become "mortal", is the stem cell, then the new paradigm should be that the first step in the carcinogenetic process must be to block "mortalization" of an immortal normal stem cell. This now sets up the discussion of the next hypothesis of carcinogenesis.

Stem Cells, the Multi-Step, Multi-Mechanism Carcinogenic Process of Initiation, Promotion and Progression

With the possible exception of the formation of teratomas, all other cancers appear to require multiple distinct events from each other, in order that a single, normal cell becomes an invasive, metastatic cancer cell, having all those "Hallmarks" associated with all cancer cells. With the early demonstration using mouse skin and rabbit ears [45, 46], it was shown that a one" hit" hypothesis of carcinogenesis was inappropriate to explain the multiple treatments an organism must get in order that a tumor appear.

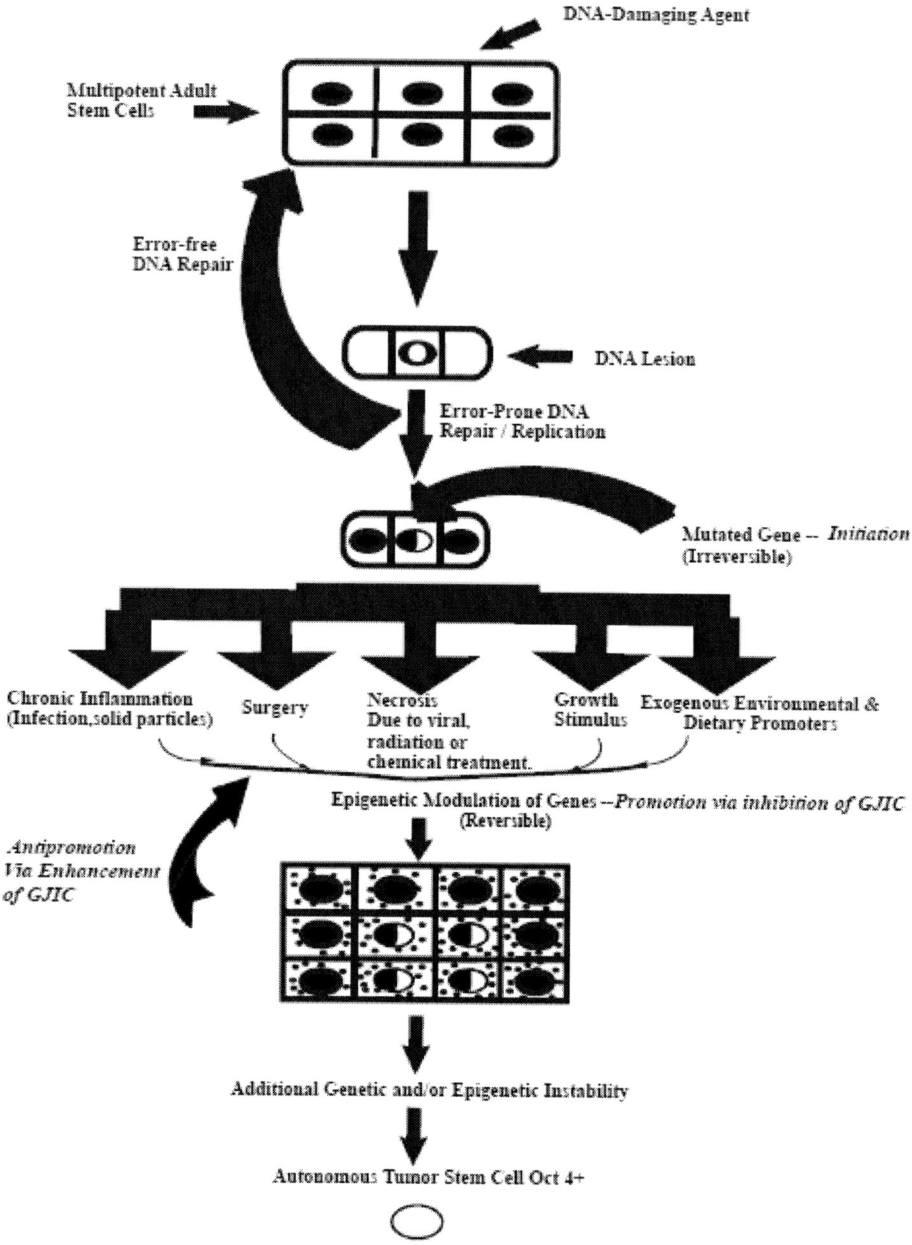

Figure 3. A diagrammatic heuristic scheme to depict the postulated mechanisms of the initiation and promotion phase of carcinogenesis. DNA lesions, induced by physical mutagens or by errors in DNA replication, are substrates in adult stem cells (Oct-4+) that can be fixed if they are not removed in an error-free manner prior to DNA replication. Promotion includes those conditions (i.e., chronic inflammation induced by infectious agents, solid particles; surgery or wounding; necrotic cell death; normal growth stimuli caused by growth factors, hormones; and exogenous epigenetic natural and synthethic epigenetic molecules), in which a pluripotent, but surviving, initiated adult stem cell (Oct-4+), can escape the nonproliferative state. The build up of initiated cells allows them to "resist" the anti-mitotic influence of neighboring non-initiated cells. In addition, the changing micro-environment within the growing benign tumor will cause some of the initiated adult stem cells to partially differentiate into cancer non-stem cells. This, together with either addition mutations or stable epigenetic changes, might allow a given initiated adult stem cell to have autonomous, invasive properties of a malignant cell.

Even with later studies on human genetic predisposing cancer syndromes, such as retinoblastoma [47], it was clearly evident that, just because all the cells of a person's body contained the cancer-predisposing gene, only a very few gave rise to a cancer.

In these early animal experiments, the concepts of "initiation", "promotion" and "progression" were coined, as "operation" terms.

Initiation was the event that occurred in only a few cells of organism that was basically *irreversible.* If the initiator was known to be associated with the induction of the target organ when given at high concentrations or doses, then at a low, non-cancer inducing concentration or dose, the animal will not form any tumors, however, if followed by the next step (promotion), one can surmise that an irreversible event had occurred in a few cells of that organism. In the case of the mouse skin or rat liver, the initiated cell could remain quiescent in the animal for months only to be stimulated later to start the carcinogenic process. The initiated cell did not die or was not "restored" to the normal state during this period. *Operationally,* initiation is only the production of a stable cell that can not terminally differentiate or apoptose easily. Consequently, initiation is that fundamental event that affects a stem cell's ability to divide, asymmetrically. This is probably the most accurate operational definition of initiation. While few studies have given us an insight as to what might be the gene or genes involved in this critical biological process of stem cells, Ko and associates have identified a gene, CoAA, that could be involved in this process [48]. A conceptual manner of viewing this initiation process in an adult stem cell in seen in Figure 4.

Promotion, on the other hand, was that process that occurred only after the animal was initiated (or as will be seen later, it could also occur on cells that were "spontaneously" initiated). In fact, especially in the case of a long-lived species such as the human being, all individuals have spontaneously-initiated cells, and the longer one lives, the greater that number of initiated stem cells. The process of tumor promotion is when the initiated animal is exposed on a regular basis, for a long period of time, at threshold and above concentrations and in the absence of "anti-promoters" causing the single initiated cell to form a tumor. In the absence of this promotion process, no tumors appear [49]. Clearly, if the promotion process is stopped or interrupted, or given together with anti-promoters, then no initiated cell can accrue the necessary characteristics needed to have all the "hallmarks" of cancer. *Operationally,* the promotion process, one that is interruptible or even reversible [50], is one where the single "initiated" cell can be clonally expanded to reach a mass of cells, in which one cell can now acquire an addition stable change to give it a move selective advance to acquire more changes. It was also noted that promotion, which leads to the expansion of initiated cells, also involves the acquisition of a resistance to apoptosis. Therefore, the increased accumulation of initiated cells by promotion could be the result of mitogenesis and an inhibition of apoptosis.

Promotion appears to be able to allow an initiated cell to escape mitotic suppression by surrounding normal cells. The literature has shown that (a) wound healing after removal of tissue by surgery, (b) chronic inflammation, (c) cell death due to burns, viruses, or non-genotoxic toxicants, such as alcohol or carbon tetrachloride, (d) growth factors and hormones, and (e) exogenous non-genotoxic chemicals, such as Phenobarbital or polybrominated biphenols, can be tumor promoters. Promotion has been shown to be induced in initiated rodent skin, ears, mammary tissue, bladder, and liver. Physical agents, such as asbestos fibers, carbon particles, and solid metal objects, such as nanoparticles, can induce chronic inflammation to act as promoters [51]. There are species and strain specific promoters.[52].

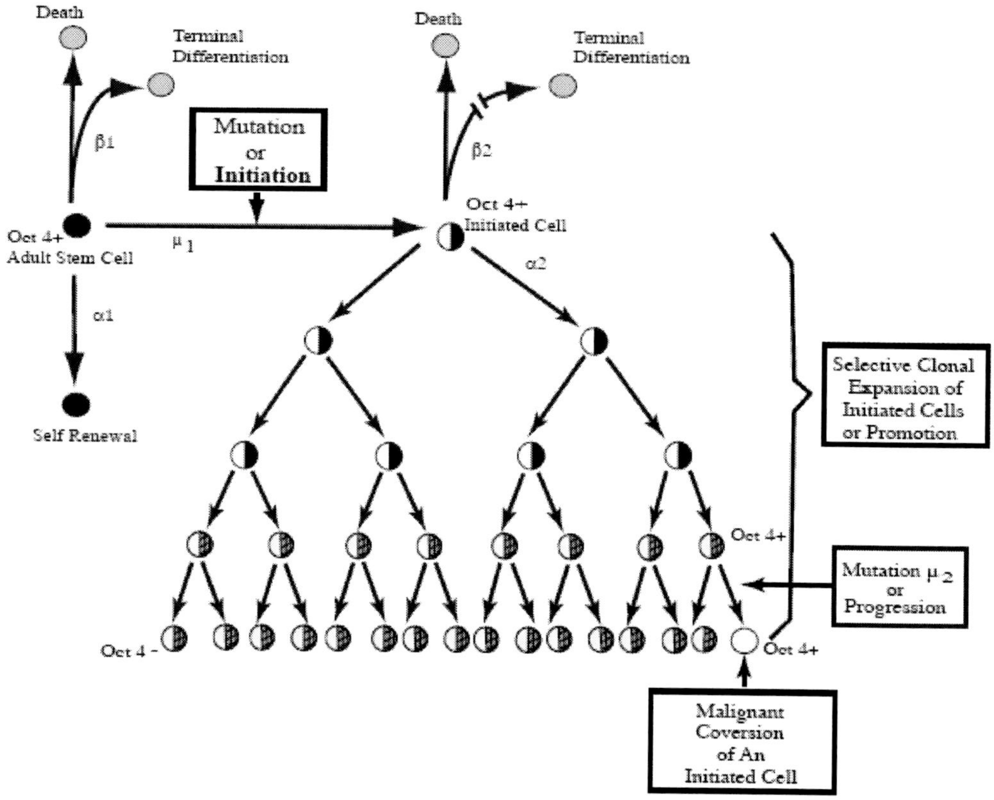

Figure 4. In this diagram, a normal adult stem cell is shown dividing asymmetrically to form one daughter that is committed to ultimately terminally differentiate. The other daughter is designated to be identical to its mother adult stem cell (Oct-4+). If that adult stem cell is exposed to some condition that prevents asymmetrical cell division, but does not suppress the Oct-4 expression, it is operationally an initiated cell. That is, if mitotically stimulated to divide, it divides symmetrically to form two initiated, non-terminally differentiated cell. Initiation is, then, defined as the process that prevents an "immortal" normal adult stem cell to terminally differentiate or become "mortal". These adult initiated stem cells are still Oct-4 positive or benign cancer stem cells. As these initiated Oct-4+ cells are stimulated to proliferate and resist apoptosis, the growing benign tumor micro-environment changes, some of these initiated Oct-4 + cells can partially differentiate into "cancer non-stem cells"[Oct-4 negative]. Evening, additional stable mutational or epigenetic events occur , providing the benign Oct-4+ cancer stem cells to become invasive, metastatic "cancer stem cells".

Although it was postulated in 1979 that tumor promoters worked, mechanistically, by inhibiting gap junctional intercellular communication [53], it still has not been integrated into the cancer field, as evidenced by the lack of references to this insight by the molecular oncologists. Most, if not all, chemical tumor promoters have been shown to inhibit, reversibly, GJIC at threshold and above concentrations which are non-cytotoxic [54]. In fact, the role of gap junctions has further been strengthened by the fact that many chemopreventive and anti-carcinogenic agents, such as green tea, [55], resveratrol [56, 57] , caffeic acid phenylester [58], or chemotherapeutic agents, such as lovastatin [59], kaempherol [60], SAHA [61], and beta-sitosterol [62], restore GJIC in cancer cells, Even various oncogenes, such as ras, src, neu, mos, have been shown to inhibit, stably, GJIC [63]. Genetic transfection of connexion genes in non-GJIC functioning cancer cells restores GJIC and normal cell growth with reduced tumorigenicity [63]. On the other hand, anti-sense connexion genes in normal cells triggered the tumorigenic phenotype of these cells [63]. Collectively, the role of GJIC must play some role, as Lowenstein and Kanno predicted in 1966 [64], in the carcinogenic process.

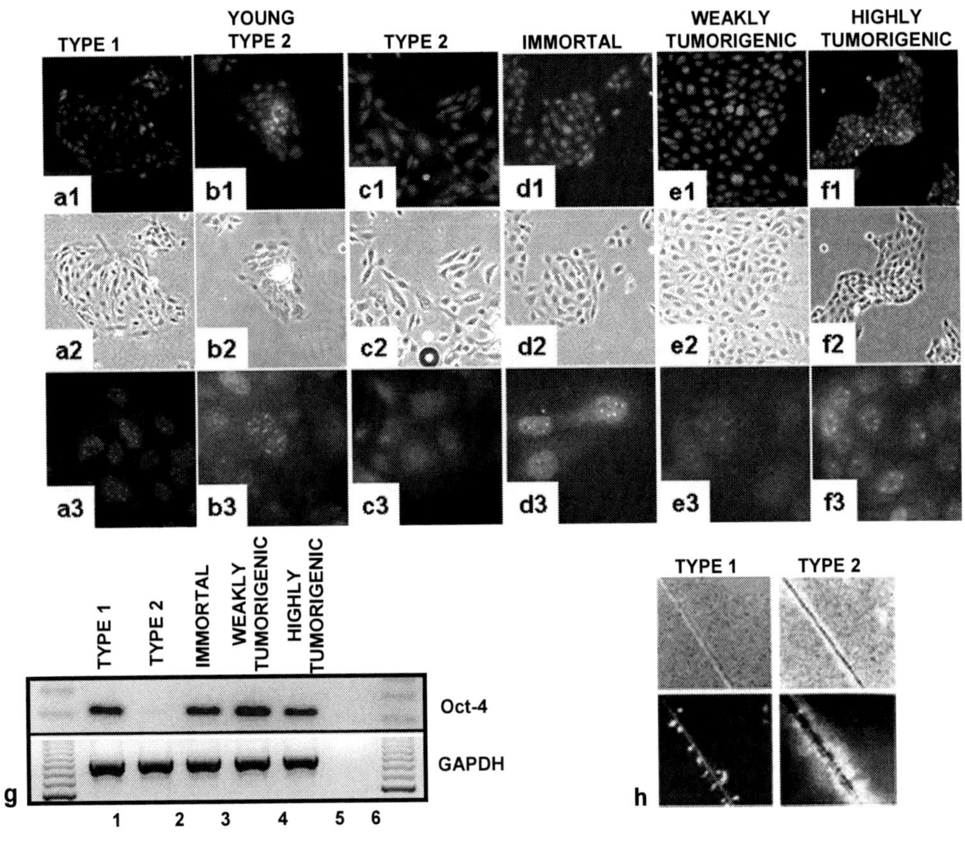

Figure 5. The composite of these three figures illustrated that (a) the clonally-derived normal human adult breast stem cells expressed Oct-4 (Figure 5.A panel) via immunohistochemical use of fluorescent antibodies to Oct-4 in the normal breast stem cells, but not in the differentiated breast cells (Figure 5.C panel), still expressed in SV40 "immortalized" normal breast stem cells which were not tumorigenic (Figure 5.D panel), still expressed in the irradiated and weakly tumorigenic breast stem cells (Figure 5.E panel) and expressed in the neu/ErB-2 highly transformed clone (Figure 5.F panel). In Figure 5.G, the RT-PCR data correlated with the immunohistochemical data of Oct-4 in this series of human breast adult stem cells. In Figure 5.H, the data clearly show that the normal breast adult stem cells have no functional gap junctional intercellular communication as measured by the fluorescent.

Progression is the final complex step (probably involving multi-events) that, *operationally*, converts one single initiated cell in the heterogeneous clone produced by promotion (e.g., a skin papilloma, liver enzyme foci, a colon polyp or a nodule in the breast).

This step, also, appears to be irreversible and leads, ultimately, to an invasive, metastatic cell with all the "hallmarks of cancer".

To try to integrate the stem cell theory into this "initiation/ promotion/progression" hypothesis, it should be obvious that, if initiation occurs in an adult normal immortal stem cell, the initiation event must be the process that inhibits asymmetric cell division, but not the symmetric cell division of an immortal adult stem cell.

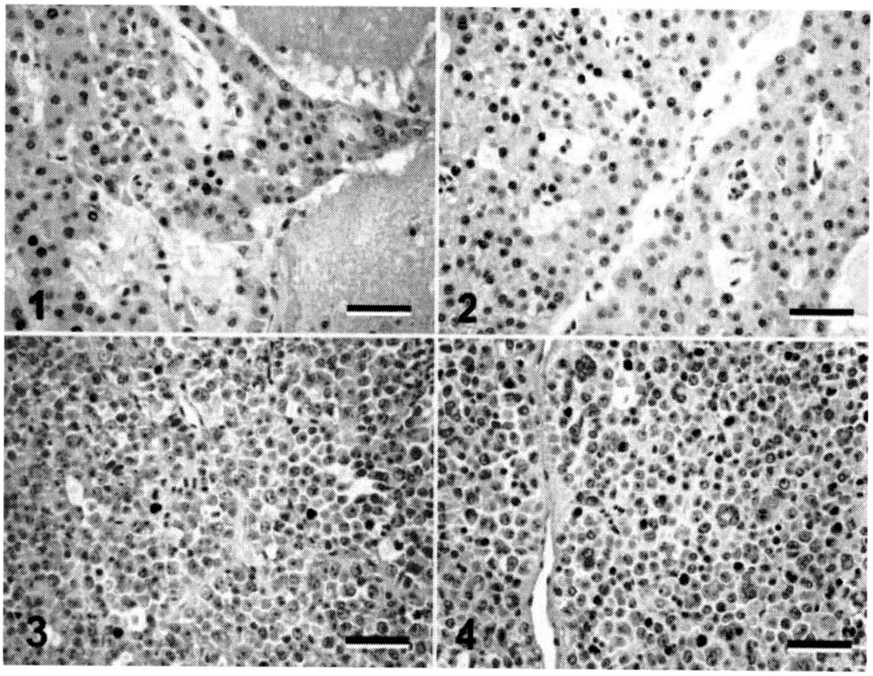

Figure 6. These photographs of Oct4 expression in spontaneous canine tumors reflect the intertumor and intratumor variation. Low (Figures 1, 3) and High (Figures 2, 4) frequencies of Oct-4 expressing cells in canine hepatocellular carcinomas (Figures 1, 2) and seminomas (Figures 3, 4 , respectively. Variation in the relative proportion of the Oct-4 –positive cells (brown nuclear precipitate) was seen in both between and within different types of spontaneous canine tumors. Immunohistochemical staining with mouse anti-human Oct-4 monoclonal antibody was visualized with the substrate 3,3'-diaminobenzidine with hematoxylin counterstain. Bar= 80 μm. Permission granted by American Society of Veterinary Pathology, Allen Press, Lawrence, Kansas, USA.

The Mutation or Epigenetic Theories of Carcinogenesis

Since inherited genes that predispose cancer in patients, such as xeroderma pigmentosum or retinoblastoma, carry a germ line mutation. In the case of cells of the skin-cancer predisposed xeroderma pigmentosum, which do not repair their DNA after ultraviolet light-induced DNA damage [65], their cells have a higher mutation frequency than their normal counterparts [13, 14]. From this, it is clear that mutations must play some role in carcinogenesis. In deed, when one examines oncogenes and tumor suppressor genes in various tumor cells, one frequently finds mutations in these genes. Especially, in the case of the mutations of the p53 gene in skin cancer patients, the mutations found correspond to that expected type if formed from unrepaired UV lesions of these cells [15]. Even in the cancer prone multi-cancer syndrome, Bloom's syndrome, the spontaneous mutation rates were found to be higher than from cells of normal patients [66].

These kinds of examples provide strong evidence that mutations, being basically an irreversible event, could be the mechanistic basis for the "initiation" event that starts the multi-stage process. This assumption has been carried over to the prominent paradigm of today's cancer research field, namely, "carcinogen as mutagen" [67]. However, the uncritical interpretation of results from in vitro studies to test if "carcinogens" are mutagens, as well as from ill-design bioassays on rodents [68], has brought massive confusion to the cancer-risk assessment field, as well as to practice assessment of new drugs and chemicals. While this does not imply that mutations do not play a role in carcinogenesis, it does question if *chemicals* (not radiation) cause mutations found in the oncogenes and tumor suppressor genes of the tumors associated with that exposure. With the demonstration that the mutation spectrum of an oncogene found in tumor cells of cigarette smokers being essentially the same as the spectrum for mutations found in the oncogenes of lung tumors of non-smokers [69], the question is raised whether the chemicals in cigarette smoke acted as promoters, rather than as initiators [68]. Animal experiments, as well as epidemiological evidence from smokers who quit smoking, suggest, strongly, that these chemicals acted more like promoters than initiators. Stopping smoking acted as stopping phorbol esters or phenobarbital on the interruption of promotion of skin and liver cancers, respectively. Must recently, Upham and co-workers [70-72] showed that the predominant chemicals in cigarette smoke performed, mechanistically, like tumor promoters, at non-cytotoxic concentrations. Promoters, by blocking intercellular communication, either by interfering with secreted growth inhibitors or their receptor-signaling, or by reversibly blocking GJIC, could block the cellular functions of "contact-inhibition", differentiation, or apoptosis. All three of these cellular phenotypes are affected by the carcinogenic process.

The important point to be made here, in trying to resolve the issue of finding DNA lesions in cells after an animal or cells in culture are exposed to chemicals associated with the appearance of tumors or neoplastic transformed cells, is that there are two sources of DNA which could be targets for DNA damage caused by electrophiles or free radicals. The first is the mitochondrial DNA where oxidative metabolism is occurring and the second is the nuclear DNA, which is sequestered away from oxidative damaging free radicals and electrophiles (except during ionizing radiation). In addition, there are three types of cells in which these two DNA targets are found, the few stem cells, the many progenitor cells with a limited life span and the terminally differentiated cells, which do not proliferate or give rise to cancers. Since very few of the studies demonstrating the existence of DNA lesions after chemical exposures separate the two sources of DNA before analysis, one can not rigorously state these lesions are those that led to mutations found in the oncogenes of tumor cells found after the chemical exposure. If one does find these DNA lesions in the nuclear DNA then, in all likelihood, the cell would have died from such massive production of electrophiles and free radicals that exceeded the cellular defence mechanisms, and traversed from the cytoplasm to the nuclear membrane. Under those conditions, the plasma membrane would be destroyed and the cell would die by necrosis. The death of these cells (usually the terminal differentiated cells, which express large amounts of metabolizing enzymes) could act as "indirect" tumor promoters by stimulating the stem cells to proliferate. If the stem cell was previously initiated by errors in replication or by UV radiation induced mutations, then the chemical could give the appearance of causing the DNA damage and mutations. In brief, while a statement suggesting that chemicals do not induce mutations that cause cancer is clearly heretical, the evidence suggesting otherwise is yet to be rigorously demonstrated. These so-called "mutagenic carcinogens" are more likely tumor promoters rather than initiators. These cancer-associated chemicals selectively promote spontaneously initiated stem cells [68].

If mutations might be the mechanistic basis for the initiation and the progression stages, one should not ignore the possibility that a stable epigenetic event could also bring about an initiation event. In the case of teratomas, it has been shown that a metastatic teratocarcinoma cell, when placed back into a blastocyst of a genetically-marked mouse, could participate in the normal development of a mosaic mouse, whereby, the teracarcimoa cells helped to generate normal tissues [73]. This could not have happened if the original teratocarcinoma cell was generated by an irreversible mutational event. The example also re-enforces the stem cell theory of cancer. The normal definition of an embryonic stem cell is that it forms a teratoma when injected into an adult animal. That implies the embryonic stem cell, when placed in a strange micro-environment, will modulate its gene expression patterns in bizarre ways, so as to differentiate but in an unorganized fashion. If a mutated cancer cell is transplanted into an adult host, it might partially differentiate or even partly apoptose, but will continue to form a tumor.

Oncogenes, Tumor Suppressor Genes, and Cancer Cells

The success of modern molecular oncology, with the discovery of oncogenes and tumor suppressor genes, easily diverted the cancer community from the classic whole animal studies to that of mutated DNA sequences in certain genes associated with a cell becoming a cancer. The emergence of the Human Genome project, with its promise to cure human diseases , such as cancer, simply by comparing sequences of cancer and non cancer patients, as well as providing new strategies for prevention or "cures", turns out not to be able to deliver on many of those promises. In fact, the insights, gained by the classic studies on carcinogenesis, as well as some of the ignored "hallmarks" of cancer [74], have already provided new insights without the need for all that Human Genomic information.

Harris has reviewed that hundreds of studies on the most common tumor suppressor gene found in human cancers (but it should be noted, not all human cancers), the p53 gene [75]. Multiple oncogenes have been identified and are still being reported [48]. In brief, the functional roles, albeit each works by different molecular/biochemical mechanisms, of these two classes of cancer-related genes is to stimulate the growth of pre-malignant (initiated) and malignant cells and to inhibit the growth of these pre-malignant cells, respectively. *Operationally*, stimulation of the increase of initiated cells can occur by either or both inhibiting "contact-inhibition" and apoptosis and by stimulating mitogenesis. In addition, this includes the fact that initiation, operationally, *prevents asymmetric cell division of the initiated adult stem cell under normal conditions*, the oncogene or tumor suppressor genes might affect the regulation of symmetric and asymmetric cell division. Few in the cancer field have addressed this as a fundamental problem to be solved. Since oncogene and tumor suppression genes affect cell proliferation and cell cycle regulation of the single cell, the molecular oncologists have ignored the fact that cell proliferation also involves cell-cell interactions, either heterogeneous, such as stromal- epithelial interactions [76, 77] by secreted factors (extra-cellular communication) or by gap junctional intercellular communication between heterologous and homologous cells within a tissue [78]. In other words, there are other genes working at a higher systems level, which transcends the reductionalists' thinking that predominates the cancer field today.

The fact that gap junction genes have been shown to be tumor suppressor genes, and the function of the these connexion genes is to affect intercellular regulation of single cell's cycle cycle control, to differentiate by receiving signals from without the cell or to apoptose by reaching signals from out side the cell, a different manner of viewing carcinogens must be gained than just from molecular or in vitro studies. As the late V.R. Potter had stated [79]:

> "The cancer problem is not merely a cell problem; it is a problem of cell interaction, not only within tissues, but also with distal cells in other tissues. But in stressing the whole organism, we must also remember that the integration of normal cells with the welfare of the whole organism is brought about by molecular messages acting on molecular receptors."

Adult Stem Cells as the Targets for Carcinogenic Initiation

Given the previous experiments that demonstrated cancer cells were "immortal", that they resisted terminal differentiation but could partially differentiate under certain conditions, that they were monoclonally derived and that they could invade and metastasize, as well as induce angiogenesis, one is struck by the similarities of these "hallmarks" of cancer with the normal properties of stem cells. Two "hallmarks" that were not identified were the stem-like nature of the cancer cell and the lack of functional cell-cell communication [74].

Conceptually, however, the initiation/promotion/progression hypothesis seems, best, to support the idea that the single cell that is initiated is a normal adult stem cell. In the case of teratomas, the single cell might be an embryonic stem cell. However, in adult cancers, since stem cells do exists for most, if not all, organs, these cells, being either multi-potent or bi-potent, could after initiation, depending on the genes affected and the micro-environment, in which the cell finds itself, causes partially differentiation of the initiated stem cell into the identifiable tumor types of that particular organ (e.g., hepatocellular, carcinomas or cholangiocellular carcinomas in the liver). In other words, for some initiated adult stem cells, these new changes in the micro-environment can induced these cells to have asymmetric cell division in order to partially differentiate.

Initiation is that operational step to cause a cell, presumably an adult stem cell, to start the complex evolutionary process for all tumors. If this cell is a normal, immortal adult stem cell, and if it is assumed that the initiation process is one that inhibits the stem cell to asymmetrically divide (i.e., it can not normally terminally differentiate), then, "Are initiated stem cells those that give rise to the so-called newly discovered *"cancer stem cells"* which have the potential to perpetuate the growth of a tumor?" [80]. Clearly, in a tumor, there are *"cancer non-stem cells",* those that appear to be partially differentiated and can not perpetuate the growth of the tumor [81]. Of course, it has not been rigorously ruled out that some differentiated progenitor cell could be "re-programmed" to de-differentiate to become "immortal" again and then start the carcinogenic process. In this case, the "initiation" step would be the so-called "immortalization" of a normal, mortal progenitor cell as the prevailing hypothesis would suggest [43].

However, there are times when "Ocham's Razor comes in handy in trying to resolve multiple scientific interpretations of observations. In the case of the "de-differentiation" or "re-programming" hypothesis of the origin of cancer cells, if an adult or somatic differentiated cell is "initiated", it must involve at least one additional step before it can utilize its new-found "immortality", compared to the normal adult step cell which is naturally immortal" at the time of initiation. Recent claims that an adult mouse skin fibroblast cell could be "re-programmed" when genetically transfected with "stemness" genes, such as oct-4, nanog, etc, would seem, at least, to keep open the possibility that "initiation" of an adult differentiated cell might happen [40-42]. However, in this case, "initiation" is operationally very different than "initiation" of a normal immortal adult stem cell. It must include two steps; one to reprogram whole sets of genes that determine the differentiation of a mature, differentiated skin fibroblast cell, which had its Oct-4 (and other "stemness" genes) transcriptionally suppressed and its senescence genes transcriptionally, operational. It, then, had to start where the normal adult get was when it was "initiated", namely already immortal but now blocked in its ability to divide asymmetrically under normal conditions.

However, there is another interpretation of these results of "re-programming" of an adult somatic, differentiated skin fibroblast cell. That is, if the original rescued genetically-engineered cell, done with a drug-resistance gene that presumably turned on the stemness genes, was originally a normal adult stem cell with it's already expressed Oct-4 and other stemness genes, then, in fact, those rescued cells were hardly a highly differentiated somatic differentiated skin fibroblast. The point being made is that adult stem cells do exist in most, if not all, adult organs, especially the skin. Many adult stem cells have been isolated from adult tissues that expressed Oct-4 and did not express the connexon genes or have functional gap junctions [82-88]. These are real multi-potential stem or bi-potential stem cells. They are not simply pluri-potential embryonic stem cells migrating throughout the body of adult organisms.

Since adult stem cells have been isolated for many years, "Is there evidence that these adult stem cells can give rise to cancer?" The answer is "yes". When human adult breast stem cells were isolated and reported in 1995 [83], it was, then, subsequently shown that SV40 could block their ability to terminally differentiate (an operational definition of initiation) [89]. These cells were unable to form tumors in an appropriated animal model. While SV40 and other viruses (i.e. human papilloma virus) have been termed, "immortalizing viruses", it appears that this might be a major misnomer. It is well known that when primary human cell cultures are infected with these viruses, the majority of the cells eventually go through "crises", while a few rare cells survive and are characterized as "immortal". The idea is that either some rare insertional mutational event had occurred in these few surviving cells or that the virus genome somehow affected the senescence genes to be re-programmed" and the immortalization process started. There is a simpler explanation, supported by the experiments with human adult breast stem cells [31]. That is, the infecting SV40 or papilloma viruses, while infecting all the cells of the primary culture, only affected the few adult stem cells of that culture. These viruses did not induce "immortalization" but, in fact, blocked "mortalization" of an already normal, immortal adult stem cell. Chang and associates showed that these cells were able to perpetuate themselves in vitro and, upon, radiation and oncogene transfection become tumorigenic, whereas, no normal, differentiated human adult breast epithelial cell became "immortal" or neoplastically transformed [89].

It's important to discuss how the original adult human kidney stem cell was isolated and reported in 1987 [82]. The idea that stem cells might be the target cell for initiating the carcinogenic process came from studies to determine the extreme variability of inducing neoplastic transformed Syrian hamster cells in vitro. Nakano and T'so were trying to discern why cultures of Syrian hamster embryo cells could be exposed to some carcinogen on one day in the lab and formed many neoplastic transformed clones, but the same cultures on another day or in another lab, no transformants were induced [90]. To make a long story short, they noticed that, only in those cultures with "contact-insensitive" populations of cells, could one obtain neoplastic transformed clones. Our lab speculated these "contact insensitive", normal embryonic cells in these cultures might be stem cells. We further reasoned that their "contact-insensitivity" was the result of not expressing connexin genes or having functional gap junctional intercellular communication. We, therefore, assumed, in all adult tissues, there existed a few adult stem cells that did not have functional GJIC. By designing an in vitro assay with lethally-irradiated human fibroblast cells, which have functional GJIC, we disassociated normal kidney tissue into single cells. This mixture of normal kidney cells contained the many progenitor cells, which have functional GJIC, the terminally differentiated cells which can not proliferate and the few adult stem cells, which we assumed had no functional GJIC. After putting these cells on the lethally irradiated monolayer of human fibroblasts, we obtained a few clones of cells, which were later shown to be the adult stem cells of the human kidney (They expressed no connexion genes or had functional GJIC but they expressed Oct-4). As controls in this experiment, 8 human carcinoma cell lines, which had no GJIC, also could be recovered on this assay system. The rationale for the selection system was that if a normal cell had functional GJIC, it would couple with the dying x ray lethally-irradiated cells and die. Only those cells with no functional GJIC would proliferate on this monolayer. All of the human adult stem cells that have been reported appear not to express any connexion genes or have functional GJIC [82-88].

The reality is that in an adult animal, including the human being, adult committed stem cells exists normally for tissue replacement and growth. These stem cells are not merely pluripotent or multi-potent stem cells floating around only to differentiate when needed in particular micro-environments. Each tissue contains these stem cells. It is these adult organ-specific stem cells that are the suspected targets for the initiation of the carcinogenic process.

Cancer Stem Cells: A Re-Discovery of an Old Idea

One of the recent paradigm-changing observations that has occurred in the cancer field happened when Al Hajj et al [80] reported that they identified a presumptive unique class of breast cancer cells within the breast tumor that had the ability to perpetuate the growth of the tumor, i.e., a breast *"cancer stem cell"*, whereas the other cancer cells within that tumor did not have this ability. These might be referred to as *cancer non-stem cells*. They are partially differentiated and ultimately senesce or apoptose. Later, Ponti et al [91] were able to show that these breast cancer stem cells to perpetuate the growth of the tumor. However, much earlier, Chang and his associates had already identified and partially characterized the normal human breast stem cell and showed that these stem cells could be "initiated" and neoplastically transformed [92]. In effect, he produced, in vitro, the human breast cancer stem cell that gave rise to a tumor when the cells were placed into an immune-compromised mouse.

Historically, when it was shown that the embryonic stem cell expressed a few unique "embryonic stem cell markers" (e.g., Oct-4, Sox 2, nanog genes) [93], Oct-4 seemed to have been correctly identified, early in the characterization of expressed genes in embryonic stem cells, as a critical "stemness-determining gene [94]. Later, observations showed that when these cells differentiated, the oct-4 gene was transcriptionally suppressed [95]. There were others that claimed that no Oct-4 expression could be found in normal differentiated tissues. Then, when a few reports saw Oct-4 expression in a few cells of some types of tumors [96, 97], it was suggested that Oct-4 must have been re-expressed or re-programmed during the neoplastic transformation process. It has been used to confirm the accepted paradigm [43] that the normal differentiated progenitor cells do not express immortalizing potential that the Oct-4 gene seems to possess.

Because our group, believers in the stem cell theory of cancer, knew the adult differentiated tissues must have a few adult stem cells, which were probably overlooked in these previous reports, we decided to examine the many isolated human adult stem cells we had in our lab (kidney, breast, liver, pancreas, mesenchyme) for the expression of Oct-4. We also assumed that these few normal adult stem cells were the target cells for the cancers seen in human organs. In addition to testing for Oct-4, we also tested for the expression of the major connexins and for functional GJIC which is required for these stem cells to differentiate. In brief, we showed that all of these normal adult stem cells expressed Oct-4 and when the stem cells differentiated, Oct-4 was repressed.

In a classic set of experiments, Dr. Chang's group obtained a series of clonally-derived cells from the normal adult breast stem cells which (a) could be differentiated into normal epithelial cells (no expression of Oct-4, but they expressed Cx43 and had functional GJIC); (b) were SV-40 transfected but non-tumorigenic and unable to terminally differentiate, had Oct-4 expressed but no GJIC; (c) after x-rayed irradiated produced a weakly tumorigenic clone with Oct-4 expressed; and (d) which after a neu/Erb2 transfection, a highly tumorigenic derivative of the weakly tumorigenic clone was obtained , which still expressed Oct-4 [98]. In essence, we showed that Oct-4 was expressed in the normal adult stem cell, stayed expressed when SV40 prevented asymmetric cell division, remained expressed during the induction of tumorigenesis by X rays and oncogene transfection. It was transcriptionally suppressed only during differentiation of the normal adult stem cells [98]. These differentiated breast epithelial cells were unable to re-program the Oct-4 gene or become immortal or tumorigenic under the conditions where the normal adult stem cell was easily blocked from differentiating and neoplastically transformed. These experiments clearly support the stem cell theory and are harder to explain using the "de-differentiation" or "re-programming" hypothesis of carcinogenesis.

It is important to note that these normal breast adult stem cells expressed the estrogen receptor, a marker found in a majority of human breast cancers. In addition, since the commonly used human breast carcinoma cell line in breast cancer studies, MCF-7, expresses the estrogen receptor, but not the connexion 43 gene [99], but does express the Oct-4 in vitro [98], one might speculate that MCF-7 was originally derived from a normal adult breast stem cell similar to our normal human isolated adult breast stem cell.

It is also important to note that MCF-7 is not a homogeneous cell population [98]. It is an immortal cell line because it contains some "cancer stem cells" that help to perpetuate the cell line indefinitely. *In vitro, as in vivo, the cells create different micro-environments for these cancer stem cells, causing some of them to partially differentiate into cancer non-stem cells or to regain some asymmetric cell division potential.* The implication from these observations is that, all tumors during their growth will be a mixture of cancer stem cells and cancer non-stem cells. The ratio of these two types of cancer cells is probably influenced by some stromal-epithelial interactions, as has been demonstrated in vivo and in vitro [76, 77, 100].

To illustrate this, we were the first to detect in vivo that 100% of 83 canine tumors from 21 different organ sites expressed Oct-4 in the tumors (the "cancer stem cells", but the ratio of the cancer stem cell to the cancer non-stem cells varied from tumor to tumor. [81] Later it was shown that 34/35 human bladder tumors expressed Oct-4, and the ratio of the two types varied widely between tumors [101]. At this point, one can only speculate that the differences in the ratio of the two types of cancer cells might be due to genetic, environmental or dietary factors that influences symmetric and asymmetric cell division of the cancer stem cell.

In a recent cautionary note, it was stated that "tumor growth need not be driven by rare cancer stem cells" [102]. The authors drew their conclusion, based on showing that isolated primary pre-B7B lymphoma cells from 3 independent Eu-myc transgenic mice could give rise to tumors in congenic mice, independent of cell injected. Their conclusion, based on everyone's assumption was that, in all tumors, the "cancer stem cells" were "rare". In the study on canine tumors, and on human bladders [81,101], the numbers of Oct-4 "cancer stem cells" varied widely. Therefore, this cautionary note might be very misleading.

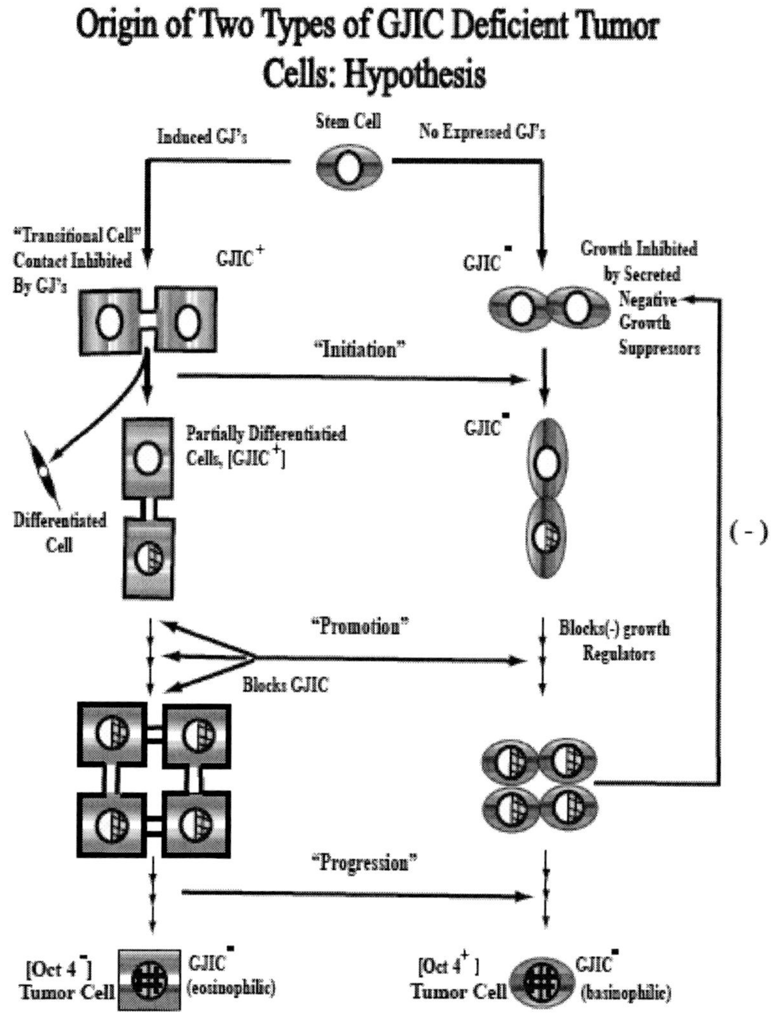

Figure 7. This figure illustrates a hypothesis to explain the existence of two types of cancer cells, namely, those that lack GJIC communication because (a) the connexin genes were never transcribed, as in HeLa or MCF-7 cancer cell lines, or (b) the expressed connexion genes could not form functional gap junctions due to oncogenes or mutations that render the connexin proteins forming functional gap junction, as in ras, raf, neu, src or mos-activated oncogene-transformed cancer cells. In other words, all cancer cells seem to be dysfunctional with regard to having GJIC, either because the connexin genes were never transcribed or if the transcribed proteins were not functional. There are several possible explanations, one being that the original stem cell, lacking expressed connexins, got initiated and subsequently promoted by agents that inhibited secreted negative growth regulators of stem cells. These might be the origin of the "cancer stem" cells. Now the cancer cells with activated oncogenes might inactivate functional GJIC by modifying, posttranslationally, the connexin proteins and gap junctions. There could be at least two explanations for this. One is that if the very early committed progenitor cells of the adult stem cell was initiated while it still expressed Oct-4 and telomerase, then its growth inhibition via gap junctions had to be inhibited by promoters that reversibly blocked GJIC, until late in promotion, when activated oncogenes stably and irreversibly inhibited gap junction proteins, such as via hyper-phosphorylation of connexins by ras, src and neu. Alternatively, these non-functional GJIC tumor cells might be derived from "cancer stem cells" but which were partially differentiated by the developing and changing microenvironments of all tumors to become "cancer non-stem cells".

The excitement seen after the reports of the existence of various “cancer stem cells” has given new insights to the reasons why past cancer therapies have failed, i.e., they failed to target the “cancer stem cells” in the tumors. In addition, one of the explanations why these various therapeutic treatments failed was because the treatments, themselves, induced drug resistance genes that allowed these drug resistant cells to re-emerge. It now seems that a more plausible explanation exists for “induced drug resistance”. The normal adult stem cell and its derived “cancer stem cell” might be naturally resistant to toxic chemotherapeutic agents. Again, the quote, “Nothing in biology makes sense except in the light of evolution”, seems appropriate here.

From an evolutionary standpoint, if, during the emergence of the multi-cellular organism and the development of both germ line stem cells and adult somatic stem cells, both the stem cells and their differentiate lineage progeny were equally sensitive to environmental toxicant, the individual, hence, species, would never have survived. Therefore, it was imperative that the stem cells evolved with some mechanism(s) to protect itself from the exposure to these toxic agents. One means was to develop mechanisms to pump out foreign chemicals before they could damage the cell. Therefore, if an organism is exposed to some toxic agent, the differentiated cells might die; however, if the adult stem cell survived, it could replace the dead, specialized, differentiated cells and the organism and species would survive.

Evidence has been reported that, when tumor cells are exposure to some toxic fluorescent agent and then passed through a cell sorter, two populations of cells are recovered. One that contains the fluorescent compound and the other, the “side population”, cells are non-fluorescent. It is these “side population” cells that seem to have stem-like properties, in that they can differentiate into the cell-lineage from which the tumor is derived [103]. One of these factors that rendered these cells to be drug resistant is because they naturally expressed various drug resistant genes, such as ABCG-2 [104].

In brief, drug resistance was not induced by the cancer chemotherapy, but it was the result of “cancer stem cells, which are naturally, expressing drug resistance genes, were selected from the mixed population of cancer cells.

A new perspective for cancer prevention and therapy is now obvious. The real target cell for prevention and treatment should be the “cancer stem cells”. Oct-4 expression appears to by a critical gene to maintain “stemness” of both the normal stem cell and “cancer stem” cell. The ultimate goal in cancer prevention and therapy will be to render, transcriptionally or posttranslationally, the Oct-4 gene inoperative.

This goal still has the same current intractable problem that has been plaguing the old therapeutic approaches. Since Oct-4 is expressed in both the normal and cancer stem cells, one must be able to target only the cancer stem cell, in order from preventing the therapy from reducing the normal stem cell pool. In addition, since the tumor contains both the cancer stem and cancer non-stem cells, which could inhibit the therapy designed to target the cancer stem cells, a dual approach might be implemented.

First, apply some therapy that can “easily” remove these cancer non-stem cells. After these are reduced, if the cancer stem cells, which express oct-4 and drug resistance genes, inhibiting the pump activity at the functional or enzymatic level, then treating with a toxic chemical, used to kill the cancer non-stem cells, would render these cancer stem cells to behave as functional cancer non-stem cells.

This approach has been tried in the past without our current knowledge of the cancer stem cell concept. Another strategy would be to target the Oct-4 gene with transcriptionally-modifying potential to block its expression, using targeting strategies that identify the organ markers for the adult stem cells, such as the estrogen receptor for adult human breast cancer stem cells and some other "cancer stem cell" marker not expressed in the normal adult stem cell.

Dietary Modulation of Normal and Cancer Stem Cell Pools: A View of How Diet, Systems View of Cell Biology, and the Risk to Cancer Interact

It is well known that genetic predispositions, gender, developmental state, caloric balance (gluttony or caloric restriction), exercise, life style, cultural, environmental , medical, or pharmacological treatments can influence the multi-stage, multi-mechanism process of carcinogenesis. What is clearly emerging is the powerful role that dietary factors play in experimental, as well as epidemiological studies, to either increase or decrease one's risk to various cancers. What has not been clearly demonstrated is, the interaction of these dietary factors and the adult normal and cancer stem cells. In fact, a new view is emerging that takes us away from only thinking, reductionalistically, about what might happen in a single adult stem cell that eventually could give rise to an initiated cancer stem cell, but how diet can involve the stem cell pool to affect the risk to increase or decrease the risk to cancer from a *systems* vantage point. In deed, this new view also will take our attention away from only viewing the cancer stem cell role as only a biological problem, but one that involves many cultural evolutionary changes.

Because of cultural evolution, which affects our dietary intake of the quantity and quality of food much more rapidly than the biological evolution needed to adapt to these changes, the long biological evolutionary adaptive balance with the diet of early humanoids, the new dietary behaviours are creating many new health problems [105-109]. Transmigration studies of humans have shown in several cases that the patterns of cancer frequencies of various ethnic groups conform to the new cultural (presumably) dietary behaviour compared to their country of origin.

Because of modern methods of altering native cultural diets to global diets, cancer patterns are changing. In fact, for a number of reasons, these new dietary habits are shaped by economic costs, availability of certain foods (depletion of tuna for sushi and sashimi), substitution of red meats for fish, agricultural genetic breeding of foods that sell or are needed for "fast food industries", and the psychological selling via mass marketing. The complexity of "diets" (calories, vitamins, nutrients, food components, processing and preparation of foods, etc.) makes epidemiological studies difficult to interpret since these studies are but a small snapshot in a dynamic time and place experience in an ever-changing dietary climate probably within every 20 years. These studies are now compounded in complexity by increasing uses of food supplements, pharmaceutical drugs, changing life styles and individual behaviours. The World Health Organization's estimation that there might be more over weight individuals than under weight in the world today suggests that global chronic (as well as acute) diseases are being affected by, on one hand, too many calories (not necessarily too many nutrients) or too few calories and nutrients [110]. Therefore, the next question has to be asked: "Which of the three stages of carcinogenesis seem to be most affected by diet modification?"

One can speculate that, since the initiation stage must take place in a single cell in a limited number of critical cancer-related genes, either by a mutational or stable epigenetic event, it will be impossible to reduce the risk to zero in the body of 100 trillion cells, most of which are not the target or adult stem cells. Initiation can occur when DNA damage is not repaired correctly (errors in DNA repair), such as in the xeroderma pigmentosum example. We can, of course, prevent the risk from being higher, such as not exposing ourselves to too much sunlight. In addition, we must recognize that mutations can be produced every time a cell replicates (errors in replication). We can never prevent this source of mutations that might initiate an adult stem cell. Cells are replicating day and night, 7 days a week and for our whole lives. Therefore, it is would seem that we will never reduce to zero the initiating event. *In fact, this source of spontaneously-originating errors in replication of DNA in stem cells might be the main source of initiated cells of the body, except for the UV-light induced initiation of skin stem cells.*

Promotion, on the other hand, takes decades, in most cases (except in children), to reach the progression stage. From a practical standpoint of designing an intervention chemoprevention strategy that would be the most efficacious, to decrease the risk to carcinogenesis, at least from the view that we, as individuals, might have some control of this process, the promotion phase would be a *life-long* process. Since the progression phase appears to occur in a single promoted initiated cell (a "pre-cancer stem cell"), that requires the phenotypes needed for invasion, metastasis and induction of angiogenesis, it might also be impossible to modify, appreciably, this phase of carcinogenesis because one might not know when to intervene. *By intervening during the promotion phase (during one's adult lifespan), diet can make a difference on the progression, hence carcinogenic transition.*

There is no question, that using the initiation, promotion and progression models of carcinogenesis, one can increase or decrease the cancer frequencies. Even using surrogate in vitro models, (transformation assays; gap junction modulation assays, etc.), one can identify dietary, as well as environmental factors, that can either increase or decrease endpoints in these models that correspond to the experimental or epidemiological evidence [111]. Of course, while there hasn't been perfect correspondence of the in vitro assay results with the experimental or epidemiological data, it should not be surprising, given the shortcomings of in vitro and in vivo animal data [68], let alone epidemiological data [112]. Most of these studies are lacking the mechanistic basis of either the assays used or the understanding of the biology of the carcinogenic process in the design or interpretation of the epidemiological studies.. The failure of the CARET study is a perfect example of this point [113]. The original design ignored previous studies on the mechanism of action of this class of natural chemicals on GJIC [114]. In addition, studies have shown that anti-oxidants can become pro-oxidants [115]. It has even been shown that some of the same class of molecules could become tumor promoters [116]. By the same interesting challenge to our understanding, many tumor promoters have been shown to be anti- carcinogens [117-119]. The conflicting and non-reproducible epidemiological studies are also not surprising, because human populations can not be controlled like rats in a laboratory. Genetic differences, exposures to unreported factors that might be additive, antagonistic or even synergistic to the factor that is under study, critical threshold concentrations, anti-oxidant proficiencies or deficiencies of the individuals, time and duration of exposures, etc., can modify the results of one study compared to another.

The critical importance of understanding the underlying mechanisms of promotion and the role of stem cells in carcinogenesis have not yet entered the cancer prevention or treatment area. A case in point is the recent TASK FORCE REPORT to suggest new approaches to identify potential cancer chemo-preventive compounds [120]. No mention was made of the mechanistically-based in vitro (and in vivo) assay, based on the prevention of tumor promoting agents from down-regulating gap junctional intercellular communication. Many agents that can, reversibly, down regulate GJIC have been shown to be potential tumor promoters by various biochemical mechanisms [121]. The consequence of inhibiting GJIC by any biochemical mechanism in normal tissues is dis-regulation of homeostasis of cell proliferation and differentiation of stem cells, progenitor and differentiated cells. Classic tumor promoters, such as phorbol esters and phenobarbital, have shown correspondence of the in vitro results with the in vivo results [52]. In deed, even the opposite case to support the role of GJIC in chemoprevention, and even chemotherapy, has been made in vitro, as well as in vivo., with a large number of dietary factors, such as green tea [55], resveratrol [56, 57], caffeic acid ethyl ester [58], beta-sitosterol [62]and lovastatin [59], SAHA [61].

Why Dogs and Cows Caused Human Prostate and Breast Cancers: The Interaction of Biological and Cultural Evolution, Diet, Adult Stem Cells and Cancer

To bring this *Commentary* to full circle, the quote made by D. Coffey should serve to provide a "systems view" of the human cancer problem. In his article comparing the similarities of breast and prostate cancers, he stated:

> "Certainly, looking for simple relation will not be sufficient, but delineating the exact mechanisms of cell cycle control and stem cell development in prostate cancer should be helpful in understanding these early preneoplastic lesions and their relations to diet." [122].

Up until now, the focus for trying to understand the complex carcinogenic process has been through the "light of biological evolution". The formation of a multi-cellular organism created a need to coordinate cell proliferation, differentiation, apoptosis, senescence and adaptive responses of adult stem cells, progenitor and terminally-differentiated cells. The need to have both somatic and germ-line stem cells served both the individual and species The fact that the DNA is not immune to DNA damage, errors in repair or in DNA replication was selected for a the production of mutations at a rate that would ensure survival of the species in an ever changing physical environment, yet not so high as to jeopardize either the individual or species' survival. Neither the somatic adult stem cells or the germ-line stem cells were immune to these mutations.

In the case of the human species, the individual was served by these somatic adult stem cells to provide growth, differentiation of highly specialized cells, and wound-healing. These were needed to allow the individual to live long enough to reach sexual maturation, to leave offspring, and to take care of the offspring until they were able to repeat this process. This ensured the survival of the species. After that period of life span (approximately mid-fourties, the individual's contribution to evolution was essentially finished. At which time, sufficient mutations had occurred in both the germ line and somatic stem cells. The geriatric individual, save for some accumulated experiences ("wisdom"), was basically a drain on limited resources for the survival of the young. As pointed out above, the adult stem cell is most likely the target cell for cancer. However, the multi-stage, multi-mechanism carcinogenic process, probably played little role as a negative selection factor for evolution, as most cancers would appear long after the median life span of most individuals in early pre-and real human biological evolutionary history.

Clues to the roles of both biological and cultural evolution, diet and breast and prostate cancers have been noted before [122,123]. Unlike the roles that biological evolution, changing physical environment and diets of non-human animals played in their evolution, human's brought with them the emergence of 4 critical new phenotypes [to consciously create symbols; to communicate with those symbols; to create new technologies using those symbols and communication skills; and to value or make choices on which technology to use or not use [124]. Unlike non-human animals, their "detritus" disappears in short time. However, as it has been stated by a philosopher, "Men build walls and walls build men". The point being that what we do to our physical and cultural environments has lasting and major impacts on future generations of both the non-human animal and the human animal.

Human beings have created a cultural environment which, among many other things, shapes both our physical environment and our diet. As noted in the subtitle of this section, early humans learned a few things that helped to rescue them from hunting and gathering and a "feast-fast"- type of dietary behaviour that shaped our biological evolution. That is, we had to have those molecular, cellular and physiological adaptive features, stored in the genome of our germ and somatic stem cells that allowed us to survive under these "feast and fast"-conditions. We inherited these from our pre-human and non-human animal ancestors. With the domestication of the cow, which provided work, food, and clothing, and of the dog, which aided human's hunting abilities, we find clues as to how these cultural evolutionary facts have impacted on human stem cells and cancer. In both of these cases, these two animals have helped to "cause" breast, colon and prostate cancers in humans. In the case of the bovine, one might note there seems not to be any significant mammary cancers associated with its existence, so why is there a link to human breast cancer? In the case of the canine, this animal seems to have a significant prostate cancer problem similar to human beings [122,123]. Can comparative oncology provide some answers or will a simple "systems" view do?

To first view how diet might affect the multi-stage, multi-mechanism process of carcinogenesis, we need to view the shared general concepts of the aforementioned integrated hypothesis, and how prostate and breast carcinogenesis might have a "higher order" or cultural component in their dietary risk factors.

When one views the current studies on the cancers found in the atomic bomb survivals of Hiroshima and Nagasaki, breast cancers seem to be one of the highest solid tumors to which could be attributed to the exposures to radiation [125]. One of the reasons it was noted is because the background frequency of breast cancers of those Japanese women was extremely low such that any attributed increase by radiation was noted to be statistically significant. While the main focus of the interpretation of these data has been the radiation exposures, little attention has been given to why the attributed increase was the level seen. In the first place, one interpretation has been that soy products which has been for generations a major component of the Japanese women's diet might have been the reason for (a) small breasts and (b) low breast cancer frequencies. Because soy contains many anti-cancer nutritional components, genistein and Bowen-Birks Inhibitor [126, 127], it has been speculated that these dietary components contributed to lowering the breast cancer frequencies of both the control and a bomb survivors. From a mechanistic perspective and our theme that adult stem cells are the target cells for carcinogenic initiation, the next question is: "How do these soy products work on the multi-stage, multi-mechanism process of breast carcinogenesis."

In the first place, human adult breast stem cells have been isolated from normal human breast tissue [83]. These breast stem cells can be neoplastically transformed in vitro.[89] Moreover, while there is no existing evidence that genistein could lower or increase the ionizing radiation genetic damage in human breast stem cells, there is compelling evidence that genistein can induce differentiation of the adult human breast stem cells. [128] Therefore, if either the mother of the daughter, exposed to the a bomb radiation, eat lots of soy products during pregnancy, the female embryo and fetus would have few breast stem cells because the breast stem cell would have been induced to asymmetrically divide rather that symmetrically divide to produce many adult breast stem cells. Further, after birth and during adolescent development, the daughter also consumed lots of soy products. Therefore, from these facts of diet on stem cells during development and adolescent growth, this dietary habit could be a chemo-preventive factor by reducing the breast stem cell pool. This alone would reduce the risk to breast cancer by reducing the number of possible initiated breast stem cells, all other factors being the same.

While radiation is assumed to be the initiators of the exposed breast stem cells, could the soy products affect the promotion of cancer? The evidence, on the whole, seems to indicate that these soy components can be chemo-preventive by their ability to interfere with the promotion process, although there is some rodent evidence it could act as a tumor promoter [129]. Again, this points out the need for better understanding of the underlying mechanisms, especially when using either animal bioassays or epidemiological studies. It should now be pointed out that, with the introduction of dairy products into the Japanese diet and the transmigration studies of Japanese, who move to Western countries, soon changed their dietary habits and frequencies of breast cancers to match to of the host country. In addition, it should also be noted that the Japanese women, who contribute to the longest median life span also pay a heavy price for their past dietary practices, namely the high frequency of osteoporosis. Could it be that the soy products which induced differentiation and asymmetrical cell division of the breast stem cell also did the same for the osteoblast precursor stem cells? This then opens up another health aspect of stem cell pool modulation, namely the reduction of stem cells via either diet or environmental agents could affect the aging process itself, as well as the diseases of aging [130,131].

To further analyze how diet can influence breast cancer and getting back to the bovine, milk, cheese, red meat, all factors associated with both breast and colon cancer, were introduced during the domestication of the bovine. Many of the components of these bovine products, aside from the caloric content, is the introduction of dietary components that are known tumor promoters in animal model systems, in vitro model systems, such as those that detect their ability to reversibly inhibit gap junctional intercellular communication [111]. Unsaturated fatty acids, insulin, insulin –like growth factors, among others factors, could cause both the symmetrical cell division in adult breast stem cells (increasing the risk to initiation) and act as tumor promoters of initiated breast stem cells. Note that, prior to the Second World War, few dairy products (cheese, meat, milk) were in the Japanese diet. Today, it is becoming a major component.

Back to the human prostate, when the early humans domesticated the canine, the hunter became more successful. The canine and the human started to share the same diet of red meat that was now grilled. While early humans did not survive long enough to manifest prostate cancers, today with the median life span in developed countries having been significantly increased over the last century, so too has the prostate cancer frequency.

An example of how both an environmental factor and the soy dietary factors play a role in prostate cancer has recently been reported. Ho et al [132] showed that pregnant rodents fed a diet contaminated with bisphenol A gave rise to male offspring that had a high incidence of prostate cancers, even though the male offspring were not exposed to the environmental non-genotoxic chemical after birth. On the other hand, if these pregnant rodents were fed both soy products and the bisphenol-A, the risk to prostate cancer in the male offspring was dramatically reduced. Clearly , if one assumes that the stem cells of the prostate are the target cells for prostate cancers, and that the effects seen occur in utero during fetal development, one can speculate that the bisphenol-A caused the prostate stem cells to symmetrical division, increasing the prostate stem cell pool. This alone, all other factors being the same, would increase the risk to cancer. On the other hand, if during fetal development the components of the soy diet cause the prostate stem cell to divide asymmetrically and to differentiate, then the stem cell pool would decrease, lowering the risk to prostate cancer.

It must be pointed out the bisphenol A is an epigenetic, not genotoxic, toxicant. Dietary chemicals, such as genistein and environmental toxicants, such as bisphenol A, TCDD, PBB, PCB, DDT, can effect, epigenetically gene expression of the offspring when agents are applied in utero. The studies by the Jirtle group showed that the genetic strain of agouti mice could have their coat color modulated by epigenetic agents [133]. The molecular alterations in methylation and histone acetylation suggest that they are associated with the altered phenotypes. However, there is another interpretation. The altered gene expression might be due to altered stem cell pools (recall that the gene patterns of particular adult stem cells will always be different from their differentiated daughter lineage cells that contribute to the agouti phenotype).

In a brief analysis of how dietary nutrients, contaminants and process of preparation, such as frying or grilling, diets, that affect either or both breast and prostate cancer (or any other kind), probably affect the promotion, rather that the initiation process. They could affect initiation, indirectly, by altering the stem cell pool that is exposed to an initiator. Most, if not all, promoters reversibly inhibit cell-cell communication to affect proliferation, differentiation and apoptosis. Promotion is the stage that would most likely be impacted by dietary factors and intervention practices to lower cancer frequencies. Several promoters and anti-promoters come to mind with the advent of cultural evolutionary changes, contributed by the bovine and canine. The animal fats, the excessive calories, the cholesterol, hormones, such as estrogens, insulin, pyrolytic polyaromatic hydrocarbons [68], which both the bovine and canine gave humans (and to the canine by us in return for its hunting and companionship attributes), we can attribute, in part, both the rise in breast cancer and prostate cancers. In the case of breast cancers, the cultural practice, now, of postponing of early marriage and children only raises the breast cancer risk.

It is interesting to note that β-sitosterol, a component of fibers of vegetables and fruits, can lower cholesterol levels [134] and inhibit the ras oncogene effect on cell-cell communication in tumor cells. [62]. It is also, a major component of olive oil [135] and this has been suggested as a possible risk reducer of both cardiovascular and prostate cancer frequencies in the Mediterranean diet. Bovine animals with large mammary glands, unlike the canine with prostate cancers due to its companionship with the humans and their diets, eats lots of plant products containing β-sitosterol (of course, they do not live long enough to develop cancers; however, it they did, it is unlikely they would have a high frequency of mammary cancers).

Conclusion

The implications of understanding the mechanisms of carcinogenesis are immense. Currently, the many known factors that must influence the mechanism of forming a tumor (e.g., genetics, developmental stage, gender, environmental agents, calories, exercise, diet, life-style and cultural behaviours, etc.) appear to prevent the generation of a coherent integrated hypothesis. However, many old ideas, such as the multi-stage, multi-mechanism hypothesis, the stem cell theory, and newer observations in molecular oncology, toxicology of chemical "carcinogens", stem cell biology , oncogene / tumor suppression gene functions ,plus the re-discovery of "cancer stem cells", have made it possible to gain a new insight.

While a tumor consists of billions of genotypically- and phenotypically-heterogeneous cells, we do know they all had a single common origin. While still debated, that single normal cell, which was altered during the "initiation" phase of carcinogens, appears to have been a normal, immortal adult stem cell. "Initiation" appears to be a process that blocks that normal stem cell's ability to divide, asymmetrically, under normal conditions of proliferation; in other words, it can not terminally differentiate senesce or apoptose. While the risk to the initiation phase, caused by either mutations or stable epigenetic mechanisms, can be minimized, it can never be reduced to zero. However, the promotion phase, which brings about the clonal expansion of these initiated stem cells or "pre-cancer stem cells", can take decades to generate an invasive and metastatic "cancer stem cell". The promotion of these initiated stem cells can be interrupted or accelerated by environmental-, dietary-, hormone-, inflammatory-, cytokine-, and growth- factors, as well as caloric restriction or gluttony. Cell-cell communication, by either secreted or gap junction-mediated factors, triggers redox-intracellular signalling to alter gene expression, can be either decreased (tumor promotion) or increased (chemo-prevention or anti-tumor promotion). The discovery that the Oct-4 gene can be a marker for both maintaining "stemness" in the normal embryonic and adult stem cells, as well as a marker for the pre-malignant and malignant " cancer stem cells", makes it possible to target these cells with new strategies for chemo-prevention and chemotherapy.

From this new integration of observations and hypotheses, comes another new important implication, namely, one's risk to cancer might be influenced during pregnancy when the mother's dietary or medical treatments could either increase or decrease the adult stem cell pools in various organs. Keeping all other cancer-influencing factors equal, just increasing or decreasing the adult stem cell pool would alter the risk to cancer in adulthood, based on the adult stem cell being the "target" for the initiation phase. On the other hand, what we as inheritors of these adult stem cells from our mothers do to any "initiated" stem cell in our body can either increase or decrease the risk to the promotion phase of carcinogenesis. In other words, *"What our mother's ate or didn't eat (or get exposed to) can influence the number of our adult stem cells; what we eat or do to these initiated stem cells can modulate our risk to cancer."*

References

[1] Dobzhansky, T. (1975) Nothing in Biology makes sense except in the light of evolution. *Am.Biol. Teachers,* 35, 125-129.

[2] Hanahan, D. and Weinberg, R.A. (2000). Hallmarks of cancer. *Cell,* 100, 57-70.

[3] Al Hajj, M., Wicha, M.S., Benito-Hernandez, A., Morrison, S.J., and Clarke, M.F. (2003). Prospective identification of tumorigenic breast cancer cells. *Proc. Nat. Acad. Sci. USA,* 100, 3983-3988.

[4] Markert, C.L. (1968). Neoplasia: A disease of differentiation. *Cancer Res.*, 28, 1908-1914.

[5] Markert, C. L. (1984). Genetic control of cell interactions in chimeras. *Develop Genet.*, 4, 267-279.

[6] Pierce, B. (1974). Neoplasms, differentiation and mutations. *Am. J. Pathol.*, 77, 103-118.

[7] Potter, V.R. (1978). Phenotypic diversity in experimental hepatomas: Concept of partially blocked ontogeny. *Br. J. Cancer,* 38, 1-23.

[8] Kerbel, R.S., Frost, P., Liteplo,R., Carlow, D.A., and Elliot, B.E. (1984). Possible epigenetic mechanisms of tumor progression: Induction of high frequency heritable but phenotypically unstable changes in the tumorigenic and metastatic properties of tumor cell populations by 5-azacytidine treatment. *J. Cell Physiol.*, 3, 87-97.

[9] Tlsty, T.D., Briot, A., Gualberto, A., Hall, I., Hess, S., Hixon, M., Kuppuswamy, D., Romanov, D., Sage, M., and White, A. (1995). Genomic instability and cancer. *Mutation Res.*, 337, 1-7.

[10] P.W.Laird. (2005). Cancer epigenetics. *Hum. Mol. Genet.,* 14, R65-R76.

[11] Boveri, T. (1914). *Zurfrage der Entstehung Maligner Tumoren.* Jena: Gustav Fisher.

[12] Cleaver, J.E. and Trosko, J.E. (1970). Absence of excision of ultraviolet-induced cyclobutane dimers in Xeroderma pigmentosum. *Photochem. Photobiol.*, 11, 547-550.

[13] Maher, V.M. and McCormick, J.J. (1976). Effect of DNA repair on the cytotoxicity and mutagenicity of UV irradiation and of chemical carcinogens in normal and xeroderma pigmentosum cells. In: J.M. Yuhas, R.W. Tennant and J.D. Regan (Eds.), *Biology of Radiation Carcinogenesis* (pp. 129-145). New York: Raven Press.

[14] Warren, S., R.A. Schultz, C.C. Chang, M.H. Wade and Trosko, J.E. (1981). Elevated spontaneous mutation rate in Bloom syndrome fibroblasts. *Proc. Natl. Acad. Science USA,* 78, 3133-3137.

[15] Brash, D. E., Rudolph, J.A., Simon, X., Lin, A. and McKenna, G.J. (1991). A role for sunlight in skin cancer: UV-induced p53 mutations in squamous cell carcinomas. *Proc. Natl. Acad. Sci. USA*, 88, 10124-10128.

[16] Ames,B.N., Durston,W. E., Yamasaki, E. and Lee, F. D. (1973). Carcinogens are mutagens a simple test system combining liver homogenates for activation and bacteria for detection. *Proc. Natl. Acad. Sci. USA*, 70, 2281-2285.

[17] Marsh, D.J. and Zori, R.T. (2002). Genetic insights into famial cancers-update and recent discoveries. *Cancer Letters,* 181, 125-164.

[18] Evans, W.H. and Martin, P.E.M. (2002).Gap junctions: Structure and Function. *Molec. Membr. Biol.*, 19, 121-136.

[19] Cruciani, V. and Mikalsen, S.-O. (2005). The connexin gene family in mammals. *Biol Chem.*, 386, 325-332.

[20] Willecke, K., Eiberger, J., Degen, J., Eckhardt, D., Romauldi, A., Guldenagel, M., Duetsch, U. and Sohl, G. (2002). Structural and functional diversity of connexion genes in the mouse and human genome. *Biol. Chem.*, 383, 725-737.

[21] Eagle, H. (1965). Growth inhibitor effects of cellular interactions. *Isreal J. Med. Sci.*, 1, 1220-1228.

[22] Revel, J.P. (1988). The oldest multicellular animal and its junctions. In: Hertzberg, E.L. and Johnson,R. (Eds.), *Gap Junction* (pp 135-149). N.Y.: Alan Liss, Inc.

[23] Loewenstein, W.R. (1966). Permeability of membrane junctions. *Ann. N.Y. Acad. Sci.*, 137, 441-472.

[24] Trosko, J.E. (2007). Stem cells and cell-cell communication in the understanding of the role of diet and nutrients in human diseases. *J. Fd. Hyg. Safety,* 22, 1-14.

[25] Takahashi, K. and Yamanaka, S. (2006). Induction of pluripotent stem cells from mouse embryonic and adult fibroblasts cultures by defined factors. *Cell,* 126, 663-676.

[26] Shi, Y. (2004). Caspase activation, inhibition, and reactivation: A mechanistic view. *Protein Science,* 13,1979-1987

[27] Wilson, M.R., Close, T.W. and Trosko, J.E. (2000). Cell population dynamics (apoptosis, mitosis and cell-cell communication) during disruption of homeostasis. *Exp. Cell Res.*, 254, 257-268.

[28] Tumbar, T., Guasch, G., Greco, V., Blanpain, C., Lowry, W.E., Rendl, M. and Fuchs, E. (2004). Defining the epithelial stem cell niche in skin. *Science,* 303, 359-363.

[29] Juckett D. A. (1987). Cellular aging (the Hayflick limit) and species longevity: a unification model based on clonal succession. *Mech Ageing Devel.,* 38, 49–71.

[30] Kalimi and Lo blastocyte lack og GJ Lo, C.W. (1996). The role of gap junction membrane channels in development. *J. Bioenerget. Biomembr.*, 28, 379-385.

[31] Trosko, J.E., Chang, C.C., Wilson, M.R., Upham, B.L., Hayashi, T. and wade, M. (2000). Gap junctions and the regulation of cellular functions of stem cells during development and differentiation. *Methods,* 20, 245-264.

[32] de Rooij, D. G., Lok, D., Wennk, D. (1985). Feedback regulation of the proliferation of the undifferentiated spermatogonia in the Chinese hamster by differentiating spermatogonia. *Cell Tissue Kinet,* 18, 71–81.

[33] Kimchi, A., Wang, X. F., Weinberg, R. A., Cheifetz, S. and Massague, J. (1988). Absence of TGF-b receptors and growth: Inhibitory responses in retinoblastoma cells. *Science*, 290,196–198.

[34] Borek, C. and Sachs, L. (1966). The difference in contact inhibition of cell replication between normal cells and cells transformed by different carcinogens. *Proc. Natl. Acad. Sci. USA,* 56, 1705-1711.

[35] Yamasaki, H. and Naus, C.C.G. (1996). Role of connexion genes in growth control. *Carcinogenesis,* 17, 1199-1213.

[36] Csete, M. (2005). Oxygen in the cultivation of stem cells. *Ann. N.Y. Acad. Sci.,* 1049, 1-8.

[37] Fialkow, P. J. (1979). Clonal origin of human tumors. *Am. Rev. Med.*, 30, 135-176.

[38] Nowell, P.C. (1976). The clonal evolution of tumour cell populations. *Science,* 194, 23-28.

[39] Sell, S. (1993). Cellular origin of cancer: De-differentiation or stem cell maturation arrest? *Environ. Health Perspect.,* 101, 15-26.

[40] Wernig, M., Meissner, A., Foreman, R., Brambrink, T., Ku, M., Hochedlinger, K., Berstein, B.E., and Jaenisch, R. (2007). In vitro reprogramming of fibroblasats into a pluripotent ES-cell-like state. *Nature,* 448, 318-323.

[41] Macerali N., Sriharan, R., Xie, W., Utikal, J., Eminli, S., Arnold, K., Stadfeld, M.,Yachechko, R., Tchieu, J. Jaenisch, R., Plath, K. and Hochedlinger, K. (2007). Directly reprogrammed fibroblast show global epigenetic remodelling and widespread tissue contribution. *Cell Stem Cell,* 1, 55-70.

[42] Okita, K., Ichisak, T. and Yamanaka, S. (2007) Generation of germline-competent induced pluripotent stem cells. *Nature,* 488, 313-319.

[43] Land, H., Parada, I.E. and Weinberg, R.A. (1983). Tumorigenic conversion of primary embryo fibroblasts requires at least two cooperating oncogenes. *Nature,* 304, 596-602.

[44] Hayflick, L. (1965). The limited in vitro lifespan of human diploid cell strains. *Exp. Cell Res.,* 37, 614-636.

[45] Berenblum, P.M. (1954). A speculative review: The probable nature of promoting action and its significance in the understanding of the mechanisms of carcinogenesis. *Cancer Res.,* 14, 471-477.

[46] Yamagiwa, K. and Ichikawa, K. (1977). Experimental study of the pathogenesis of carcinoma. *CA Cancer J. Clin.,* 27, 174-181.

[47] Knudson, A.G. (1971). Mutations and cancer: statistical study of retinoblastoma. *Proc. Natl. Acad. Sci. USA,* 68, 820-823.

[48] Yang, Z., Sui, Y., Xiong, S., Liour, S.S., Phillips, A.C. and Ko, L. (2007). Switched alternative splicing of oncogene CoAA during embryonal carcinoma stem cell differentiation. *Nucleic Acid Res.,* 35(6),1919-1932.

[49] Trosko, J.E. (2001). Is the concept of tumor promotion a useful paradigm? *Molec. Carcinogen.*, 39, 131-137.

[50] Goodman, J.A. (2001). Operational reversibility is a key aspect of carcinogenesis. *Toxicol. Sci.,* 64, 147-148.

[51] Trosko, J.E. and Tai, M.-H. (2006). Adult stem cell theory of the multi-stage, multi-mechanism theory of carcinogenesis: Role of inflammation on the promotion of initiated cells. In Dittmar, T., Zaeker, K.S. and Schmidt, XXX (Eds.), *Infections and Inflammation: Impacts on Oncogenesis* (Contributions to *Microbiology,* Vol. 13, pp. 45-65). K. Karger AG.

[52] Klaunig, J. and Ruch, R.J. (1987). Strain and species effects on the inhibition of hepatocyte intercellular communication by liver tumor promoters. *Cancer Letters,* 36, 161-168.

[53] Yotti, L.P., Chang, C.C. and Trosko, J.E. (1979). Elimination of metabolic cooperation in Chinese hamster cells by a tumor promoter. *Science,* 206, 1089-1091.

[54] Trosko, J.E. and Chang, C.C. (1988). Nongenotoxic Mechanisms in carcinogenesis: role of inhibited intercellular communication. In: Hart, R.W. and Hoerger, F.D. (Eds), Banbury Report 31: Carcinogen Risk Assessment: New Directions in the Qualitative and Quantitative Aspects (pp. 139-170). Cold Spring Harbor, N.Y.: Cold Spring Harbor Laboratory.

[55] Sai, K., Kanno, J., Hasegawa, R., Trosko, J.E., and Inoue, T. (2000). Prevention of the down regulation of gap junctional intercellular communication by green tea in the liver of mice fed pentachlorophenol. *Carcinogenesis,* 21, 1671-1676.

[56] Nielson, M., Ruch, R.J., and Vang, O. (2000). Reservatrol reverses tumor-promoter-induced inhibition of gap junctional intercellular communication. *Biochem. Biophys. Res. Commun.*, 275, 804-809.

[57] Upham, B.L. Guˇzvic, M., Scott, J., Carbone, J.M., Blaha, L., Coe, C.Li, L. L., Rummel, A.M., and Trosko, J.E. (2007). Inhibition of Gap Junctional Intercellular Communication and Activation of Mitogen-Activated Protein Kinase by Tumor-Promoting Organic Peroxides and Protection by Resveratrol. *Nutrition and Cancer, 57*(1), 38–47.

[58] Na, H.-K., Wilson, M.R., Kang, K.S., Chang, C.C., Grunberger, D. and Trosko, J.E. (2000). Restoration of gap junctional intercellular communication by caffeic acid phenethyl ester (CAPE) in a ras-transformed rat liver epithelial cell line. *Cancer Letters,* 157, 31-38.

[59] Ruch, R.J., Madhukar, B.V., Trosko, J.E., and Klaunig, J.E. (1993). Reversal of ras-induced inhibition of gap junctional intercellular communication, transformation and tumorigenesis by lovastatin. *Molec. Carcinogen.*, 7, 50-59.

[60] Nakamura, Y., Chang, C.C., Mori, T., Sato, K., Ohtsuki, K., Upham, B.L., and Trosko, J.E. (2005). Augmentation of differentiation and gap junction fubction by kaempferol in partially-differentiation colon cancer cells. *Carcinogenesis,* 26, 665-671.

[61] Ogawa, T., Hayashi, T., Tokunou, M., Nakachi, K., Trosko, J.E., Chang, C.C., and Yorioka, N., (2005). Suberoylanilide hydroxamic acid enhances gap junctional intercellular communication via acetylation of histone containing connexin43 gene locus. *Cancer Res*., 65, 9771-9778.

[62] Nakamura, Y., Yoshikawa, N., Hiroki, I., Sato, K., Ohtsuki,K., Chang, C.C., Upham, B.L., and Trosko, J.E. (2005). β- Sitosterol, From Psyllium Seed Husk (Plantago ovata Forsk), Restores Gap Junctional Intercellular Communication in Ha-ras Transfected Rat Liver Cells. *Nutrition Cancer,* 5, 218-225.

[63] Trosko, J.E. and Ruch, R.J. (1998). Cell-cell communication in carcinogenesis. *Front. Biosci.*, 3, 208-236.

[64] Loewenstein, W.R and Kanno, Y. (1966). Intercellular communication and the control of tissue growth: Lack of communication between cancer cells. *Nature,* 209, 1248-1249.

[65] Cleaver, J.E. (1978). Xeroderma pigmentosum: genetic and environmental influences in skin carcinogenesis. *International Journa of Dermatology,* 17, 435-444.

[66] Warren, S., Schultz, R.A., Chang, C.C., Wade, M.H. and Trosko, J.E. (1981). Elevated spontaneous mutation rate in Bloom syndrome fibroblasts. *Proc. Natl. Acad. Science USA,* 78, 3133-3137.

[67] Ames, B.N., Lois, Swirsky, Gold, L.S., and Shigenaga, M.K. (1996). *Cancer Prevention, Rodent High-Dose Cancer Tests, And Risk AssessmentRisk Analysis,* 16, 613-617.

[68] Trosko, J.E. and Upham, B.L. (2005). The emperor wears no clothes in the field of carcinogen risk assessment: Ignored concepts in cancer risk assessment. *Mutagenesis,* 20, 81-92.

[69] Thilly, W.G. (2003). Have environmental mutagens caused oncomutations in people? *Nat. Genet.,* 34, 255- 259.

[70] Upham, B.L., Weis, L.M. and Trosko, J.E. (1998). Modulated gap junctional intercellular communication as a biomarker of PAH epigenetic toxicity: structure--function relationship. *Environ. Health Perspect.* 106(Suppl 4), 975--981.

[71] Weis,L.M., Rummel,A.M., Masten,S.J., Trosko,J.E. and Upham,B.L.(1998). Bay or baylike regions of polycyclic aromatic hydrocarbons were potent inhibitors of gap junctional intercellular communication. *Environ.Health Perspect.,* 106, 17--22.

[72] Tai, M.H., Upham, B.L., Olson, L.K., Tsao, M.S., Reed, D.N., and Trosko, J.E. (2007). Cigarette smoke condensate inhibited intercellular communication and differentiation in human pancreatic ductal epithelial cells. *Int. J. Cancer,* 120, 1855-1862.

[73] Minsk, B. and Illensee, K. (1975). Normal genetically mosaic mice produced from malignant teratocarcinoma cells. *Proc. Natl. Acad. Sci. USA,* 72, 3585-3589.

[74] Trosko, J. E. (2006). From adult stem cells to cancer stem cells: Oct-4 gene, cell-cell communication and hormones during tumor promotion. *Ann. N.Y. Acad. Sci.,* 1089, 36-58.

[75] Wang X. and Harris, C. (1997). p53 tumor- suppressor gene: clues to molecular carcinogenesis. *J. Cell Physiol.,* 173, 247-255.

[76] Barcellos-Hoff, M.H. (2001). Three down and counting: The transformation of human mammary cells from normal to malignant in three steps. *Trends Molec. Med.*, 7, 142-143.

[77] Bissell, M.J. and Radisky, D. (2001). Putting tumors in context. *Nature Rev. Cancer,* 1, 46-54.

[78] Trosko, J.E., Chang, C.C., Upham, B. and Wilson, M. (1998). Epigenetic toxicology as toxicant-induced changes in intracellular signalling leading to altered gap junctional intercellular communication. *Toxicol. Lett.,* 102—103, 71--78.

[79] Potter, V.R. (1973). Biochemistry of cancer. In Holland, J. and Frei, E (Eds.), *Cancer Medicine* (pp. 178-192). Philadelphia: Lea, E. and Febiger.

[80] Al Hajj, M., Wicha, M.S., Benito-Hernandez, A., Morrison, S.I. and Clarke, M.F. (2003). Prospective identification of tumorigenic breast cancer cells. *Proc. Natl. Acad. Sci. USA,* 100, 3983-3988.

[81] Webster, J.D., Yusbasiyan-Gurkan, V., Trosko, J.E., Chang, C.C., and Kiupel, M. (2007). Expression of the embryonic transcription factor Oct4 in Canine neoplasms: A potential marker for stem cell subpopulations in neoplasia. *Vet. Pathol.,* 44, in press.

[82] Chang, C.C., Trosko, J.E., El-Fouly, M.H., Gibson, D.R. and D'Ambrosio, S.M. (1987). Contact insensitivity of a subpopulation of normal human fetal kidney epithelial cells and of human carcinoma cell lines. *Cancer Res.*, 47, 1634-1645.

[83] Kao, C.Y., Nomata, K., Okley, C.S., Welsch, C.W. and Chang, C.C. (1995). Two types of normal human breast epithelial cells derived from reduction mammoplasty: Phenotypic characterization and response to SV40 transfection. *Carcinogenesis,* 16, 531-538.

[84] Linning, K.D., Tai, M.H., Madhukar, B.V., Chang, C.C., Reed, D.N., Ferber, S., Trosko, J.E., and Olson, L.K. (2004). Redox-mediated enrichment of self-renewing adult human pancreatic cells which possess endocrine differentiation potential. *Pancreas,* 29, e64-e76.

[85] Lin, T.-M., Tsai, J.-L., Lin, S.-D., Lai, C.-S., and Chang, C-C. (2005). Accelerated Growth and prolonged lifespan of adipose tissue-derived human mesenchymal stem cells in a medium using reduced calcium and antioxidants. *Stem Cells Devel.,* 14, 92–102.

[86] Yang, Y.C., S.W. Wang, H. Y.Hung, C.C. Chang, I.C. Wu, Y.L. Huang, T. M. Lin, J. L. Tsai, A. Chen, F.C. Kuo, W.M. Wang and D.C. Wu. (2007). Isolation and characterization of human gastric cell lines with stem cell phenotypes. *J. Gastroenterology Hepatology,* doi:1111/j.1440-1746.2007.05031.x.

[87] Matic, M., Evans, W.H., Brink, P.R. and Simon, M. (2002). Epidermal cells do not communicate through gap junctions. *J. Invest. Dermat.*, 118,110-116.

[88] Matic, M., Petrov, I.N., Chen, S., Wang, C., Dimitrijevich, S.D., and Wolosin, J.M. (1997). Stem cells of the corneal epithelium lack connexins and metabolic transfer capacity. *Different.,* 61, 251-260.

[89] Kang, K.S., Sun, W., Nomata, K., Morita, I., Cruz, A., Liu, C.J., Trosko, J.E. and Chang, C.C. (1998). Involvement of tyrosine phosphorylation of p185 c-erB2/neu in tumorigenicity by X rays and neu-oncogene in human breast epithelial cells. *Molec. Carcinogen.,* 21, 225-233.

[90] Nakano, S., Ueo, H., Bruce, S.A. and Ts'o, P.O.P. (1985). A contact-insensitive subpopulation in Syrian hamster cell cultures with a greater susceptibility to chemically induced neoplastic transformation. *Proc. Natl. Acad. Sci. USA,* 82, 5005-5009.

[91] Ponti, D., Costa, A., Zaffaroni, N., Pratesi, G., Petrangolini, G., Coradini, D., Pilotti, S., Pierotti, M.A. and Daidone, M.A. (2005). Isolation and In vitro propagation of tumorigenic breast cancer cells with stem/progenitor cell properties. *Cancer Res.,* 65, 5506-5511.

[92] Chang, C.C., Sun, W., Cruz, A., Saitoh, M., Tai, M.H. and Trosko, J.E. (2001). A human breast epithelial cell type with stem cell characteristics as targets for carcinogenesis. *Radiat. Res.,* 155, 201-207.

[93] Takahashi, K. and Yamanaka, S. (2006). Induction of pluripotent stem cells from mouse embryonic and adult fibroblast cultures by defined factors. *Cell,* 126, 663-676.

[94] Okamoto, K., Okazawa, H., Okuda, A., Sakai, M., Muramatsu, M. and Hamada, H. (1990). A novel octamer binding transcription factor is differentially expressed in mouse embryonic cells. *Cell,* 60, 461-472.

[95] Niwa, H., Miyazaki, J. and Smith, A.G. (2000). Quantitative expression of 0ct3/4 defines differentiation, de-differentiation or self-renewal of ES cells. *Nat. Genet.* 24, 372-376.

[96] Rosner, M.H., Vigano, M.A., Ozato, K., Timmons, P.M., Poirier, F., Rigby, P.W. and Staudt, L.M. (1990). A POU-domain transcription factor in early stem cells and germ cells of the mammalian embryo. *Nature,* 345, 686-692.

[97] Monk, M and Holding, C. (2001). Human embryonic genes re-expressed in cancer cells. *Oncogene,* 20(20), 8085-8091.

[98] Tai, M.H., Chang, C.C., Kiupel, M., Webster, J.D. and Trosko, J.E. (2005). Oct-4 expression in adult stem cells: Evidence in support of the stem cell theory of carcinogenesis. *Carcinogenesis,* 26, 495-502.

[99] Momiyama, M., Omori, Y., Isizaki, Y., Nishikawa, Y., Tokairin, T., Ogawa, J. and Enomoto, E. (2003). Connexin 26 mediated gap junctional communication reverses the malignant phenotype of MCF-7 breast cancer cells. *Cancer Sci.,* 94: 501-507.

[100] Barcellos-Hoff, M.H. (2001). It takes a tissue to make a tumor: epigenetics, cancer and the microenvironment. *J. Mammary Gland Neoplasm,* 6, 213-221.

[101] Atlasi, Y., Mowla, S.T., Ziaee, S.A. and Bahrami, A.R. (2007). Oct-4, an embryonic stem cell maker is highly expressed in bladder cancer. *Internatl. J. Cancer,* 120, 1598-1602.

[102] Kelly, P.N., Dakic, A., Adams, J.M., Nutt, S.L. and Strasser, A. (2007). Tumor growth need not be driven by rare cancer stem cells. *Science,* 317, 337.

[103] Umemoto, T. Yamato, M., Nishida, K., Yang, J., Tano, Y. and Okano, T. (2005). Limbal epithelial side-population cells have stem cell-like properties, including quiescent state. *Stem Cells,* 24, 86-94.

[104] Kim; M., Turnquist, H., Jackson, J., Sgaglas, M., Yan, Y., Gong, M., Dean, M., Sharp, J.G., and Cowan, K. (2002). The multidrug resistance transporter ABCG2 (Breast cancer resistance protein 1) effluxes Hoechst 33342 and is overexpressed in hematopoietic stem cells. *Clinical Cancer Res.*, 8, 22-28.

[105] Trosko, J.E. (2007). Stem cells and cell-cell communication in the understanding of the role of diet and nutrients in human diseases. *J. Fd. Hyg. Safety,* 1-14.

[106] Milton, K. (2000). Back to basics: Why foods of wild primates have relevance for modern human health. *Nutrition,* 16, 480-483.

[107] Kiple, K.F. (Ed). (2000). *The Cambridge World History of Food.* Cambridge University Press.

[108] Teaford, M.F. and Ungar, P.S. (2000). Diet and the evolution of the earliest human ancestors. *Proc. Natl. Acad. Sci. USA,* 97, 13506-13511.

[109] Mariani-Constantini, A. (2000). Natural and cultural influences on the evolution of the human diet: Background of the multifactorial processes that shaped the eating habits of Western societies. *Nutrition,* 16, 483-486.

[110] Popkin, B.M. (2007). The world is fat. *Sci. Amer.,* 297, 88-95

[111] Trosko, J.E. and Ruch, R. J. (2002). Gap junctions as therapeutic targets. *Curr. Drug Targets,* 3, 465-482.

[112] Franco,E.L., Correa,P., Santella,R.M., Wu,X., Goodman,S.N. and Petersen,G.M. (2004). Role and limitations of epidemiology in establishing a casual association. *Semin. Cancer Biol.,* 14, 413--426.

[113] Goodman G.E., Thornquist, M.D., Balmes, J., Cullen, R.M., Meysken, F.L., Omenn, G.S., Valanis, G.S. and Williams, J.H. (2004). The beta-carotene and retinol efficacy trial: Incidence of lung cancer and cardiovascular disease mortality during 6 year follow-up after stopping beta-carotene and retinol supplements. *J. Natl. Cancer Instit.,* 96, 1743-1750.

[114] Shuin, T., Nishimura, R., Noda, K., Umeda, M., and Ono, T. (1983) Concentration-dependent differential effect of retinoid acid on intercellular metabolic cooperation. *Gann,* 74, 100-105.

[115] He,K., Nukada, H., Urakami, T. and Murphy, M.P. (2003). Antioxidant and pro-oxidant properties of pyrroloquinoline quinine (PQQ): Implications for its function in biological systems. *Biochem.Pharmocol.,* 65, 67-74.

[116] Henning, H., Wenk, M.L., Dohahoe, R. (1982). Retinoic acid promotion of papilloma formation in mouse skin. *Cancer Letters,* 16, 1-5.

[117] Cohen, G.M., Bracken, W.H., Iyer, R.P., Berry, D.L., Selkirk, J.K., and Slaga, T. J. Anticarcinogenic effects of 2,3,7,8-tetrachlorodibenzo –p-dioxin on benzo(a) pyrene and 7,12-dimethylbenz (a) anthrcene tumor initiation and its relationship to DNA binding. *Cancer Res.,* 39, 4027-4033.

[118] Kushida, M., Sukata, T., Uwagawa, S., Ozaki, K., Kinoshita, A., Wanibusbuchi, H., Morimura, K., Okuno, Y. and Fukushima, S. (2005). Low dose DDT inhibition of hepatocarcinogenesis by diethylnitrosamine in male rats: Possible mechanisms. *Toxicol. Appl. Pharmacol.,* 208, 285-294.

[119] Lee, G.H. (2000). Paradoxical effects of Phenobarbital on mouse hepatocarcinogenesis. *Toxicol. Pathol.,* 28, 215-225.

[120] Kelloff,G.J., Lippman,S.M., Dannenberg, A.J., Sigman, C.C.H.L., Reid, B.J., Szabo, E., Jordan, V.C., Spitz, M.R., Mills,G.B., Papadimitrakopoulou, V.A., Lotan,R., Aggarwal,B.B., Bresalier, R.S., Banu Arun, J.K., Lu,K.H., Thomas, M.E., Rhodes, H.E., Brewer, M.A., Follen, M., Shin,D.M., Parnes, H.L., Siegfried, J.M., Evans, A.A., Blot, W.J., Chow, W.-H., Blount, P.L., Maley, C.C., Wang, K.K., Lam, S., Lee, J.J., Dubinett, S.M., Engstrom, P.F., Meyskens, Jr. F.L., O'Shaughnessy, J., Hawk, E.T., Levin, B., Nelson, W.G., Hong, W. K. (2006). Progress in Chemoprevention Drug

Development: The Promise of Molecular Biomarkers for Prevention of Intraepithelial Neoplasia and Cancer—A Plan to Move Forward. *Clin. Cancer Res.,* 12, 3661-3697.

[121] Upham, B.L., K.-S. Kang, H.-Y Cho, J.E. Trosko (1997). Hydrogen peroxide inhibits gap junction intercellular communication in glutathione sufficient but not glutathione deficient cells. *Carcinogenesis.,* 18, 37-42.

[122] Coffey, D.S. (2001). Similarities of prostate and breast cancer: Evolution, diet and estrogens. *Urology,* 57, 31-38.

[123] Grover, P.L. and Martin, F.L. (2002). The initiation of breast and prostate cancer. *Carcinogenesis,* 23, 1095-1102.

[124] Trosko, J.E. (1984). Scientific views of human nature: Implications for the ethics of technological intervention. In D. H. Brock (Ed). *The Culture of Biomedicine (*Vol. 1., pp. 70-97) Newark: University of Delaware Press.

[125] Thompson, D.E., Mabuchi, K., Ron, E., Soda, M., Tokunaga, M., Ochikubo, S., Sugimoto, S., Ikeda, T., Terasaki, M., Preston, D.L. (1994). Cancer incidence in atom bomb survivors. Part II: Solid tumors 1958-1987. *Radiat. Res.,* 137, S17-S67.

[126] Murrill, W. B., Brown, N., Zhang, J.X., Manzolillo, A., Barnes, S. and Lamartiniere, C.A. (1996). Prepubertal genistein exposure suppresses mammary cancer and enhances gland differentiation in rats. *Carcinogenesis,* 17, 1451-1457.

[127] Kennedy, A.R. (1998). The Bowman-Birk inhibitor from soy beans as an anticarcinogenic agent. Am. *J. Clin. Nutr.*, 68,1406s-1412s.

[128] Hsieh C.Y. and Chang, C.C. (1999) Stem cell differentiation and reduction as a potential mechanism for chemoprevention of breast cancer. *Chinese Pharm. J.,* 51, 15-30.

[129] Ju, Y. H., Allred, C.D., Allred, K.F., Karko, K.L., Doerge, D.R. and Helferich, W.G. (2001). Physiological concentrations of dietary genistein dose-dependently stimulate growth of estrogen-dependent human breast cancer (MCF-7) tumors implanted in athymic mice. *J. Nutr.,* 131, 2957-2962.

[130] Trosko, J.E. (2003) Human stem cells as targets for the aging and diseases of aging processes. *Medical Hypo*., 60, 439-447.

[131] Trosko, J.E. (2007). Aging as the 'System's' Breakdown of Communication between the Quality and Quantity of Stem Cells. In *The "Manifesto" For a Long Life*. In Press.

[132] Ho, S.M., Tang, W.Y., de Frauto, J.B., and Prins, G.S. (2006). Developmental exposures to estradiol and bisphenol A increases susceptibility to prostate carcinogenesis and epigenetically regulates phosphodiesterase Type 4 Variant 4. *Cancer Res.,* 66, 5624-5632.

[133] Dolinoy, D.C., Weidman, J.R., Waterland, R.A. and Jirtle, R. I. (2006). Maternal genistein alters coat color and protects AVY mouse offspring from obesity by modifying the fetal epigenome. *Environ. Health Perspect.,* 114, 567-572.

[134] Moghadasian, M.H. and Frohlich, J.J. (1999). Effects of dietary phytoterols on cholesterol metabolism and atherosclerosis: Clinical and experimental evidence. *American J. Med.,* 107, 588-94.

[135] De la Puerta, R., Martinez-Dominguez, E., and Riuz-Gutierrez,V. (2000). Effect of minor componbents of virgin olive oil on topical antiinflammatory sassays. *Z. Naturforsch. C.*, 55, 814-819.

In: Cancer and Stem Cells
Eds: Thomas Dittmar and Kurt S. Zänker
ISBN 978-1-60456-478-5

Chapter 10

Targeting Cancer Stem Cells

Thomas Dittmar*[*] *and Kurt S. Zänker
Institute of Immunology, Witten/ Herdecke University,
Stockumer Str. 10, 58448 Witten, Germany

Abstract

Cancer stem cells (CSCs) have been described as a rare population of cells within the tumor bulk exhibiting stem-cell properties such as self-renewal, differentiation, tissue reconstitution, and drug resistance. Due to their tissue restoration capacity it is now widely assumed that CSCs initiate primary tumor growth as well as metastases at distant organ sites. This in turn presupposes that CSCs must fulfill the hallmarks of metastatic cancer cells including i) to get accession to the circulatory system, ii) to survive within the blood stream, and ii) to perform endothelial cell adhesion and transendothelial migration. In addition to primary tumor and metastasis formation CSCs, due to drug resistance, have also been associated with tumor recurrence after cancer therapy. Interestingly, recurrent cancers often differ from the original disease by being resistant to cancer therapy indicating that the multidrug resistance is no longer restricted to the stem cell population, but to the entire tumor mass. Additionally, multidrug resistance of recurrent tumors is often associated with a highly aggressive cancer phenotype. We therefore postulate the existence of the recurrence cancer stem cell (rCSC) representing a certain type of cancer therapy resistant CSCs capable to initiate the re-growth of a more malignant tumor clone. We further summarize possible CSC eradication strategies.

Thereby we will focus on the rate-limiting step of extravasation, the inhibition of multidrug resistance transporters and cell fusion, which has been described as one possible mechanism for the origin of CSCs.

[*] Corresponding authors: Prof. Dr. Thomas Dittmar, Prof. Dr. Dr. Kurt S. Zänker, Institute of Immunology, Witten/ Herdecke University, Stockumer Str. 10, 58448 Witten, Germany. Phone: +49 2302 926 165 (TD), +49 2302 916 159 (KSZ), FAX: +49 2302 916 158, E-mail: thomasd@uni-wh.de (TD), ksz@uni-wh.de (KSZ).

Let's Talk about Cancer Stem Cells

When we are talking about cancer stem cells (CSCs) we simply define them as a rare population of cancer cells with stem cell properties such self-renewing, differentiation, and tissue reconstitution capacities [1, 2], which in case of CSCs leads to tumor initiation and metastasis formation. Although this rather simple view of CSCs is sufficient for most studies, and because of that it will be used in this chapter, the reality is a little bit more complex. An excellent overview about the complexity of cancer stem cells and how they should be defined – either stringent (by the CSC phenotype) or rather functional (by serial transplantation assay) – is given by Jichao Qin and Dean G. Tang in their chapter.

Interestingly, it is generally assumed that the disease cancer, consisting of the primary tumor and its metastases (and relapse), can be reduced to a summary of events that leads to the evolution of a single cancer stem cell (which in fact is the most stringent definition for a cancer stem cell). Although the possibility of such a scenario can not be ruled out we believe that cancer, including primary tumor formation as well as metastatic spreading as well as tumor recurrence, is not the result of a single CSC but is rather attributed to a pool of tumor stem cells exhibiting different properties. This hypothesis is partially in view with assumptions of Li and colleagues [2] (also see the appropriate chapter of Benjamin Tiede and Yibin Kang) postulating the existence of primary tumor CSCs (pCSCs) and dubbed metastatic CSCs (mCSCs). The population of pCSCs initiates primary tumor growth, but fail to induce metastasis formation, which in turn is facilitated by mCSCs ([2]; and see appropriate chapter in this book). Thus mCSC must fulfill the hallmarks of metastasis formation including the ability to migrate through the connective tissue, to intravasate into blood vessels as well as to adhere to and transmigrate across the endothelial lining [3]. The existence of different types of CSCs makes sense since cancer is not a steady-state but rather a dynamic disease. Tumor tissue is heterogenous and resembles chronic inflamed tissue and therefore tumors are often described as wounds that do not heal [4]. The chronically inflamed tumor microenvironment represents an explosive mixture for dividing cells since it promotes both cell proliferation due to secretion of various growth factors, chemokines and cytokines as well as causing DNA and protein damages due to elevated levels of reactive oxygen species provided by recruited immunocompetent cells [5]. Thus it is conceivable that the heterogeneous tumor microenvironment may be the maternity room for a second generation of cancer stem cells (e.g. mCSCs), which may arise from not yet transformed tissue stem cells or committed progenitor tumor cells. In this context, the role of bone marrow-derived stem cells (BMDCs) and its recruitment to (chronically) inflamed tissue can not be ruled out since data of Houghton and colleagues impressively demonstrated that bone marrow-derived stem cells (BMDCs) can be the inducers of gastric cancer after chronic *Helicobacter* infection [6]. These findings together with other data demonstrating the *in-vivo* tumor-initiating capacity of *in-vitro* transformed BMDCs [7] suggest that CSCs might originate from transformed BMDCs. Rizivi et al. showed recently that BMDCs fuse with neoplastic intestine epithelium [8], indicating that BMDCs are recruited by neoplastic tissues. In addition to this, it is also conceivable that recruited BMDCs trans-differentiate in accordance to the blueprint given by the surrounding neoplastic tissue without cell fusion [5]. In accordance with Rizivi and colleagues we observed that breast stem cells spontaneously fuse with breast cancer cells, thereby giving rise to hybrid cells [9, 10]. However, what will be the fate of hybrid cells comprising of tumor cells and BMDCs as well as tumor cells and tissue stem cells still remains unknown. Cell fusion has been postulated as one mechanism leading to CSC formation. Since fusion between stem cells and cancer cells occur in present tumor tissue it might be speculated that such cells (either BMDC/ tumor cell hybrid or tissue stem cell/ tumor cell hybrids or mis-trans-differentiated BMDCs) could give rise to CSCs possessing the capacity to drive metastasis formation.

Our results show that breast stem cell/ breast cancer cell hybrids possess a higher chromosomal number, proliferatory capacity, and expression level of ATP-binding cassette (ABC) family multidrug resistance transporters in comparison to the parental breast stem and breast cancer cells [9]. ABC family members are phenotypic markers and functional regulators of various stem cells [11] including tumor stem cells [12]. Of pivotal interest in CSC research is ABCG2 (also named breast cancer resistance protein, BCRP), which is commonly used as a marker molecule for the so-called side-population (SP) [13-16], whereby also other members of the ABC family play a role in the determination of this phenotype [14]. This is in agreement with observations that both ABCG2^{+} and ABCG2^{-} cancer cells exhibit similar tumorigenic levels [17] indicating that SP cells are tumor-initiating cells [13, 15]. What we know so far is that SP cells are enriched in tumorigenic, stem-like cancer cells [15, 17]. Whether SP cells are CSCs or solely represent a subpopulation of CSCs, or vice versa, is not yet clear. Nonetheless, drug resistance has been postulated to be a hallmark of cancer stem cells and is associated with tumor recurrence after therapy.

In this context we would like to postulate a third kind of cancer stem cell, namely that type of drug-resistant tumor-initiating cells that induce tumor formation after cancer therapy. These recurrence CSCs, or rCSCs, must differ from pCSCs - and possibly - mCSCs. If recurrent cancers would arise from the original pCSCs, which would have survived tumor therapy, than one would expect a similar progression of the “second” cancer disease in comparison to the progression of the “first/ original” cancer disease. As a consequence of that it would be able to treat the recurrent cancer with the same regiment of chemotherapeutic agents and/ radiation for several times. This, however, is mostly not the case since cancer relapse is often associated with the so-called oncogenic resistance [18], which means that the tumor became resistant to the first line therapy. Furthermore, oncogenic resistance is often associated with a highly aggressive cancer phenotype [18]. Thus the tumor stem cell type (rCSC) that causes cancer relapses must possess the following characteristics: i) rCSCs and its derivatives must be drug resistant e.g. due to stable up-regulation of drug transporters, ii) rCSCs and its derivatives should exhibit a higher proliferatory activity, and iii) rCSCs and its derivatives should be capable to induce metastases, which in turn suggests that also mCSCs could arise from a recurrent cancer.

The findings that breast stem cell/ breast cancer cells hybrids express higher levels of ABC transporters and possess a higher proliferatory activity than the parental cells [9] might indicate that rCSCs might have been evolved, which, however, has to be investigated in future studies.

What Are the Best Strategies to Target Cancer Stem Cells?

Due to their capacity to initiate primary tumor formation (and most likely be responsible for metastatic spreading and relapses after cancer therapy), CSCs have been postulated to be the most attractive candidates for novel anti-cancer strategies since eradication of this pivotal cell type would mean to get down to the root of the trouble [19].

But what are the best strategies to eradicate this pivotal cell type, which has not yet been completely characterized. Moreover, if certain types of CSCs exist, e.g. pCSC [2], mCSC [2], and rCSC, is it recommended to develop CSC type specific eradication strategies or is it possible to appropriate eradication strategies that will target all possible types of cancer stem cells? However, the answers to these questions cannot be given so far. Nonetheless, by checking the recent literature (as well as the excellent chapter of Benjamin Tiede and Yibin Kang in this book), various strategies have been postulated to target and eradicate CSCs. Since Tiede and Kang give an excellent summary about the possible targets: *self-renewal and differentiation, metastasis niche, reactivation and CSC clearance*, we will not go into details here. However, we would like to add this list by introducing three additional possible CSC target molecules/ mechanisms.

The first strategy targets integrins and chemokine/ chemokine receptor pairs. Both integrins and chemokine/ chemokine receptor pairs play pivotal roles in the organ-specific metastatic spreading of various tumors [20]. For instance, the $\alpha_v\beta_3$-integrin has been associated with the organ-specific spreading of melanomas into the lung [21, 22] and bone [23], whereas $\alpha_v\beta_3$-integrin expression in colon cancer cells is correlated with liver metastases [24, 25]. Furthermore, progression and organ-specific metastatic spreading of various cancer types have mostly been associated with the CXCL12/CXCR4 axis [20]. In accordance with the hypothesis that both the primary tumor as well as its metastases arise from cancer stem cells it can be concluded that CSCs must get accession to the circulatory system and must be capable to perform endothelial cell adhesion and transendothelial migration likely indicating that CSCs and non-CSCs use the same molecules for the rate-limiting step of extravasation [20]. This would be in view with a recent report of Miki and colleagues showing that hTERT-immortalized malignant RC-92a tumor-derived prostate epithelial cells, which retain stem cell properties, responded to CXCL12 stimulation with an increased locomotory activity, which was inhibited using an anti-CXCR4 antibody [26]. Since both integrin antagonists (e.g. RGD-peptides (Cilengitide) or blocking antibodies (Vitaxin)) and chemokine receptor antagonists (e.g. AMD3100) reduce metastasis formation it can be assumed that also CSCs (most likely mCSCs [2]) can be targeted by these compounds [20].

As mentioned above, side populations (SP) cells belong to the group of tumor-initiating cells. However, it still remains unclear whether SP cells are true CSCs or solely represent a subpopulation of CSCs, or vice versa. Nonetheless, drug transporters of the ABC family have been chosen to be appropriate targets for eradicating this particular type of tumor initiating cells (and possibly CSCs). Of pivotal interest is ABCG2 (also named breast cancer resistance protein; BCRP), which is the major mediator for SP cells and which effectively efflux a broad range of cytotoxic compounds such as mitoxantone, doxorubicin, daunorubicin and methotrexate [12], thus mediating drug resistance. However, in addition to ABCG2 other ABC family members are expressed by SP cells such as ABCB1 (multidrug resistance protein 1 (MDR1); also named p-glycoprotein) and ABCA3, which also determine the SP phenotype [14]. Thus, elimination of SP cells (and possibly CSCs) should be achieved by blocking more than one member of the ABC drug resistance transporter family.

An example for such purposes might be Gefitinib (also named Iressa), which is a well-known EGFR inhibitor [27]. In addition to its tyrosine kinase inhibiting activity Gefitinib also reverses the ABCG2/BCRP-mediated drug resistance, thus being a potent inhibitor of this drug transporter [28]. Gefitinib enhances the antitumor activity and oral bioavailability of irinotecan and topotecan in mice [29, 30]. Moreover, studies on ABCG2 and ABCB1 knock-out mice revealed that Gefitinib increased the oral absorption and decreased the systemic clearance of topotecan in these animals, indicating that additional transporters were inhibited [29]. This in turn suggests that Gefitinib seems to be a potent inhibitor of various multidrug resistance proteins. Similar results have been recently reported for the EGFR tyrosine kinase inhibitor Erlotinib (Tarceva, OSI-774), which efficiently antagonizes the ABCB1 and ABCG2 mediated drug resistance [31]. Thus drug resistance transporter inhibitors might be suitable compounds to target at least SP cells (and possibly CSCs). Moreover, since all postulated types of cancer stem cells (pCSCs [2], mCSCs [2], and rCSCs) should express multidrug resistance transporters the inhibition of these molecules should lead to an eradication of all possible cancer stem cell types. However, ABC transporters are expressed by a variety of tissues, including stem cells [11], which recommends the necessity of further studies to understand the pharmacologic interactions between ABC transporters and its inhibitors alone and in combination with other anti-cancer agents.

Although the role of cell fusion in CSC origin is not yet clear this process might represent a possible target for future therapeutical strategies. In Caenorhabditis elegans, fusogenic factors have been studied in detail and there are a large number of molecules that both promote and inhibit cell fusion [32]. By contrast, considerably less is known about the mechanism of mammalian cell fusion including those proteins that direct the amalgamation of two cells. Till now, solely a handful of molecules have been identified that might be involved in mammalian cell fusion including CD44, CD47, the macrophage fusion receptor PTPNS1 [33], interleukin-4 (IL-4) and IL-4 receptor [34, 35], and SDF-1α and CXCR4 [36]. Most of these molecules and receptor-ligand pairs have been well characterized [37] and appropriate inhibitors are already available. As mentioned above cell fusion has been considered to be one possible mechanism explaining the origin of cancer stem cells. Since cell-fusion leading to CSC formation can occur in non-tumorous and tumorous tissue it is conceivable that all types of postulated cancer stem cell types can arise by this mechanism, which in turn suggests that inhibition of cell fusion might prevent CSC formation. However, cell fusion plays a crucial role in the homeostasis of various tissues such as placenta, bone, nerve, and bone [38] and to date considerably less is known about the molecules that direct this process. Thus further studies are strictly recommended to identify additional fusogenic proteins and protein pairs as well as clarify whether CSCs arise from rare cell fusion events.

Conclusions

In this book the role of stem cells in cancer was excellently summarized and we would like to thank all authors who contributed to this excellent work. It became clear that although big efforts have already been made in cancer research considerably less is still known about this disease. Nevertheless, from day-to-day, from month-to-month we learn more about the complexity of cancer, which will help us to find the targets where cancer cells and cancer stem cells are vulnerable. What was once believed as a disease that has its origin in transformed somatic cells is now considered to be a stem cell-based disease, which has its origin in the generation of cancer stem cells. Cancer stem cells share several similarities with normal stem cells including the capacity to self-renew, to differentiate, to be drug-resistant due to expression of membrane transporters of the ABC family, and to "restore tissue integrity" at low cell numbers. The latter properties of CSCs have been associated with two hallmarks of cancer, namely metastasis formation and tumor recurrence.

Currently, various hypotheses are debated to explain the origin of cancer stem cells. It is conceivable that cancer stem cells might derive directly from tissue stem cells and/or BMDCs or indirectly from committed progenitor cells that have regained self-renewal capacity. It is also postulated that cancer stem cells might originate from rare cell fusion events, whereby several different (stem) cell types have been suggested a fusion partners.

Due to their tumor-initiating capacity as well as their feature to be drug-resistant the future of cancer research will focus on these cells. Till now, the primary cause (>95%) of death in cancer disease is not attributed to primary tumor formation, but to secondary tumor growth at distant organ sites as well as to tumor recurrence after conventional cancer therapy. Thus the challenge of future cancer research will be to identify and to characterize cancer stem cells. However, it should be noted that CSCs and normal stem cells share several similarities. Thus, the identification and characterization of unique features of CSCs that discriminate them from normal stem cells will be pivotal for devising specific therapies that would spare normal stem cells [2]. Which of the presented strategies will win the race against CSCs has to be elucidated in the near future. But: "the winner takes it all" and if it would be possible to take away cancer stem cells we would have a realistic hope to really cure cancer.

Acknowledgements

This work was supported by the Fritz-Bender-Foundation, Munich, Germany and the Verein zur Förderung der Krebsforschung Deutschland e.V., Heidelberg, Germany.

References

[1] Clarke MF; Fuller M. Stem cells and cancer: two faces of eve. *Cell*, 2006 124, 1111-1115.

[2] Li F; Tiede B; Massague J; Kang Y. Beyond tumorigenesis: cancer stem cells in metastasis. *Cell Res.*, 2007 17, 3-14.

[3] Heyder C; Gloria-Maercker E; Hatzmann W; Niggemann B; Zanker KS; Dittmar T. Role of the beta1-integrin subunit in the adhesion, extravasation and migration of T24 human bladder carcinoma cells. *Clin. Exp. Metastasis*, 2005 22, 99-106.

[4] Dvorak HF. Tumors: wounds that do not heal. Similarities between tumor stroma generation and wound healing. *N. Engl. J. Med.*, 1986 315, 1650-1659.

[5] Dittmar T; Seidel J; Zaenker KS; Niggemann B. Carcinogenesis driven by bone marrow-derived stem cells. *Contrib. Microbiol.*, 2006 13, 156-169.

[6] Houghton J; Stoicov C; Nomura S; Rogers AB; Carlson J; Li H; Cai X; Fox JG; Goldenring JR; Wang TC. Gastric cancer originating from bone marrow-derived cells. *Science*, 2004 306, 1568-1571.

[7] Liu C; Chen Z; Chen Z; Zhang T; Lu Y. Multiple tumor types may originate from bone marrow-derived cells. *Neoplasia*, 2006 8, 716-724.

[8] Rizvi AZ; Swain JR; Davies PS; Bailey AS; Decker AD; Willenbring H; Grompe M; Fleming WH; Wong MH. Bone marrow-derived cells fuse with normal and transformed intestinal stem cells. *Proc. Natl. Acad. Sci. USA*, 2006 103, 6321-6325.

[9] Schwitalla S; Keil S; Zänker KS; Dittmar T. Cell fusion: the origin of cancer stem cells?. *Regenerative Med.*, 2007 2, S46.

[10] Seidel J; Batistin E; Schwitalla S; Niggemann B; Zänker KS; Dittmar T. Cancer Cell + Stem Cell = Cancer Stem Cell? In: Saitama H. *New Cell Differentiation Research Topics*. Hauppauge, NY: Nova Science Publishers; 2007; in press.

[11] Bunting KD. ABC transporters as phenotypic markers and functional regulators of stem cells. *Stem Cells*, 2002 20, 11-20.

[12] Dean M; Fojo T; Bates S. Tumour stem cells and drug resistance. *Nat. Rev. Cancer*, 2005 5, 275-284.

[13] Hadnagy A; Gaboury L; Beaulieu R; Balicki D. SP analysis may be used to identify cancer stem cell populations. *Exp. Cell Res.*, 2006 312, 3701-3710.

[14] Hirschmann-Jax C; Foster AE; Wulf GG; Nuchtern JG; Jax TW; Gobel U; Goodell MA; Brenner MK. A distinct "side population" of cells with high drug efflux capacity in human tumor cells. *Proc. Natl. Acad. Sci. USA*, 2004 101, 14228-14233.

[15] Ho MM; Ng AV; Lam S; Hung JY. Side population in human lung cancer cell lines and tumors is enriched with stem-like cancer cells. *Cancer Res.*, 2007 67, 4827-4833.

[16] Zhou S; Schuetz JD; Bunting KD; Colapietro AM; Sampath J; Morris JJ; Lagutina I; Grosveld GC; Osawa M; Nakauchi H; Sorrentino BP. The ABC transporter Bcrp1/ABCG2 is expressed in a wide variety of stem cells and is a molecular determinant of the side-population phenotype. *Nat. Med.*, 2001 7, 1028-1034.

[17] Patrawala L; Calhoun T; Schneider-Broussard R; Zhou J; Claypool K; Tang DG. Side population is enriched in tumorigenic, stem-like cancer cells, whereas ABCG2+ and ABCG2- cancer cells are similarly tumorigenic. *Cancer Res.*, 2005 65, 6207-6219.

[18] Blagosklonny MV. Why therapeutic response may not prolong the life of a cancer patient: selection for oncogenic resistance. *Cell Cycle*, 2005 4, 1693-1698.

[19] Reya T; Morrison SJ; Clarke MF; Weissman IL. Stem cells, cancer, and cancer stem cells. *Nature*, 2001 414, 105-111.

[20] Dittmar T; Heyder C; Gloria-Maercker E; Hatzmann W; Zanker KS. Adhesion molecules and chemokines: the navigation system for circulating tumor (stem) cells to metastasize in an organ-specific manner. *Clin. Exp. Metastasis*, 2007.

[21] Hieken TJ; Ronan SG; Farolan M; Shilkaitis AL; Das Gupta TK. Molecular prognostic markers in intermediate-thickness cutaneous malignant melanoma. *Cancer*, 1999 85, 375-382.

[22] Vink J; Thomas L; Etoh T; Bruijn JA; Mihm MC, Jr.; Gattoni-Celli S; Byers HR. Role of beta-1 integrins in organ specific adhesion of melanoma cells in vitro. *Lab. Invest.*, 1993 68, 192-203.

[23] Byzova TV; Kim W; Midura RJ; Plow EF. Activation of integrin alpha(V)beta(3) regulates cell adhesion and migration to bone sialoprotein. *Exp. Cell Res.*, 2000 254, 299-308.

[24] Kikkawa H; Kaihou M; Horaguchi N; Uchida T; Imafuku H; Takiguchi A; Yamazaki Y; Koike C; Kuruto R; Kakiuchi T; Tsukada H; Takada Y; Matsuura N; Oku N. Role of integrin alpha(v)beta3 in the early phase of liver metastasis: PET and IVM analyses. *Clin. Exp. Metastasis*, 2002 19, 717-725.

[25] Enns A; Korb T; Schluter K; Gassmann P; Spiegel HU; Senninger N; Mitjans F; Haier J. Alphavbeta5-integrins mediate early steps of metastasis formation. *Eur. J. Cancer*, 2005 41, 1065-1072.

[26] Miki J; Furusato B; Li H; Gu Y; Takahashi H; Egawa S; Sesterhenn IA; McLeod DG; Srivastava S; Rhim JS. Identification of putative stem cell markers, CD133 and CXCR4, in hTERT-immortalized primary nonmalignant and malignant tumor-derived human prostate epithelial cell lines and in prostate cancer specimens. *Cancer Res.*, 2007 67, 3153-3161.

[27] Rocha-Lima CM; Soares HP; Raez LE; Singal R. EGFR targeting of solid tumors. *Cancer Control*, 2007 14, 295-304.

[28] Yanase K; Tsukahara S; Asada S; Ishikawa E; Imai Y; Sugimoto Y. Gefitinib reverses breast cancer resistance protein-mediated drug resistance. *Mol. Cancer Ther.*, 2004 3, 1119-1125.

[29] Leggas M; Panetta JC; Zhuang Y; Schuetz JD; Johnston B; Bai F; Sorrentino B; Zhou S; Houghton PJ; Stewart CF. Gefitinib modulates the function of multiple ATP-binding cassette transporters in vivo. *Cancer Res.*, 2006 66, 4802-4807.

[30] Stewart CF; Leggas M; Schuetz JD; Panetta JC; Cheshire PJ; Peterson J; Daw N; Jenkins JJ, 3rd; Gilbertson R; Germain GS; Harwood FC; Houghton PJ. Gefitinib enhances the antitumor activity and oral bioavailability of irinotecan in mice. *Cancer Res.*, 2004 64, 7491-7499.

[31] Shi Z; Peng XX; Kim IW; Shukla S; Si QS; Robey RW; Bates SE; Shen T; Ashby CR, Jr.; Fu LW; Ambudkar SV; Chen ZS. Erlotinib (Tarceva, OSI-774) antagonizes ATP-binding cassette subfamily B member 1 and ATP-binding cassette subfamily G member 2-mediated drug resistance. *Cancer Res.*, 2007 67, 11012-11020.

[32] Bjerkvig R; Tysnes BB; Aboody KS; Najbauer J; Terzis AJ. Opinion: the origin of the cancer stem cell: current controversies and new insights. *Nat. Rev. Cancer*, 2005 5, 899-904.

[33] Vignery A. Osteoclasts and giant cells: macrophage-macrophage fusion mechanism. *Int J. Exp. Pathol.*, 2000 81, 291-304.

[34] Horsley V; Jansen KM; Mills ST; Pavlath GK. IL-4 acts as a myoblast recruitment factor during mammalian muscle growth. *Cell*, 2003 113, 483-494.

[35] Horsley V; Pavlath GK. Forming a multinucleated cell: molecules that regulate myoblast fusion. *Cells Tissues Organs*, 2004 176, 67-78.

[36] Wright LM; Maloney W; Yu X; Kindle L; Collin-Osdoby P; Osdoby P. Stromal cell-derived factor-1 binding to its chemokine receptor CXCR4 on precursor cells promotes the chemotactic recruitment, development and survival of human osteoclasts. *Bone*, 2005 36, 840-853.

[37] Chen EH; Olson EN. Unveiling the mechanisms of cell-cell fusion. *Science*, 2005 308, 369-373.

[38] Ogle BM; Cascalho M; Platt JL. Biological implications of cell fusion. *Nat. Rev. Mol. Cell Biol.*, 2005 6, 567-575.

Index

A

B

C

D

E

F

G

H

I

J

K

N

Q

R

S

T

U

V

W

X

Y

Z